Pathophysiology of Respiration

Wiley Pathophysiology Series

Neville Bittar, M.D., *Series Editor*
University of Wisconsin School of Medicine, Madison

Pathophysiology of Respiration

Meir H. Kryger

Renal Pathophysiology

Avery R. Harrington
Stephen W. Zimmerman

Pathophysiology of Respiration

Edited by

Meir H. Kryger, M.D., F.R.C.P.(C)

Assistant Professor
Department of Medicine
University of Manitoba
Winnipeg, Manitoba
Canada

A WILEY MEDICAL PUBLICATION
JOHN WILEY & SONS
New York • Chichester • Brisbane • Toronto

Cover design: Wanda Lubelska
Production editor: Eileen Tommaso
Copy editor: Teresa Buford

Library of Congress Cataloging in Publication Data:
Main entry under title:

Pathophysiology of respiration.

(A Wiley medical publication) (Wiley pathophysiology series)
Includes index.
1. Respiratory organs—Diseases. 2. Respiration. 3. Physiology, Pathological. I. Kryger, Meir. II. Series: Wiley medical publication. III. Series: Wiley pathophysiology series. [DNLM: 1. Respiratory tract diseases—Physiopathology. WF 140 P298]
RC732.P37 616.2 81-2113
ISBN 0-471-05923-4 AACR2

Printed in the United States of America

10 9 8 7 6 5 4 3 2 1

To my wife Barbara and my mother Rose

Contributors

Victor Chernick, M.D., F.R.C.P.(C)
Professor
Department of Pediatrics
University of Manitoba
Health Sciences Centre
Winnipeg, Manitoba
Canada

Howard S. Goldberg, M.D.
Assistant Professor
Department of Medicine
University of Manitoba
Health Sciences Centre
Winnipeg, Manitoba
Canada

Wayne Kepron, M.D., F.C.C.P.
Assistant Professor
Department of Medicine
University of Manitoba
Respiratory Centre
Winnipeg, Manitoba
Canada

Meir H. Kryger, M.D., F.R.C.P.(C)
Assistant Professor
Department of Medicine
University of Manitoba
Director, Respiratory Medicine
St. Boniface General Hospital
Winnipeg, Manitoba
Canada

Bruce Light, M.D.
Research Fellow in Infectious Diseases
Department of Respiratory Diseases
Health Sciences Centre
Winnipeg, Manitoba
Canada

Donal S. McCarthy, M.D., Ph.D., F.R.C.P.(C)
Associate Professor
Department of Medicine
University of Manitoba
Respiratory Centre
Winnipeg, Manitoba

David Ostrow, M.D., F.R.C.P.(C), F.C.C.P.
Assistant Professor
Department of Medicine
University of British Columbia
Vancouver General Hospital
Vancouver, British Columbia
Canada

Thomas L. Petty, M.D.
Professor and Head
Division of Pulmonary Sciences
University of Colorado
Health Sciences Centre
Denver, Colorado

C. P. W. Warren, M.B., F.R.C.P.(C)
Associate Professor
Department of Medicine
University of Manitoba
Respiratory Centre
Winnipeg, Manitoba
Canada

Series Preface

It has come to be generally appreciated that knowledge concerning the pathophysiology of organ dysfunction serves as the basis for our understanding of the underlying mechanisms of disease. The phenomenal growth of pathophysiology as a discipline during the past ten years and its efficacy in medical education have prompted the preparation of the Wiley Pathophysiology Series.

Until recently, the traditional method of instructing first- and second-year medical students has been to teach the basic sciences including pharmacology and biochemistry separately. Today, however, an increasing number of medical schools have come to favor a multidisciplinary course of study where the pathophysiology of each organ system is examined and dealt with in its entirety. It has been found that this provides medical students with a firm bases of knowledge concerning cellular biology and basic science and their relevance to the practice of medicine. The purpose of this series is to offer an accompaniment to such a curriculum that is both thorough and up-to-date.

The first book in the series, *Pathophysiology of Respiration,* deals with the disordered function of the respiratory system. Dr. Kryger and his colleagues at the University of Manitoba Medical School present a concise multidisciplinary treatment of the subject that touches on all aspects of the altered performance of the diseased lung. It is felt that this work adds a valuable perspective to current medical knowledge, and it is hoped that teachers and practitioners of medicine as well as second-year students will find it stimulating and useful.

The unfailing support and courtesy of the staff of John Wiley & Sons is gratefully acknowledged.

Neville Bittar, M.D.
University of Wisconsin, Madison

Preface

This book was written for those who are interested in how function is disturbed when respiratory disease is present. Our approach is to link pathology and physiology, and we assume the reader has some familiarity with both. Thus, this volume will be of greatest value to medical students who have completed their basic sciences and are beginning their clinical studies. Others who will find this volume useful are house staff, trainees in respiratory medicine, and respiratory technology students.

Our goal is to help the reader understand respiratory disease as seen through the eyes of the contributors. All the contributors, besides being scientists and teachers, are clinicians: they take care of patients. Thus, this book is very clinically oriented in that it deals with the problems *commonly* encountered by chest physicians. The chapter titles are evidence of this clinical approach. In spite of the clinical emphasis, the approach in each chapter is to review the pertinent physiology, starting with very basic principles.

This book is meant to be used in two ways. First, it can be read from cover to cover. Second, the reader can pick up the book and read, and hopefully understand, a chapter somewhere in the middle of the book without necessarily having read the preceding chapters. This results in a certain amount of duplication, which we think is more helpful than not.

There have been several recent exciting developments in our understanding of respiratory disease. These include the natural history of chronic airflow obstruction, the pathogenesis of asthma, the infantile respiratory distress syndrome, and sleep apnea. We wish to share these developments with the reader.

M.K.

Acknowledgments

My Teachers

I have been fortunate to have been associated with some of the most innovative men in respiratory medicine: Nicholas Anthonisen, Peter Macklem, Tom Petty, and John Weil. What they have taught me is found throughout the book.

Joan Young

I cannot thank my secretary enough for all the work she did in the preparation of this manuscript. Her care and patience were extraordinary.

Laurie Richardson

The illustrations were prepared by Laurie Richardson of the Instructional Media Department of the University of Manitoba, Winnipeg. It is a pleasure to work with a craftsman.

My Colleagues

Many of my colleagues reviewed chapters and offered excellent suggestions. In particular, I wish to thank Neil Donen, John Fleetham, Jacques Savoy, Jacques Malo, Jacques Wacker, Ram Abdullah, Christine Bradley, Ian Fraser, John Acres, Frederik Santman, Peter West, Alan Mutch, and Laurence Brownell.

M.K.

Contents

1

Introduction to Respiratory Pathophysiology

Meir H. Kryger

All living systems ranging in size from our planet Earth down to individual cells must be able to capture and use energy from their environment. Mammalian cells obtain energy by coupling their metabolism to the breakdown of foodstuffs. The most important of these energy-producing reactions require oxygen and generate a waste product, carbon dioxide.

The word *respiration* has two meanings. The first refers to the energy-liberating chemical reactions that require oxygen and produce carbon dioxide. The second refers to the act of breathing. These two processes are, of course, linked. Breathing exchanges oxygen and carbon dioxide between the body and its environment. In this book, we are concerned with the breathing process and with what happens when there is disease of the organ of gas exchange, the lung.

Overview of the Normal Respiratory System

When the respiratory muscles contract, the pressure around the lungs becomes negative compared to the atmospheric pressure. This causes alveolar pressure to become negative. When the alveolar pressure is less than the atmospheric pressure, fresh air flows via the airways into the alveoli (Figure 1.1).

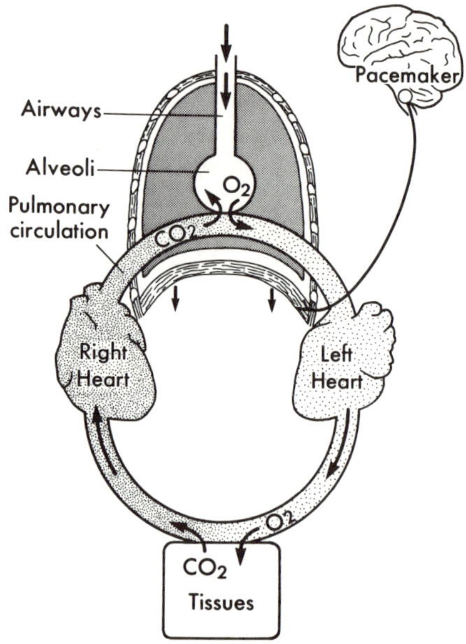

Figure 1.1. The components of the respiratory system. Abnormalities in each of these components can disturb normal respiratory function.

Gas exchange in the lung requires the coming together of large volumes of both fresh air and blood. The alveoli supply a huge surface area for oxygen uptake and carbon dioxide excretion to occur. The quantity of air pumped into the lungs is controlled by a "pacemaker" located in the brainstem. After carbon dioxide is unloaded into alveolar gas and oxygen is loaded onto the blood, the oxygenated blood is pumped into the left side of the circulation to the tissues. In the tissues, oxygen is unloaded from the blood and used in metabolic reactions. The metabolic waste product, carbon dioxide, is then taken by the blood, which returns to the right ventricle to be pumped into the network of pulmonary capillaries that envelop the alveoli.

Overview of the Abnormal Respiratory System

Disease is present when the functions of the respiratory system are disturbed or deranged. The disordered function is determined by the response of the entire organism to some form of injury. All or any part of the respiratory system, airways, alveoli, capillaries, respiratory muscles, and even the pacemaker, may suffer injury or be abnormal. In this book, we stress the disordered function as seen in diseases of the respiratory system—what happens when disease is present.

When studying a patient's disease, we are concerned with the cause of the disease, the pathological process that is present, the disease interference with normal function, and finally how the disease is treated. There are several approaches to disease classification: etiological, pathological, and functional.

Classification by etiology (cause) is ideal. However, we do not often know the etiological factor in lung disease; thus the word *idiopathic* looms large in such classification. Etiological classification is most useful when an infectious disease is present.

Classification by pathological process is a means of categorizing diseases into the following groups: inflammatory (infectious and immunological), neoplastic, vascular, hemorrhagic, traumatic, developmental, etc. This type of classification often is not useful to the clinician for two reasons. First, tissue is seldom obtained to make a diagnosis. Second, clinical diagnostic procedures are oriented toward evaluating the function of the system. Classification by pathological process is most useful for neoplastic and inflammatory disease.

Classification stressing abnormal physiological function is used by most clinicians who take care of patients with respiratory disease. This system of classification also has problems, because some diseases such as cancer may be lethal and yet not interfere significantly with the respiratory system function. However, such a classification is useful, because most of the time it helps us to understand how the disease interferes with the patient's normal physiology.

When disease of the respiratory system is present, one or more of the following patterns of physiological abnormalities emerge as the dominant feature:

Airflow obstruction: when airways are abnormal.

Lung restriction: when expansion of lungs is impaired.

Respiratory distress syndrome: when the gas exchanging interface is diffusely injured.

Pulmonary vascular disease: when pressure in the pulmonary circulation is elevated.

Abnormal control of breathing: when the system regulating ventilation is abnormal.

Respiratory failure: when failure of gas exchange has occurred.

Neoplasia: when uncontrolled cell growth occurs.

The above list includes the vast majority of problems seen by respiratory physicians. Often, there may be an overlap of two or more patterns, or one problem may cause another to occur. For example, patients with airflow obstruction may develop respiratory failure, pulmonary vascular disease, and abnormal control of breathing. Some disorders do not fit neatly into the above pigeon holes. Infections and immune disorders may present with different functional disorders. Although this type of classification is the most widely used, it is imperfect; it is only a step in clinical evaluation. After abnormal function is documented, an attempt is still made to unravel the etiology or the pathological process involved. However, learning the major patterns is very useful, allowing the student to obtain the building blocks necessary for his or her understanding of respiratory disease. When we understand how a disease interferes with function, we are better able to treat our patients.

SYSTÈME INTERNATIONAL (SI) UNITS*

There has been a movement in recent years to standardize the units of measurement used in all the sciences. For example, pressure is a force per unit area whether measured by a physicist, engineer, physiologist, or nurse. Why should each discipline use its own unit? Indeed there is much logic (and in some nations, legislation) in attempting to adopt SI units. However, there has been some resistance, particularly among physiologists. They often prefer to use units based on their calibrating procedures. In addition, virtually everything written in medicine uses the "older" units. Hence, we were faced with a dilemma in this text—to use SI or not to use SI units. There are two measurements in which there is a major problem—pressure and amount of gas.

Gas pressure and vascular pressure are represented in mmHg and pleural pressure in cmH_2O in the older system. Using SI units kilopascals (kPa) are used.

Amount of gas is represented in ml (STPD) in the older units and mmole in the SI units.

Because the adoption of SI units is still in a state of flux, and because the majority of physiologists, physicians, laboratories, and medical schools still use the older units, we decided that for the body of the text at present it is more helpful to use the more familiar units. We have included an appendix that contains conversion tables for pressure and amount of gas, which will be useful for the student who has learned SI units.

GENERAL BIBLIOGRAPHY

Respiratory Physiology

Bates DV, Macklem PT, Christie RV: *Respiratory Function in Health and Disease*, ed 2. Philadelphia, WB Saunders, 1971.

Comroe JH, Forster RE, Dubois AB, et al: *The Lung*. Chicago, Year Book Medical Publishers, 1962.

Comroe JH: *Physiology of Respiration*, ed 2. Chicago, Year Book Medical Publishers, 1974.

Fenn WO, Rahn H (eds): Respiration, in *Handbook of Physiology*, I and II. Washington, American Physiological Society, 1964, 1965.

Murray JF: *The Normal Lung*. Philadelphia, WB Saunders, 1976.

Nunn JF: *Applied Respiratory Physiology*, ed 2. London, Butterworths, 1977.

West JB: *Respiratory Physiology—The Essentials*. Baltimore, Williams and Wilkins, 1974.

*See Appendix 1

Bates et al. emphasizes the use of the pulmonary function laboratory. Comroe et al. and Comroe are excellent physiological textbooks. Comroe et al., although now two decades old, is a classic; its clear language and figures make it still one of the best texts available. Fenn et al. is the encyclopedia of respiratory physiology. A new edition is in preparation. Murray and Nunn are modern reviews of the respiratory physiology of normal man. West is a clearly written and illustrated introductory textbook.

Respiratory Medicine Textbooks

Fraser RG, Paré JAF: *Diagnosis of Diseases of the Chest*, ed 2, Vols 1–4. Philadelphia, WB Saunders, 1977.

Fishman AP (ed): *Pulmonary Diseases and Disorders.* New York, McGraw-Hill, 1980.

Guenter CA (ed): *Pulmonary Medicine.* Philadelphia, JB Lippincott, 1977.

Hinshaw HC, Murray JF: *Diseases of the Chest*, ed 4. Philadelphia, WB Saunders, 1980.

Series of Special Interest

Basics of RD is an excellent series of short articles that are published 5 times a year and cover the major topics in respiratory medicine and physiology. This series is published by the American Thoracic Society, the medical section of the American Lung Association, 1740 Broadway, New York, N.Y. 10019, U.S.A.

Lung Biology in Health and Disease is a series of comprehensive volumes on various subjects of respiratory physiology and medicine. Some of the volumes are pure basic science, while some are clinically oriented. By mid 1981, 17 volumes were published. The executive editor is Claude Lenfant. The publisher is Marcel Dekker, New York.

MEDICINE North America reviews topics in internal medicine. Volumes 21, 22 and 23 (March, April, and May 1982) are devoted to a state of the art review of respiratory disorders.

2

Airflow Obstruction

Donal S. McCarthy

STRUCTURE AND FUNCTION OF THE CONDUCTING AIRWAYS
Mechanisms of Breathing
Anatomical Considerations
  Upper airway
  Bronchi
  Bronchioli
  Ciliated cells
  Alveoli
Physiological Considerations
  Lung compliance or distensibility
  Airflow resistance
  Distribution of airflow resistance
  Flow during forced expiration: The equal pressure point
  Influence of "effort" on forced expiration
  Airway closure
  Distribution of ventilation
  Collateral ventilation

TESTS OF AIRWAY FUNCTION
Measurement of Airflow Obstruction
  Spirogram
  Flow-volume curve
  Airway resistance
  Lung volumes
  Lung compliance (distensibility)
Early Diagnosis of Airflow Obstruction
  Frequency-dependence of compliance
  Closing volume
  Slope of Phase III
  Maximum expiratory flow-volume curves on air and helium

Airflow obstruction refers to a disturbance of physiology in which there is an impediment to the flow through the conducting passages leading from the atmosphere to the gas-exchanging units of the lung. Airflow obstruction is the most common problem confronted by pulmonary physicians. A variety of disease processes can adversely affect airflow within the lungs: inflammation and mucus hypersecretion of the airways, bronchitis; destruction of elastic tissue of the lung, emphysema; and airway smooth muscle constriction, asthma. In this chapter, we will review the physiology of airways and the effect of disease on airway function.

STRUCTURE AND FUNCTION OF THE CONDUCTING AIRWAYS

The essential function of the lungs is the exchange of oxygen and carbon dioxide between pulmonary capillary blood and atmospheric air across the alveolar-capillary membrane. This requires the to and fro movement of large volumes of air through a system of tubes or airways (Figure 2.1).

Mechanisms of Breathing

Air moves into the lungs because the pressure in the alveoli or air sacs becomes negative relative to the atmospheric pressure. This differential in

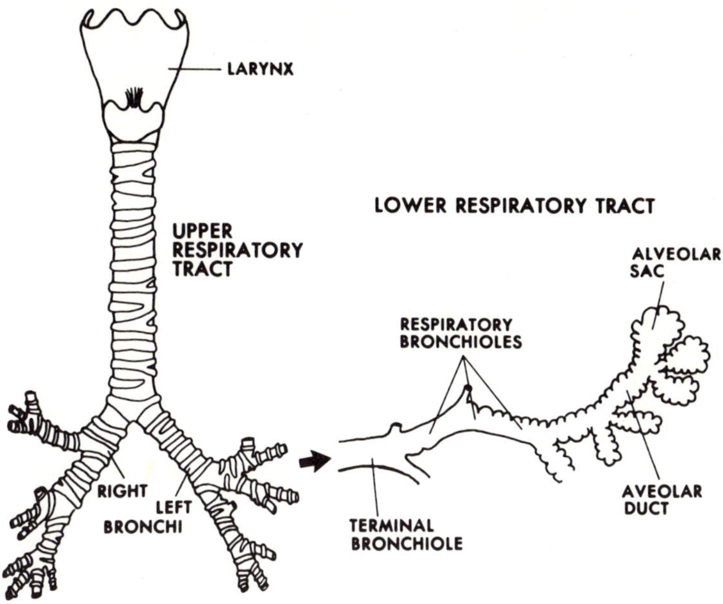

Figure 2.1. After entering the trachea, inspired air traverses successive divisions of airways before reaching the alveoli.

pressure is achieved by the contraction of the inspiratory muscles (the diaphragm and intercostals), which expand the thorax and the lungs thereby reducing alveolar pressure. At the end of inspiration, the inspiratory muscles relax and the thorax and lungs return to their resting position.

Expiration during quiet breathing is achieved by relaxation of the muscles of inspiration, thereby allowing the stretched elastic lungs to collapse under the influence of stored inspiratory energy. During expiration, air is expelled from the lungs because alveolar pressure briefly exceeds atmospheric pressure. Thus, the pattern of quiet breathing is active inspiratory muscle contraction and passive expiration. On forced or labored breathing, additional muscles are employed; the sternocleidomastoids are used to facilitate inspiration, while the abdominal muscles increase abdominal pressure, which pushes up the diaphragm and accelerates expiration.

Anatomical Considerations

Upper Airway

Air moving in and out of the lungs travels in the conducting airways. Inspired air enters the body via the nose or mouth, where it is humidified and warmed to body temperature. The gas then passes through the larynx and enters the trachea. The *trachea* has cartilaginous horseshoe-shaped "rings," which support its anterior and lateral walls. The posterior wall of the trachea is made up of relatively thin, flaccid trachealis muscle. When there is an increase in pressure around the trachea such as occurs during coughing, this posterior segment billows forward reducing the lumen of the trachea to a U-shaped slit. This results in a high linear velocity of airflow, which produces a shearing effect facilitating the clearance of any excess secretions.

Bronchi

The trachea divides into two main airways or *bronchi.* The left main bronchus is longer than the right and comes off at a more abrupt angle. The right mainstem bronchus is more directly in line with the trachea so that inhaled material tends to enter the right lung rather than the left. The mainstem bronchi then divide into lobar and then into segmental bronchi as shown in Figure 2.1. Further divisions occur in an uneven fashion; that is, branches at a division are not necessarily of the same size.

The bronchi have irregular plates of cartilage in their walls. Smooth muscle is arranged in a spiral fashion internal to the cartilaginous plates and attached to them. This configuration contributes to the bronchial lumen stability. Further down the bronchi, the cartilaginous plates become more scant while the muscle component increases. The epithelial lining of the bronchi is ciliated. The larger bronchi have mucus secretory glands in the submucosa. Hypertrophy of these secretory glands occurs when the airways are chronically inflamed.

Bronchioli

Bronchioli are smaller airways further out on the bronchial tree that do not contain cartilage in their walls. The bronchioli immediately proximal to the appearance of alveoli are called the *terminal bronchioli.* When alveoli do appear in the wall of the bronchioli, they are called *respiratory bronchioli.* The number of divisions between the bifurcation of the trachea and the terminal bronchioli varies between 9 and 32. Though these airways have no cartilage in their walls, they have instead a well-organized smooth muscle layer. Peripherally the muscular layer thins out, and at the level of the respiratory bronchioles, only strands of muscle fibers persist. The epithelium is a single layer of ciliated cells with very occasional "goblet cells" that are mucus-secreting cells.

Ciliated Cells

Ciliated epithelial cells in the tracheobronchial tree possess about 200 cilia per cell, each cilia 3 to 6 μm in length. Cilia beat with a whiplike action mouthward at a frequency of up to 1000 times per minute in organized waves of contraction passing from cell to cell. The cilia beat in a layer of thin mucus secreted by the goblet cells and mucus glands of the tracheobronchial tree forming the so-called "mucus blanket" or "mucus escalator." In the trachea, the mucus layer carrying cellular debris and particles moves upward. The role of mucociliary clearance is discussed in Chapter 15.

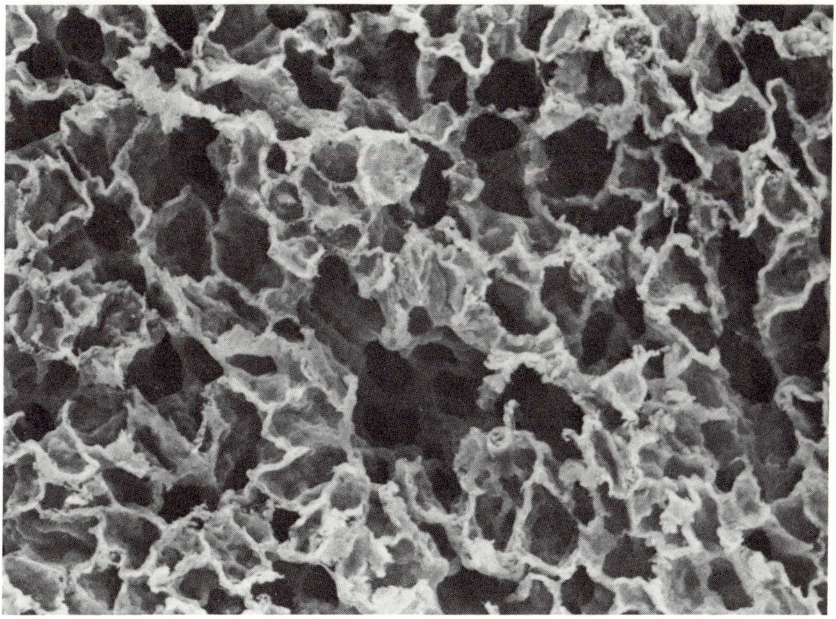

Figure 2.2. The alveoli act like a three-dimensional mosaic, such that each individual unit inflates and deflates in concert with the adjacent units (magnification ×200). (The author acknowledges the work of Dr. J.M. Papadimitriou, Pathologist, Sir Charles Gairdner Hospital, The Queen Elizabeth II Medical Centre, Nedlands, Western Australia, 6009.)

Alveoli

There are about 8 million *alveoli* in adult human lungs. Each alveolus is .1 to .5 mm in diameter and takes on a variety of shapes depending on the arrangement of adjacent alveoli and the state of lung inflation. Since the wall of an alveolus is in fact connected to the walls of the adjacent alveoli, when one alveolus increases its volume, this will tend to increase the volume of the adjacent alveoli. This interaction is called *interdependence* and contributes to stability and uniformity of lung expansion (Figure 2.2). In addition, peripheral airways are surrounded by alveoli, which tend to tether open these airways. Increasing alveolar volume will thus increase the lumen of these airways.

The alveoli are lined by an epithelial layer made up of two cell types. The *type I alveolar cells* have extensive flattened processes that cover most of the internal surface of the alveolus (Figure 2.3). The *type II alveolar cells* are less numerous and more globular in shape. On electron microscopy, these cells can be seen to contain bodies with a concentric laminated structure—"lamellar bodies." These bodies appear to be involved in the manufacture,

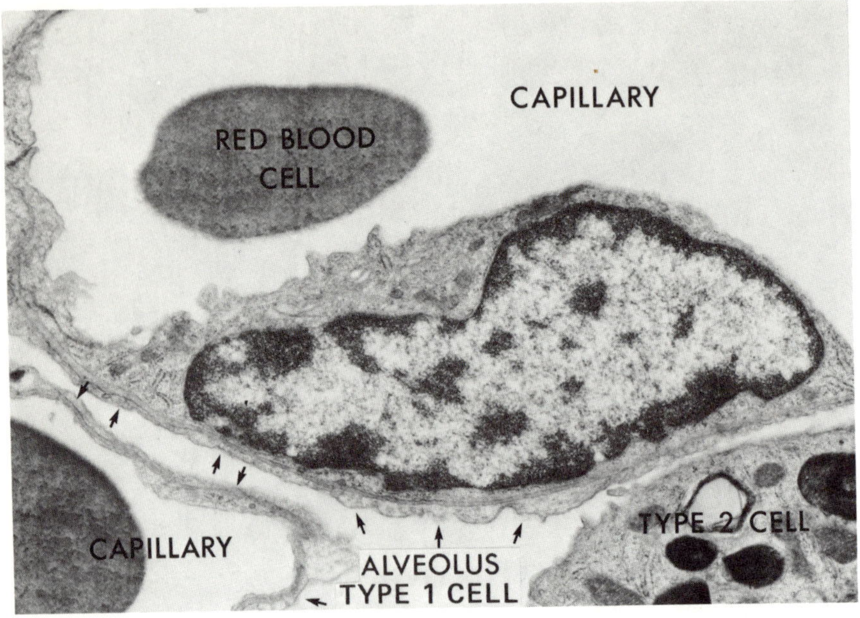

Figure 2.3. The flattened type I cell (indicated by arrows) covers most of the internal surface of the alveolus. Type II cells contain lamellar inclusion bodies (bottom right), which are probably the site of surfactant formation. Above and to the bottom left are pulmonary capillaries showing an endothelial cell and red cells (magnification × 17,000). (The author acknowledges the work of Dr. J.M. Papadimitriou, Pathologist, Sir Charles Gairdner Hospital, The Queen Elizabeth II Medical Centre, Nedlands, Western Australia, 6009.)

storage, and secretion of surfactant, a substance that enhances the stability of alveoli (see Chapter 13). The alveoli also contain phagocytic macrophages.

Holes in the alveolar walls, the *pores of Kohn* (Figure 2.4), allow communication between adjacent alveoli, which may be supplied by different respiratory bronchioli. Thus, any individual alveolus may be ventilated via the subtending airway or through the collateral channels from its neighboring alveoli. This latter process is called *collateral ventilation*. In emphysema, there is an increase in the size and number of these pores. This facilitates collateral ventilation, which probably plays an important role in gas exchange in patients with emphysema. There are other routes for collateral ventilation that are short pathways between distal bronchioles and neighboring alveoli.

The *interstitial space* between the alveolar epithelium and the capillary endothelium is more a potential space that only becomes apparent in disease states. This space is continuous with the interstitial space surrounding airways and larger blood vessels. Fluid in the interstitial space readily accumulates around the airways and blood vessels (peribronchial and perivascular cuffing) and may account for increased flow resistance in these structures in the presence of pulmonary edema.

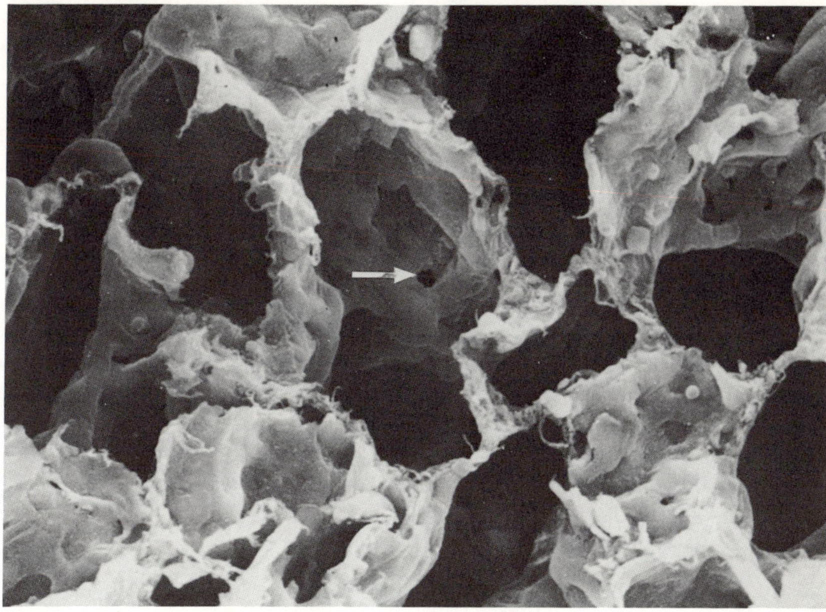

Figure 2.4. The pores of Kohn (indicated by arrow), are about 3 to 5 μm in diameter and form a communication with neighboring alveoli, and enable collateral ventilation to occur (magnification ×1000). (The author acknowledges the work of Dr. J.M. Papadimitriou, Pathologist, Sir Charles Gairdner Hospital, The Queen Elizabeth II Medical Centre, Nedlands, Western Australia, 6009.)

Lymphatic channels, which are present in the interstitial space, transport fluid from this compartment to the venous system. Lymph vessels accompany the bronchial tree but are also found in the interlobular septae and are abundant beneath the pleural surface.

Physiological Considerations

Lung Compliance or Distensibility

The lungs are elastic structures. Since they are encased in a closed and relatively rigid thorax, they tend to retract from the chest wall causing a negative pressure in the space between the lungs and the chest wall, i.e., the pleural space. This is really a potential space because under normal conditions the visceral pleura that covers the lung and the parietal pleura that lines the thoracic wall are separated by a very thin film of lubricating fluid.

The strength of retraction of the lung, the *elastic recoil,* is related to the degree of stretching of the lungs. That is, the greater the lung volume, the greater is the elastic recoil; therefore, the more negative is the intrapleural pressure.

The slope of the line relating the change in lung volume to a unit change in

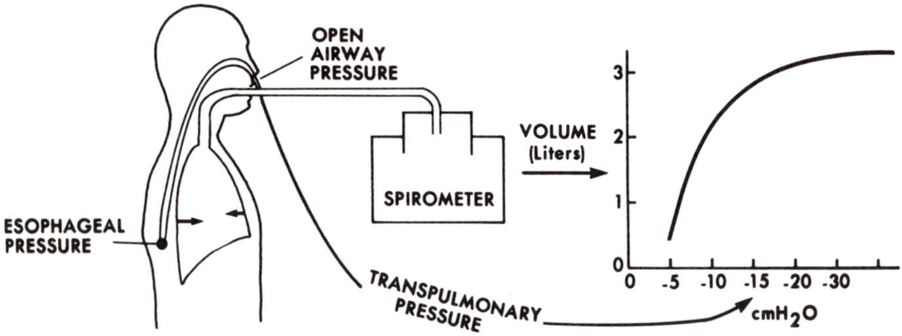

Figure 2.5. The pressure-volume relationship of the lung is obtained by plotting esophageal pressure (an index of pleural pressure) at different lung volumes measured with a spirometer. Lung compliance, the change in lung volume for unit change in transpulmonary pressure, can be calculated from the slope of the pressure-volume relationship. Notice that compliance ($\Delta V/\Delta P$) is high at lower and midlung volumes and very low at higher lung volumes.

the distending or transpulmonary pressure ($\Delta V/\Delta P$) is termed lung compliance or distensibility (Figure 2.5). The units employed are L/cmH_2O. The relationship between lung volume and pressure is not constant. At lower lung volumes, a large volume change is associated with a small pressure change—the compliance ($\Delta V/\Delta P$) is high; that is, the lung is distensible. At high lung volumes, a small volume change is associated with a huge pressure change—the compliance ($\Delta V/\Delta P$) is low; that is, the lung is stiff.

Airflow Resistance

When pressure is measured during breathing, there is a greater pressure change than is required to overcome the elasticity of the lung alone (Figure 2.6) because pressure is required to overcome the friction between molecules of the gas and the friction between the gas molecules and the airway wall. Thus, friction determines the resistance to airflow offered by the airways. The additional pressure required to produce airflow is a function of flow rate, caliber of the airways, the nature of the gas breathed, and the type of flow (turbulent or laminar, which are described below) that is present. In the simplest terms, resistance to the flow of gas through an airway is described by an equation that relates the flow per unit time to the pressure difference or gradient between the ends of the tube ($P_1 - P_2$)

$$\text{Airflow resistance} = \frac{P_1 - P_2}{\text{flow per unit time}}$$

Air flows because of the pressure difference between these two points. Thus, the unit for resistance is pressure/flow and is cmH_2O/L/sec.

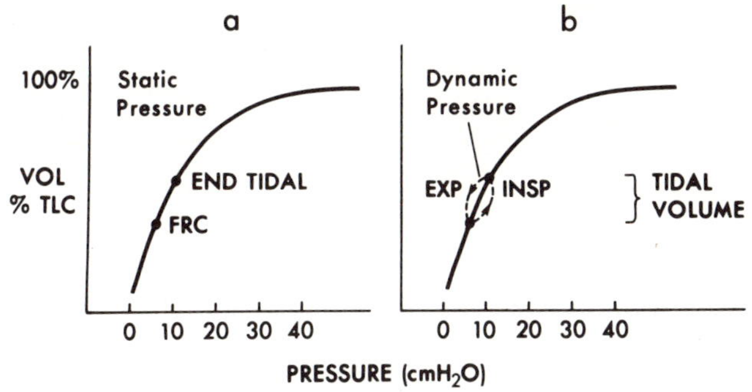

Figure 2.6. (*a*) The entire pressure-volume relationship of the lung when there is no flow. The dots indicate the points obtained at end expiration and end tidal; both are situations when no flow is occurring. (*b*) During breathing, pressure must be used to overcome the elasticity of the lung and the resistance to flow. The dashed line represents the continuous recording of pressure during a respiratory cycle. The displacement of the dashed line from the continuous line at any given lung volume during tidal breathing demonstrates the pressure required to produce airflow.

Distribution of Airflow Resistance

The cross-sectional area of the upper respiratory tract is quite narrow immediately above the vocal cords and in the larynx and trachea (Figure 2.7). Since the whole of the tidal volume passes through this area, the velocity of flow is high, and since there are many irregularities in the upper respiratory tract, secondary eddies are formed. This produces disorganized or *turbulent flow*

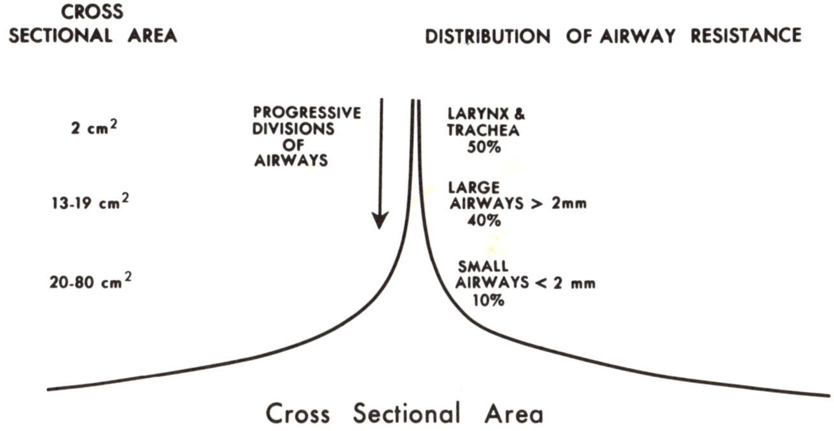

Figure 2.7. The distribution of airway resistance in the respiratory tract. The major component of airflow resistance resides in the larynx, trachea, and large airways where the cross-sectional area is small as compared to the progressively increasing cross-sectional area of the "small" peripheral airways.

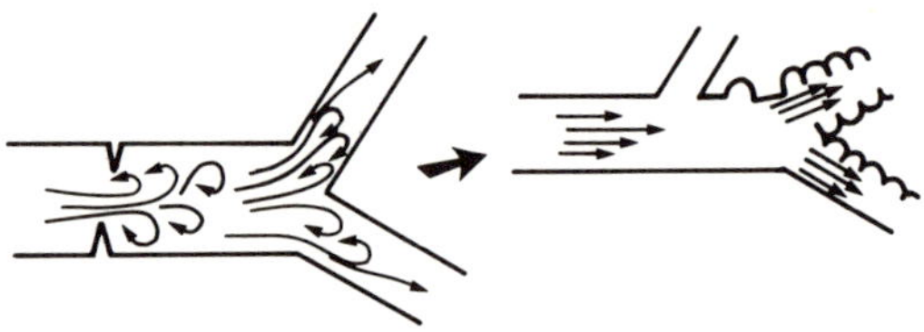

Figure 2.8. In turbulent flow, eddy currents occur where the flow rate is relatively high and where there are either irregularities in airway caliber or branches. In laminar flow, the gas molecules are arranged in concentric layers and slide smoothly over each other in an orderly manner.

(Figure 2.8). With this type of flow, while the gas molecules are traveling, they are also bumping into each other and off the walls of the airway, increasing the friction between gas molecules and the airway wall, so some of the energy used to drive the molecules is wasted. More energy is lost with the bouncing of heavy molecules than light ones. Thus, turbulent flow is dependent on the density of the gas. When turbulent flow is present, the resistance to airflow is reduced when breathing a low density gas such as helium. This has been applied in the pulmonary function laboratory—an increase in flow rates while the subject is breathing helium implies that turbulent flow is being examined. The resistance to airflow is high with turbulent flow; that is, the pressure required to maintain such a flow is high. The pressure required for such flow is summarized by the equation $P \propto d\dot{V}^2$; the pressure is directly proportional to the density of the gas and the square of the flow.

As flow proceeds through the trachea and the lower airways, the cross-sectional area increases progressively with each succeeding branching of the bronchi, leading to a progressive diminution of the linear velocity of the gas flow. In the terminal airways, flow rates are very low because of the huge cross-sectional area of the airways. The flow can now assume an orderly pattern, streamlined or *laminar flow*—the molecules seem to slide over each other. There is little friction between the gas molecules and the airway wall. The pressure required is proportional to the flow but *is not* dependent on the density of the gas breathed. The resistance to flow in this situation is very low compared with turbulent flow.

Total airway resistance in normal subjects may be divided into that which resides in the central airways with turbulent flow (80 to 90% of total resistance) and that due to the laminar flow in the peripheral airways, which are defined as those with internal diameter of less than 2 mm (10 to 20% of the total resistance). Obstructive lesions in the central air passages such as the larynx, trachea, or large bronchi will produce a marked increase in total

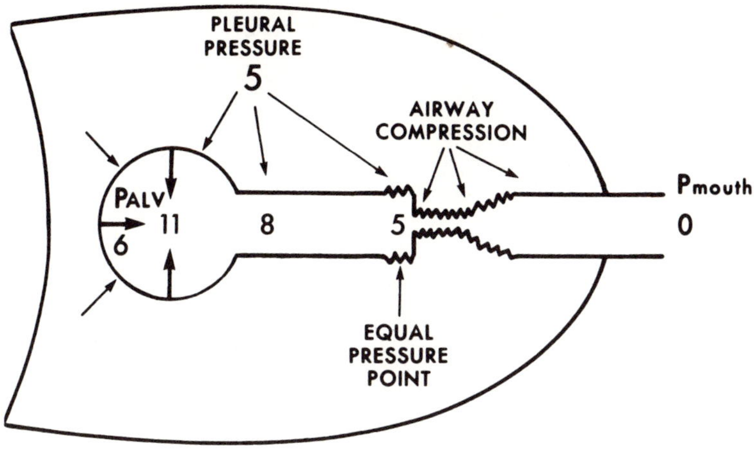

Figure 2.9. Dynamic airway compression during forced expiration. The pressures are given in cmH_2O. Alveolar pressure, Palv, equals the elastic recoil pressure (6) plus the pleural pressure (5). At a point in the airway, the pressure inside the airway equals the pressure outside the airway. This is the equal pressure point.

airway resistance, while extensive occlusion of peripheral airways may have only a small effect on total resistance. To restate: peripheral airway resistance makes up such a small portion of the total airway resistance that widespread disease involving the peripheral airways might raise the peripheral airway resistance by 500%, yet would only increase the total airway resistance by about 50%.

Flow During Forced Expiration: The Equal Pressure Point

The factors governing flow in forced expiration are complex, but consideration of a simplified *model* may be helpful. In Figure 2.9, the balloon represents the elastic alveolar tissue, and the long tube represents the intrathoracic airway. These are surrounded by the thoracic cage.

During forced expiration, the positive pressure in the pleural space acts not only on the alveoli but also on the outer side of the airway walls promoting airway compression or closure.

The airways near the alveoli do not collapse, because the pressure due to alveolar elastic recoil that promoted airflow produces a pressure within the airway lumen. However, as flow proceeds, pressure is expended against resistance; and so pressure drops along the airways, being high near the alveoli and reaching atmospheric pressure at the mouth. The pressure within the airway lumen falls progressively until a point is reached where the pressure within the airway is the same as that around the outside of the airway—this has been called the equal pressure point (EPP).

Mouthward from this point, the pressure outside the airway is greater than

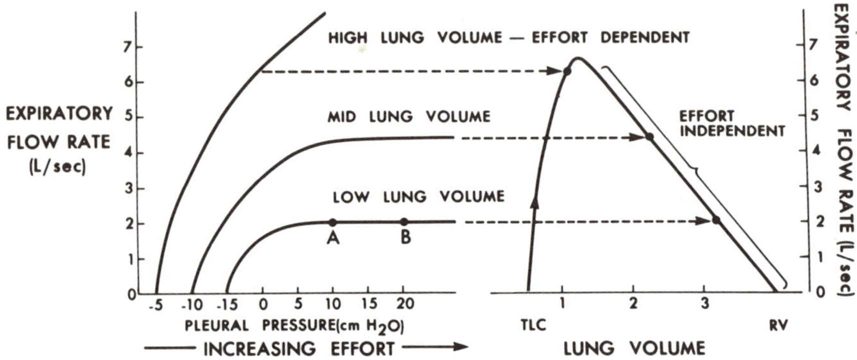

Figure 2.10. Influence of effort on forced expiration. The left graph shows the effect of increasing expiratory effort (pleural pressure) on expiratory flow rates. At high lung volumes, increasing effort increases flow. At lower lung volumes, flow plateaus; with increasing effort, there is no further increase in flow; flow is now effort independent. The effort-independent portion of the flow-volume curve is shown in the right figure.

that within the airway, and this may cause the airway to collapse ("dynamic compression") and limit further increase in flow rate.

On reflection, it can be appreciated that the advantage gained by increasing pleural pressure by increasing expiratory muscle effort in an attempt to increase airflow is canceled by the effect of this pressure exerting a collapsing pressure on the airways walls. Since alveolar pressure is made up of the sum of elastic recoil pressure and pleural pressure, and since the effect of increasing pleural pressure is canceled by its effect on increasing compression, it is the elastic recoil of the alveolar wall that is the pressure actually producing airflow, the driving pressure for airflow.

Influence of "Effort" on Forced Expiration

During forced expiration, flow is greater at larger lung volumes (Figure 2.10). At high lung volumes, the airways are widely patent, tethered open by the high elastic recoil; therefore, flow is a direct reflection of voluntary effort. At lower lung volumes, flow rate during forced expiration increases to a maximum after which increasing effort does not produce increasing flow rates—flow has plateaued and is independent of effort. Thus, flow rates at 50% and 25% of the vital capacity are "effort independent."

The mechanism underlying this "effort independence" is related to several factors. The forces contributing to airway patency and caliber are the pressure within the lumen of the airways, the intrinsic properties of the airway wall, and the tethering function of the surrounding lung on the airways.

At very high lung volume, airway collapse does not occur, because at high lung volume the equal pressure point is in large cartilaginous airways, which resist compression. As lung volume decreases during forced expiration, air-

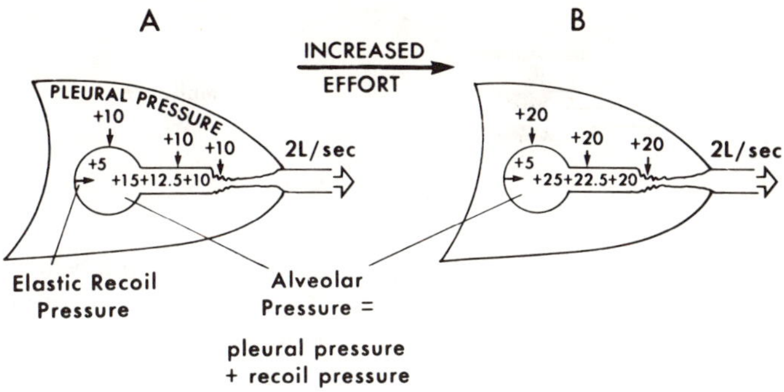

Figure 2.11. Effort independence of flow. Once dynamic compression is occurring, increasing effort does not increase flow rate. Between A and B there has been an increase in expiratory effort with pleural pressure increasing from 10 cmH_2O to 20 cmH_2O. The increased effort has resulted in the same pressure change in and around the airways; hence there is no change in the equal pressure point; the same portion of airway is being compressed. There has been no increase in flow.

way resistance increases as the airway caliber narrows. This is in part due to the reduction in tethering of the airways by the lung tissue, which occurs as lung volume decreases. Concurrently, the lung recoil pressure which is directly related to lung volume is also decreasing; therefore, alveolar pressure and intraluminal pressure also fall. Since the airway intraluminal pressure is decreasing in the course of a forced expiratory maneuver, the EPP moves down the airways toward the alveoli as lung volume decreases. In this way, the major resistance to airflow at low lung volumes is located in the smaller, more compliant (compressible) peripheral airways. Once airway compression is occurring, increasing effort simply accentuates the collapse and is not accompanied by an increase in flow rate (Figure 2.11).

Airway Closure

Airway closure is a phenomenon associated primarily with the expiratory phase of the respiratory cycle. Two factors contribute to airway patency during inspiration. First, during inspiration, the pressure around the airways (pleural pressure) is less than the pressure in the airways. This will promote airway dilatation. Second, the attachment of alveolar and lung elastic tissue to the smaller more compliant airways increases the size of these airways with increasing lung volume (the tethering effect).

The situation during expiration is quite different. At the beginning of an expiration, the airways remain patent because the pressure surrounding the airway (pleural pressure) still remains negative relative to the pressure within the airway lumen. However, during expiration below the resting lung volume, when expiratory muscles contract, the intrapleural pressure may become positive. This pressure may exceed the intraluminal pressure and thus promote

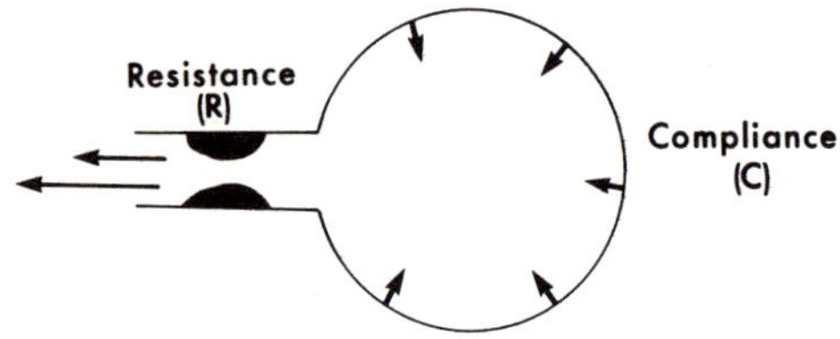

Figure 2.12. The facility with which the model of a lung unit will ventilate will depend on the product of the resistance (R) and the distensibility or compliance (C) of the unit; this is termed the *time constant* (TC) of the unit.

airway collapse. In addition, during expiration the traction on the airway wall diminishes as lung volume and elastic recoil diminish. In these circumstances, the airways may close and trap gas in the subjacent alveoli. Methods of measurement of the degree of airway closure are reviewed below.

Distribution of Ventilation

The facility with which a lung unit will ventilate depends on the resistance to airflow into that unit (R) and the compliance or distensibility of the unit (C). The product of resistance and compliance (R × C) has the dimension of time and is called the *time constant* (Figure 2.12). The greater the time constant of a lung unit, the lower its ventilation. The lung can be considered as being made up of millions of lung units, each with its own time constant. When the lungs are normal, all the units will have similar short time constants. When disease is present, not all units are affected to the same degree—some units will have relatively normal time constants, whereas others will have abnormal time constants. Thus with disease, because not all units have the same time constant, ventilation will be unevenly distributed.

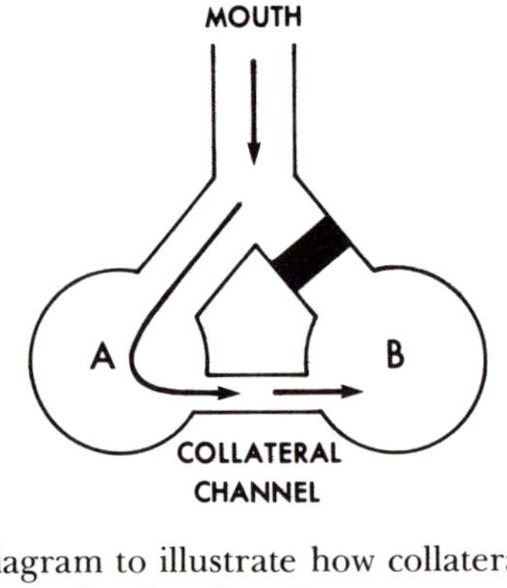

Figure 2.13. Schematic diagram to illustrate how collateral ventilation may occur in the lung. Air is inspired into alveolus A and traverses to alveolus B via a collateral channel, probably the pores of Kohn or some other communication.

Collateral Ventilation

Access of gas to airspaces beyond collapsed or closed airways in chronic airflow obstruction may be possible through collateral channels such as the pores of Kohn (Figure 2.13). This mechanism, presumably, accounts for the rarity of atelectasis in chronic airflow obstruction. However, ventilation via the collateral channels is inefficient because of the increased distance required for molecular diffusion. This results in impaired gas mixing. In addition, the air going into the collaterally ventilated unit has also traversed the normal unit and so has already taken part in gas exchange. Thus, the air going *into* the collaterally ventilated unit will have a higher P_{CO_2} and a low P_{O_2}. This unit thus appears to be hypoventilating relative to the normal unit.

TESTS OF AIRWAY FUNCTION

The simplest, safest, and most reproducible lung function tests should be chosen in a given situation. In this section, we review the lung function tests commonly used to diagnose and manage airflow obstruction.

Measurement of Airflow Obstruction

Data obtained during a forced expired vital capacity (FEVC) are the most widely used tests of airflow obstruction. This test is simple to perform; the equipment is portable and widely available, and the time necessary for analysis of the data is minimal.

Spirogram

The simple timed spirogram (Figure 2.14) is suitable for diagnosis and management of patients with overt airflow obstruction. This is the pulmonary function test most frequently done. Measurements commonly obtained from this plot of volume against time include:

- Forced vital capacity (FVC) in liters.
- Forced expired volume in the first second (FEV_1) in liters.
- FEV_1/FVC ratio. In normals this ratio exceeds 80%; with severe airflow obstruction it may be less than 30%.
- Maximum midexpiratory flow rate (MMEFR) in liters per second; derived by measuring the time required for expiration of the middle half of the FEVC.

Flow-Volume Curve

The plot of the flow-volume curve is obtained from the same maneuver (FEVC) as the spirogram; only this time the flow rate in liters per second is measured directly and plotted against the lung volume (Figure 2.14).

Additional information obtained from the flow-volume curve includes the

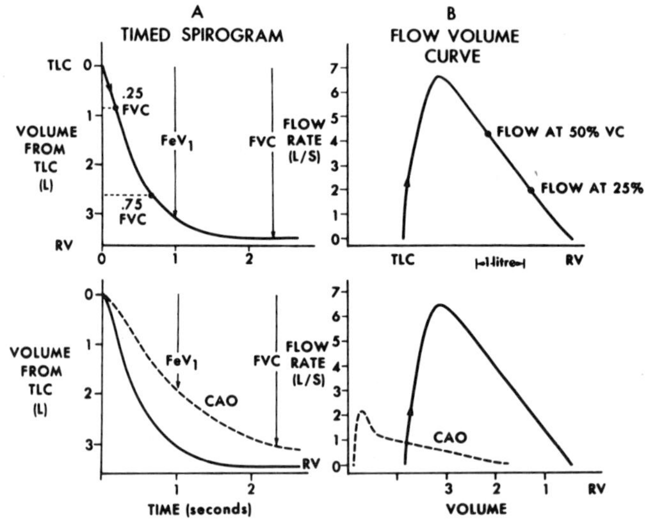

Figure 2.14. (*a*) Forced expired vital capacity (FEVC) in liters is plotted against time in seconds. The forced expired volume in the first second of expiration (FEV_1) can readily be measured. MMEFR is the slope of the line joining .25 and .75 FVC. The solid line is typical of a normal subject, while the dashed line is typical of a patient with airflow obstruction. (*b*) From the same maneuver the flow-volume curve can be obtained. Flow in liters per second is plotted against forced expired vital capacity in liters. This is the maximum expiratory flow-volume curve (MEFV). Peak expiratory flow rate (PEFR) and flows at 50% and 25% of FEVC can be read off this plot.

peak expiratory flow rate (PEFR) and the instantaneous flow rates at 50% and 25% of FEVC. The examination of the shape of this curve is also useful. Subjects with early lung disease may have normal FEV_1 and PEFR, but the flow-volume curve may be concave (Figure 2.15) to the volume axis at low lung volumes. In such people, flow rates at 50% and 25% of FEVC may be reduced. This information has been employed in epidemiological studies to identify asymptomatic smokers with normal FEV_1 and PEFR who may be destined to develop chronic airflow obstruction.

Airway Resistance

Resistance can be calculated by using the equation $(P_1 - P_2)$/Flow. The driving pressure $(P_1 - P_2)$ is the difference between alveolar pressure and the airway-opening pressure. Alveolar pressure can be estimated using a body plethysmograph. Another approach is to measure pressure in the esophagus. This is a good approximation of intrapleural pressure. The difference between the pleural and airway-opening pressure, the transpulmonary pressure, and flow are measured simultaneously, and resistance is calculated. Resistance measured in this way is the sum of airway resistance (80%) and

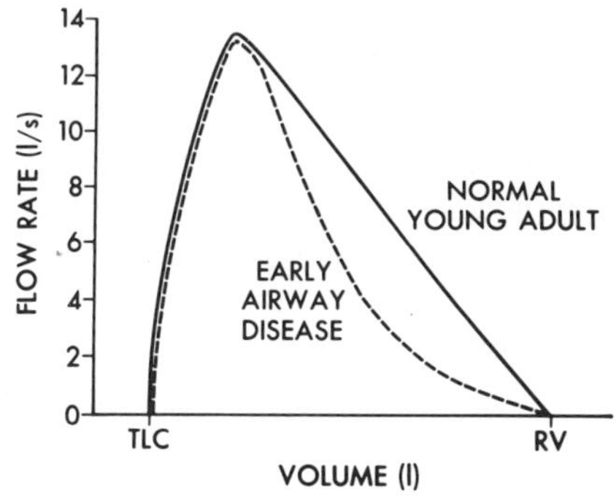

Figure 2.15. Shape information. Inspection of the MEFV curve may yield further information. In normal subjects the flow rates over most of the FEVC are linearly related to lung volume, but in subjects with early airway disease the configuration of the curve may become concave.

tissue resistance (20%). There are two reasons why resistance measurements are not as frequently used as other tests. First, the test is difficult to perform and uncomfortable to the patient. Second, as previously mentioned, total resistance that is mainly due to the turbulent flow of larger airways may be normal in the face of widespread peripheral airway disease.

Lung Volumes

The factors determining the lung volumes are described in more detail in the following chapter. *Functional residual capacity* (FRC) is the "rest position" between tidal breaths (Figure 2.16). No conscious effort is required to achieve or maintain this lung volume, which is the point of equilibrium between the elastic recoil of the lungs acting inward and that of the chest wall acting outward. The FRC is thus an "effort independent" lung volume, whereas other subdivisions of lung volume require subject cooperation and for that reason may be less reliable. In the presence of disease, the FRC may change due to changes in the mechanical properties of the lungs or chest wall. With severe loss of elastic recoil of the lung, there occurs an increase in FRC, hyperinflation. This finding is common in emphysema.

Functional residual capacity (FRC) is best measured in a body plethysmograph. This measurement is based on Boyle's Law, which states that the volume of a gas varies inversely as the pressure applied to the gas. Thus, if a gas of pressure Px and volume Vx changes to pressure Py and volume Vy, then $PxVx = PyVy$. The patient is put into an airtight box. While the subject is breathing, the mouthpiece is occluded at end expiration then the mouth pressure Px is measured; the volume Vx in the lungs is unknown. Let us call the product $PxVx$. The subject then tries to inspire against the occluded airway—the thorax enlarges by ΔV, which can be measured by the plethysmograph, and this reduces the pressure of the intrathoracic gas, which is also measured. If the new pressure is Py and the new volume is Vy, then $PxVx = PyVy$. Remember that $Vy = Vx + \Delta V$, and ΔV can be measured. Thus, $PxVx = Py(Vx + \Delta V)$. All the variables in this equation except Vx, the FRC, are measured, so that this equation is used to solve for Vx.

Where body plethysmography is unavailable or unsuitable, lung volumes may be measured by a helium dilution technique. Helium has been employed because it is an inert gas and is not appreciably absorbed from the alveolar gas. When the patient is at end expiration, his airway is connected to a spirometer of known volume containing a measured concentration of helium. While the patient is breathing, the helium will equilibrate; that is, the helium concentration in the lung will rise, while that in the spirometer will fall until the concentrations are equal. Since the amount of helium is unchanged, its dilution (the reduction in concentration) is a function of the volume of FRC. However, when lung units have long time constants, or where airway closure is present, helium dilution may underestimate lung volume, since the helium may not reach into these units.

Total lung capacity (TLC) is obtained by having the subject perform an inspiratory capacity (IC) maneuver immediately following the FRC measurement. With the increased compliance of emphysema, TLC may be markedly increased. Residual volume (RV) is calculated by subtracting the vital capacity (VC) from total lung capacity (Figure 2.16). Residual volume is usually increased when airflow obstruction is present, because airways close at higher lung volume than in normals. Since TLC and RV are both elevated in emphysema, when the flow-volume curve is plotted using absolute lung volume, the entire curve will be shifted to a higher volume. This is indicated by the dashed line in Figure 2.14B.

Lung Compliance

Lung compliance (distensibility) is also described in more detail in the next chapter. Measurement of lung compliance, distensibility, is not routinely required, but it may be helpful in further elucidating the mechanism of

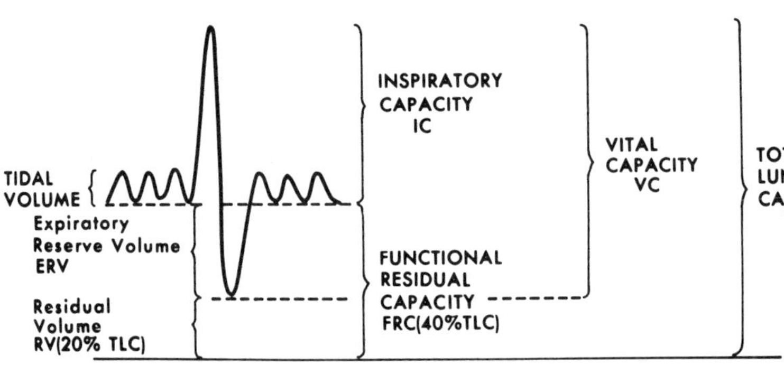

Figure 2.16. Total lung capacity (TLC) and its subdivisions.

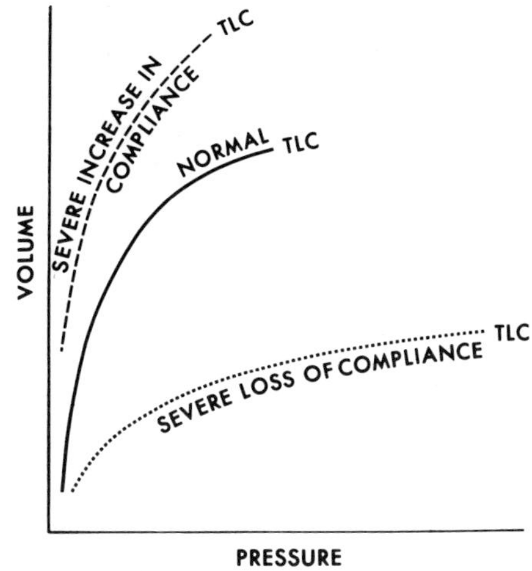

Figure 2.17. Pressure-volume diagram of the lungs. Volume is in liters, and transpulmonary pressure is in cmH_2O. In restrictive lung disease, the lungs have a severe loss of compliance and are "stiff"; they require large increments of pressure to achieve modest volume increase. TLC is reduced. In emphysema, for a given increase in transpulmonary pressure, there is a large volume change. Both TLC and lung compliance are increased.

disease in selected patients. An index of lung distensibility is referred to as lung compliance or the relationship of a given change of volume to a given change in pressure. Emphysema is the classic example of a disease in which the lungs have reduced recoil (high compliance). Conversely, where there is an increase in elastic recoil (low compliance or distensibility), the lungs are said to be "stiff" or restricted (see Chapter 3). Any disease process causing interstitial lung disease or leading to pulmonary fibrosis produces "stiff lungs" (Figure 2.17).

Early Diagnosis of Airflow Obstruction

Lung function tests have been developed that may detect abnormalities of peripheral lung units in asymptomatic subjects with normal routine spirometry. These tests have been designated "sensitive tests" of lung function and may predict the ultimate development of chronic airflow obstruction (CAO).

Frequency-Dependence of Compliance

The classic example of such a sensitive test is frequency-dependence of compliance. In the early stages of airflow obstruction, some airways are obstructed, while others are normal. The alveoli distal to the obstructed airways have long time constants; they fill and empty slowly. At slow breathing frequencies, there is sufficient time for these units to fill and empty a given tidal volume. As breathing frequency increases, the time required to empty and fill these abnormal units is too short, and they will get less and less air; the volume going in and out of the normal units, however, will increase. In this situation, if we measure compliance ($\Delta V/\Delta P$), it will be found that compliance decreases with increasing breathing rate. Thus, compliance will fall progressively as breathing frequency increases. This measurement, *dynamic compliance,* requires the measurement of pleural pressure with an esophageal balloon and, therefore, is uncomfortable to the patient and so is seldom used clinically. Thus, other tests were developed in an attempt to diagnose airflow obstruction in its early phases.

Closing Volume

Closing volume may be defined as the lung volume at which the airways in the dependent part of the lungs begin to close.

Because the pleural pressure in the top of the pleural space is more negative than the pleural pressure in the bottom, the alveoli in the dependent part of the lung are at a lower distending pressure at residual volume and, therefore, are actually smaller than the alveoli in the upper zone that operate at a higher transpulmonary pressure (Figure 2.18). When a maximal inspiration has been attained, all alveoli are the same size. The change in volume is, therefore, greater in A (the lower zone) compared to B. Thus, if a subject inspires maximally from residual volume with pure oxygen, the dependent lung regions will increase volume more and so receive more oxygen than the upper lung regions. This larger volume of oxygen will reduce the nitrogen concentration of the lower zones.

After an inspiration with O_2, the N_2 concentration at the mouth is measured during expiration. At first, phase I is seen, which contains only oxygen; this is followed by a rise in N_2, phase II, a transition to a plateau, phase III. This plateau represents the emptying of alveoli and is discussed in greater detail in the following sections. As expiration proceeds, the factors that can promote airway collapse (the increasingly positive pleural pressure and the loss of tethering with decreasing lung volume) become important. Because the pressure is always greater in the bottom than the top of the pleural space, as expiration proceeds, the pleural pressure acting on the dependent part of the lung becomes positive first, so it is here that airway closure occurs first. When the dependent airways close, we suddenly are looking at the N_2-rich upper lung regions, explaining the abrupt increase in N_2 concentration, the onset of phase IV.

Causes of Increased Closing Volume. Factors that resist airway closure are the intrinsic properties (stiffness) of the airways themselves and the tethering influence of the surrounding lung parenchyma that is related to lung elastic recoil, and so is dependent on lung volume. As lung volume decreases, the tethering force diminishes and the airways tend to close. Disorders in which

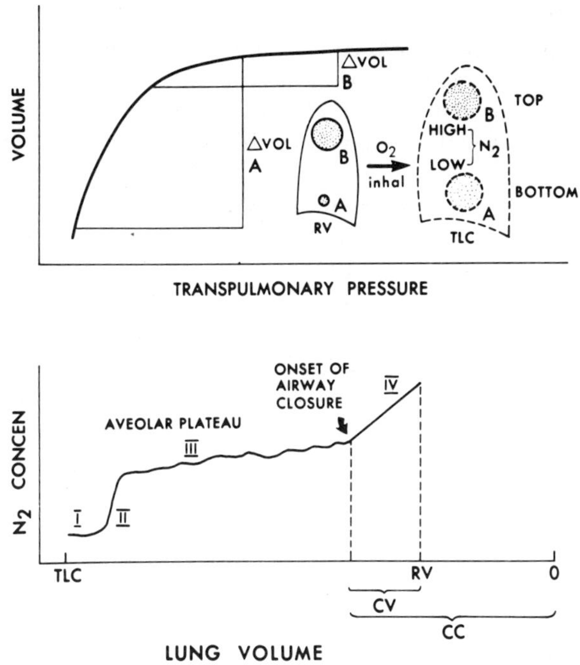

Figure 2.18. (*Top*) pressure-volume curve of the lung. At RV, because of the gravity-oriented gradient of pleural pressure (0.2 cmH_2O/cm down the lung) down the lung, the lower zones are subjected to a lower transpulmonary pressure than the upper zones. Since A and B will have a similar volume at TLC, after inhalation of O_2, the lower unit will have increased its volume more and thus reduced its N_2 concentration more than the upper unit B. Thus B has a high N_2 concentration compared to A. The density of the dots indicates N_2 concentration.
(*Bottom*) Closing volume trace. Following a vital capacity inspiration of 100% oxygen, the subject expires slowly to RV, during which volume on the abscissa is plotted against nitrogen concentrations on the ordinate. A trace with four phases is generated. Phase I, which is the dead space, contains oxygen only and is flat. Phase II contains mixed dead space and alveolar gas, which contains some nitrogen. This accounts for the rapid rise in N_2 concentration. Phase III contains alveolar gas, which shows a slowly rising concentration of N_2. Phase IV has an abrupt rise in nitrogen concentration indicating airway closure in the dependent regions of the lung. Closing volume is the lung volume, extending from the junction between phases III and IV and residual volume. Closing capacity (CC) is made up of closing volume (CV) and residual volume (RV).

abnormal airways are the cause of increased closing volume are *chronic bronchitis* (airways are inflamed and contain secretions) and asthma (airways are constricted). Conditions in which reduced lung elastic recoil (reduced tethering) cause increased closing volume are emphysema and aging. The closing volume test is so sensitive that it is not used in patients with overt airflow obstruction. The test's main use is as a screening tool in an attempt to detect airway disease in the earliest stages.

Slope of Phase III

The slope of phase III (Figure 2.19) is an index of the evenness of distribution of ventilation in the lungs. Because of disease of the airways (increased airflow resistance) or alveolar walls (loss of elastic recoil), the volume of air in abnormal lung units is greater than the volume in the more normal units at residual volume.

Following maximal inspiration of 100% oxygen, the change in volume in the normal unit will be greater than that of the abnormal unit, assuming that both have the same volume at TLC. At TLC, the concentration of nitrogen will be lower in the normal unit A, which has had a greater volume change than the abnormal unit B, which had a smaller volume change. During the subsequent expiration, the normal unit with the lower N_2 concentration will empty earlier, contributing to the earlier part of phase III, and the slower unit with the higher N_2 concentration empties later, contributing to the rising slope of phase III as expiration continues. The greater the unevenness of the distribution of ventilation, the greater the slope of phase III.

Maximum Expiratory Flow-Volume Curves on Air and Helium

Because airflow in the central airways is turbulent, the pressure required to produce a unit increase in flow is directly related to the density of the gas breathed. Conversely, in the peripheral airways where there is fully developed laminar flow, the pressure required to increase flow is independent of gas density.

It therefore follows that in normal subjects breathing a low density gas (80%

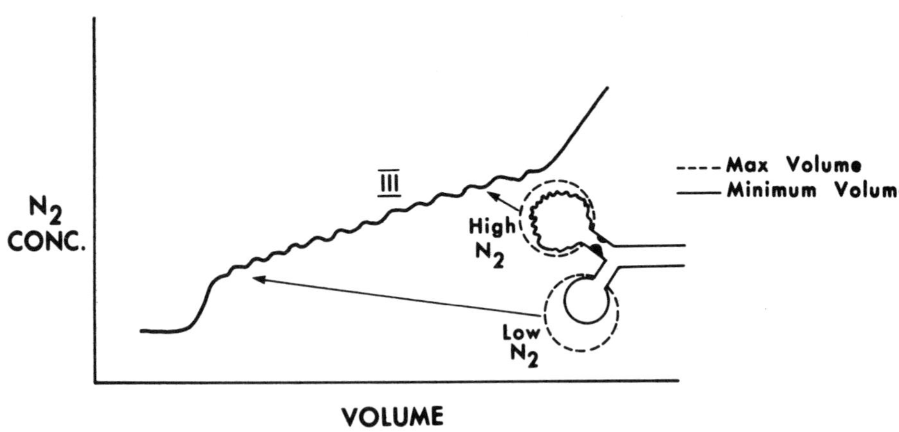

Figure 2.19. Slope of phase III. The slope of phase III is increased, because after O_2 inhalation, lung units containing different concentrations of nitrogen empty out of phase or asynchronously. The normal units empty first and have a lower N_2 concentration. The long time constant units empty later and have a higher N_2 concentration. The greater the difference between normal and abnormal units, the greater the slope.

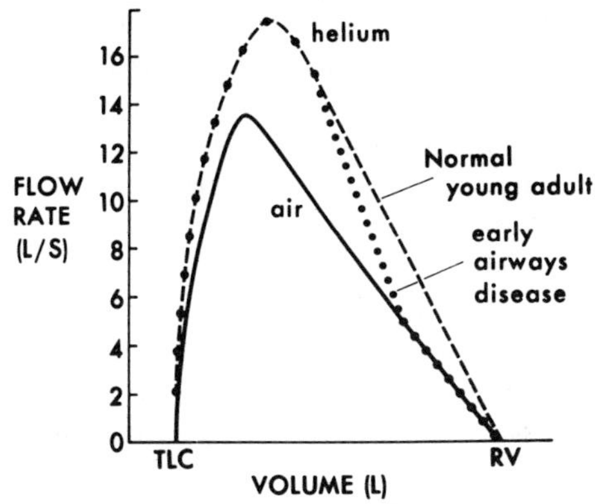

Figure 2.20. Helium air flow-volume curves. An FEVC is first performed on air (solid line). Following a brief equilibration with two vital capacities of 80% helium in 20% oxygen, an FEVC is performed following a maximal inspiration of this mixture. The dashed line shown is data of a normal response, and the dotted line is the type of data seen with early airways disease. Note that in early airways disease, flow on helium is the same as on air at low lung volume.

helium, 20% oxygen) who then perform an FEVC, there will be a substantial increase in flow rate because of a fall in total pulmonary resistance, since most of the resistance resides in the larger central airways where flow is density dependent (Figure 2.20)

In patients in whom the small peripheral airways are the predominant region of abnormality, the flow rate changes little on the helium-oxygen mixture because the flow regime in these airways is density independent. This test has proven valuable in detecting early airways disease in asymptomatic subjects. This test has the special advantage of being sensitive to abnormality of airways as distinct from lung parenchyma.

CHRONIC AIRFLOW OBSTRUCTION

Prevalance and Risk Factors

Airflow obstruction is by far the most common problem confronted by the chest physician. It has been estimated that 2.5 million Americans have restricted activities because of chronic airflow obstruction, and about 50,000 patients die each year as a direct consequence of the disease. The social consequences of chronic airflow obstruction are considerable, and the annual cost in terms of time lost from work and in medical treatment exceeds a billion dollars. It has been estimated that chronic airflow obstruction accounts for more than 10% of all disability claims.

Many other terms are commonly used to describe chronic airflow obstruction including: *chronic obstructive pulmonary disease* (COPD), *chronic obstructive lung disease* (COLD), *chronic obstructive airway disease* (COAD), and simply *airways obstruction.* The patients are even called "chronic lungers."

The sufferers are generally men (male/female ratio 4 : 1). The vast majority of patients who die of CAO have a history of cigarette smoking. The risk of dying of CAO is about 20 times greater in a heavy smoker than a nonsmoker. Yet many cigarette smokers do not develop CAO. Thus, some people are much more prone to the harmful effects of cigarettes. In most instances, the factors making a person more susceptible are unknown. In a minority of patients with emphysema, a deficiency of α_1-antitrypsin has been demonstrated.

Pathophysiology of CAO

In chronic airflow obstruction, the disease process involves the airways (bronchitis) or the alveolar tissue (emphysema). By far the most common situation is that the disease process involves both the airways and alveolar tissue (Figure 2.21).

Chronic Bronchitis

Chronic bronchitis is a clinical entity that is defined empirically as a chronic cough with production of sputum on most days for at least 3 months in the year for at least 2 years. The term excludes conditions such as bronchiectasis in which localized lesions in the lungs lead to chronic sputum production. The disorder is characterized by hypersecretion and inflammation of the bronchial walls which are caused by exposure to such chronic irritants as cigarette smoke. This results in increased resistance to airflow due to narrowing of the bronchial lumen and excess intraluminal secretions. The source of these se-

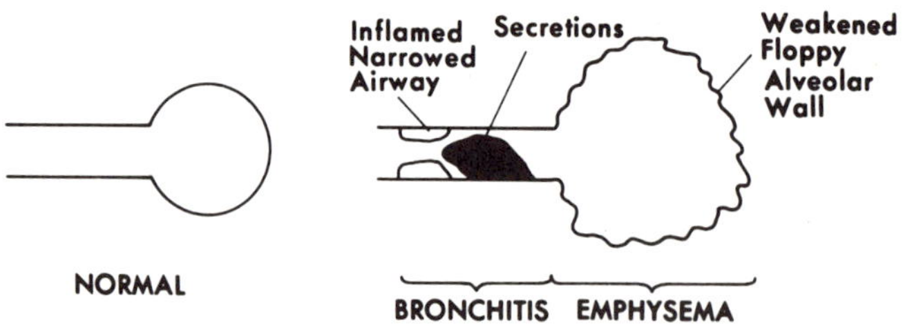

Figure 2.21. Schematic diagram to illustrate the distribution of bronchitis and emphysema. In bronchitis, there is thickening, inflammation, and narrowing of the airway lumen leading to increased airflow resistance. There is also hypersecretion and secretions within the airway lumen contributing to increased flow resistance. In emphysema, there is weakening, "floppiness," and destruction with disappearance of alveolar walls.

cretions is the bronchial mucus glands, which undergo hypertrophy and hyperplasia, and the bronchiolar goblet cells, which increase in number in chronic bronchitis.

Emphysema

Emphysema refers to a form of lung parenchymal damage and destruction and is not a clinical syndrome or symptom-complex such as chronic bronchitis. Emphysema is a pathological diagnosis and is difficult to diagnose reliably in life. The presence of emphysema can be inferred from tests that show a loss of elastic recoil. Because of the destructive nature of the disease it is irreversible. Emphysema is always accompanied by evidence of airflow obstruction, because the airway wall is poorly supported by the damaged lung and it readily collapses during expiration (Figure 2.22).

The mechanism of the alveolar destruction that causes emphysema is not clear. It appears to be related to the balance of enzyme systems in the lung. One enzyme system (elastase) tends to degrade the elastic tissue of the lung, while another enzyme system ("antielastase") tends to keep the elastase in check. A deficiency of the "antielastase" will thus allow the effect of elastase to dominate. α_1-antitrypsin seems to act as an antielastase, and so its deficiency can result in emphysema. Cigarette smoke may inactivate the "antielastase" and also cause the effect of the elastase to dominate.

Emphysema can be pathologically classified according to the location of the disease. In *centrilobular emphysema,* there is distension and damage primarily of

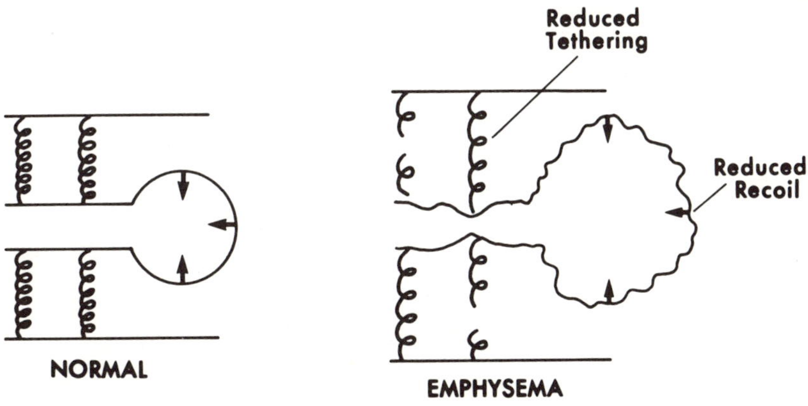

Figure 2.22. Mechanism of increased airflow obstruction in emphysema. Schematic diagram of an alveolus that has lost elastic recoil because of emphysema. Flow rates are reduced for two reasons: first, the elastic recoil of the alveolus, which produces flow, is decreased; second, the tethering effect of alveolar tissues adjacent to airways is reduced, so that airway collapse more readily occurs during expiration.

the respiratory bronchioles. The more distal alveolar ducts and alveolar sacs are well preserved (Figure 2.23).

Moderate centrilobular emphysema is common in chronic airflow obstruction and is not necessarily associated with disability. More severe centrilobular emphysema is associated with prominent symptoms.

Significant centrilobular emphysema is associated with disturbance of ventilation-perfusion relationships and hypoxia due to preservation of perfusion to poorly ventilated alveoli beyond the bronchiolar dilatation.

In *panlobular emphysema,* there is distenstion and destruction of the entire acinus, the gas-exchanging part of the lung. The elastic network of the lungs is disorganized, and the lungs lose recoil. This leads to collapse and closure of airways during expiration (Figure 2.22). Disturbance of gas exchange is often surprisingly mild, because the blood supply to damaged areas of the lung is reduced in proportion to the reduced ventilation of these areas.

Natural History of CAO

Most patients who develop CAO have smoked cigarettes for 20 or more years. They may have had a cough productive of mucoid or clear sputum for many years. At first, the cough may be present only in the morning; after several years, the coughing may occur throughout the day. When they develop infections of

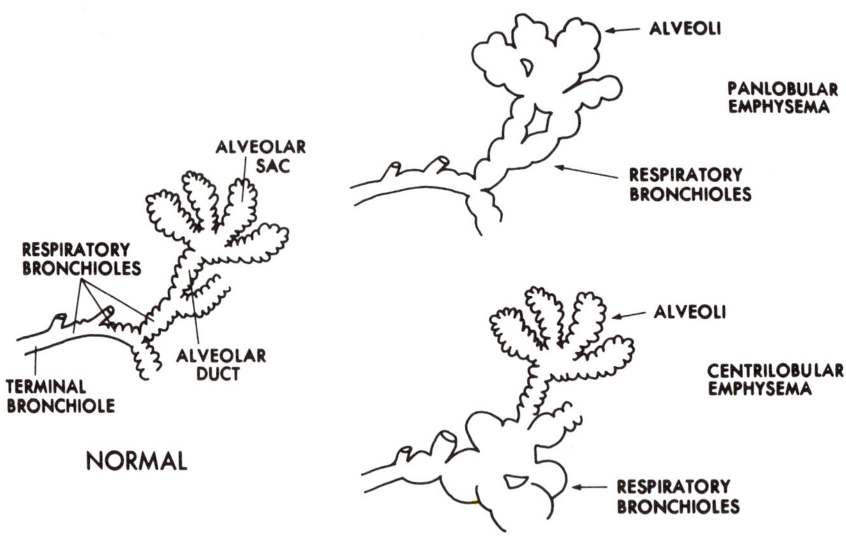

Figure 2.23. In panlobular emphysema, the entire lobule may be destroyed and replaced by dilated irregular airspaces. In centrilobular emphysema, the dilatation occurs at the level of the bronchioli, the alveoli being relatively normal. The terms *centriacinar* and *panacinar* emphysema have been used synonymously with centrilobular and panlobular emphysema.

the lower respiratory tract, infective exacerbations, the sputum may become yellow or green (purulent), and they may be short of breath. After 15 to 20 years, shortness of breath in the absence of infections becomes apparent, at first on exercise but later even at rest. In some patients, cough is not prominent but severe shortness of breath develops insidiously. With severe CAO, the infective exacerbations may lead to acute severe respiratory failure. Finally, cardiac failure (cor pulmonale) supervenes, and the patient dies in slow progressive deterioration of function. The FEV_1, the test most commonly done to document obstruction, decreases by 50 to 80 ml/year. Patients with an FEV_1 of about half predicted live on the average about 10 years; those with an FEV_1 of about a third predicted live 4 years. Once the FEV_1 is about one litre (1L), patients usually become dyspneic on exertion. When the FEV_1 is reduced below this level the patients are usually very disabled; walking and the chores of everyday life become difficult.

Clinical Evaluation of CAO

Symptoms of CAO

The cardinal symptoms of chronic airflow obstruction are cough, sputum production, shortness of breath at rest or on exertion and with far advanced disease swelling of the ankles (see Chapter 17).

The shortness of breath may be accompanied by wheezing indicating that there is increased airflow resistance. The patient may complain of "whistling noises" in the chest. Wheezing is usually more pronounced during expiration because the airways are becoming narrower as lung volume decreases. Thickening and inflammation of the airway wall, secretions in the bronchial lumen, or spasm of bronchial muscle (bronchospasm) may contribute to airway narrowing. Headache caused by the cerebral vasodilation of hypercapnia may be a prominent complaint. The occurrence of swelling of the ankles is an ominous feature since it indicates that cor pulmonale has supervened (p. 35).

Signs of CAO

Patients with CAO often have a rapid breathing frequency, appear to be struggling to breathe, and use their accessory respiratory muscles. Cyanosis, indicating hypoxemia, may be present. Evidence of right ventricular failure may be present (see below).

In the presence of minimal disease, no physical signs may be detected. Wheezing, especially during expiration, is a striking feature in moderate disease where reasonable airflow is preserved; severe disease is characterized by the "silent chest" because of the grossly reduced airflow rate.

The degree of hyperinflation, which is a reflection of the severity of the underlying lung disease, is indicated by the shape of the chest and by the shape and motion of the diaphragm. This is often best appreciated by radiographic examination.

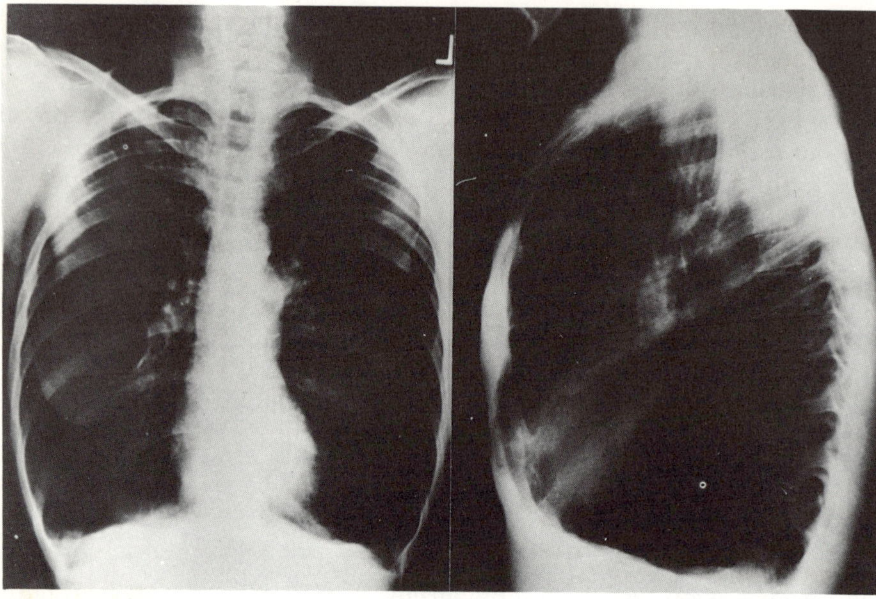

Figure 2.24. Anteroposterior and left lateral chest radiograph of a patient with severe CAO. Flattening of the diaphragm increased translucency of the lungs and pearlike configuration of the heart shadow are present in this patient, who has hyperinflated lungs and severe airflow obstruction. The lateral projection confirms the low flat position of the diaphragm and demonstrates an increased retrosternal airspace.

Radiological Examination in CAO

The radiological examination of the chest in CAO may be quite misleading in that it is insensitive in mild or moderate CAO. In severe cases of CAO, the chest radiograph confirms the presence of hyperinflation as indicated by low, flat diaphragmatic shadows and increased airspace between the sternum and the cardiovascular silhouette. When emphysema is advanced, hyperinflation may be extreme, and the diaphragms may in fact be inverted downward (Figure 2.24). Bullae, which are totally avascular, may be noted and the lung fields generally appear relatively avascular. In the presence of cor pulmonale, the proximal pulmonary arteries are enlarged.

Laboratory Assessment of CAO

The main purpose of lung function measurements in CAO is to provide an objective estimate of the degree of respiratory dysfunction. The measurements may provide information that aid in the treatment, management, and continued follow-up of the patient.

In the lung function evaluation of CAO, it is desirable to measure:

1. Airflow rates and the influence of an aerosol bronchodilator on the measurement. Simple tests such as the FEV_1 are adequate for managing patients with overt CAO and are often the only tests required for follow-up.
2. Lung volumes with special attention to estimation of trapped gas (residual volume) and total lung capacity and functional residual capacity.
3. Gas transfer using CO as the marker gas. This test (described in more detail in Chapter 9) is always low in established emphysema, but may be near normal in bronchitis indicating a special sensitivity of this test to the surface area curtailment in the former disease.
4. Distribution of ventilation. The slope of phase III following a VC of pure oxygen is suitable for this purpose.
5. Lung compliance: Severe loss of lung elastic recoil is indicative of emphysema rather than bronchitis or asthma.

Tests 1, 2, and 3 are done in most modern pulmonary function laboratories. Tests 4 and 5 are not done frequently in clinical evaluations.

Gas Exchange in CAO

The principles of gas exchange and the mechanisms of hypoxemia and hypercapnia are presented in Chapters 9 and 10. Briefly, the major abnormalities found are hypoxemia with or without hypercapnia. These abnormalities can be caused by ventilation-perfusion mismatching, with or without hypoventilation.

Cor pulmonale

Airway hypoxia and hypercapnia each cause pulmonary arterial vasoconstriction. Thus, pulmonary vasoconstriction is especially severe when both hypoxia and hypercapnia are present. In order to pump blood through these constricted vessels, greater pressure is required. This increased pressure in the pulmonary arteries, pulmonary hypertension, increases the afterload of the right ventricle, the load that the right ventricle works against. Thus, the ventricle works harder to maintain cardiac output and may fail. When this occurs, right ventricular end-diastolic pressure and, therefore, right atrial and venous pressure increase. When venous pressure is elevated, edema may develop in the dependent portions of the body.

Work of Breathing and Drive to Breathe

There are two factors that impede or "hinder" airflow into the lungs. The first is the elasticity of the lungs, and the second is the resistance of the conducting airways. The respiratory muscles do the necessary work to overcome these factors.

When the lungs are stiff (as in restrictive lung disease described in the next chapter), much energy is used in trying to expand the lungs. Thus, a breathing pattern with a low tidal volume and rapid frequency would minimize work by the respiratory muscles.

With CAO, the major impediment to airflow lies with the resistance to flow. The greater the flow rates, the more work has to be done to overcome resistance. Thus, having a low breathing frequency with large tidal volume and low flow rates would minimize the work of the respiratory muscles with CAO.

In reality, there is no "work sensor," and the breathing pattern is "chosen" by the respiratory control system. In other words, the actual breathing pattern is determined by the factors that influence the drive to breathe (see Chapter 6)—chemical drives, lung reflexes, and inputs from the cerebral cortex. Fortuitously, in restrictive lung disease, reflexes arising from the lungs predominate; there is rapid shallow breathing, an efficient pattern. In CAO, breathing frequency may be rapid or slow. Inflammation may stimulate irritant receptors in the airways, and the resultant rapid shallow breathing pattern results in wasted work by the respiratory muscles.

The drive to breathe is a critical factor in CAO. When airways are obstructed, to maintain ventilation, drive must be increased. In CAO, ventilation-perfusion mismatching can cause hypercapnia (Chapter 10); depressed chemical drive may allow the hypercapnia to persist. Increased drive can maintain blood gases at fairly normal levels in spite of severe disease.

Clinical Patterns in Severe CAO

Two clinical types of CAO, the "pink puffer" and the "blue bloater," have been described (Figure 2.25). In reality, these stereotypes represent both extremes of the spectrum of CAO. Only a tiny fraction of CAO patients can be categorized as "pure" pink puffers and blue bloaters. Between these two extremes are the vast majority of patients who may have features of both. We even occasionally see "blue puffers" and "pink bloaters."

The pink puffer is intensely dyspneic (puffing) but well oxygenated (pink) (Table 2.1). He is thin and has no right ventricular failure. The blue bloater has little or no dyspnea, is cyanotic (blue), and has peripheral edema (bloated)

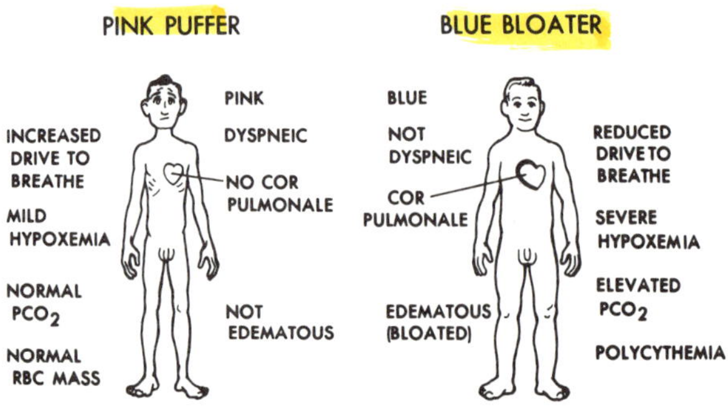

Figure 2.25. The pink puffer and blue bloater stereotypes of severe CAO.

Table 2.1. Features of the Pink Puffer

Ventilatory drive well preserved.
Intense dyspnea often with pursed-lip breathing.
The patient is thin and pink.
Small sputum volume.
Rarely develop edema and overt heart failure.
The predominant disease is panlobular emphysema.
Laboratory investigations
Severe expiratory airflow obstruction.
Severe hyperinflation and gas trapping.
Mild or moderate hypoxemia without hypercapnia.
Marked impairment of gas transfer (DL_{CO}).
Radiological evidence of hyperinflation.

as evidence of right heart failure (Table 2.2). Our understanding of these two stereotypes has evolved and is likely to further evolve in the future.

It used to be thought that the major difference between these types was the nature of the underlying lung disease with the pink puffer having panlobular emphysema, while the blue bloater was thought to have centrilobular emphysema or chronic bronchitis. The type of lung disease does not adequately explain why some patients with adequate ventilatory reserve "decide" to increase ventilation in an attempt to maintain normal PCO_2, while others permit the PCO_2 to rise. It is, therefore, likely that the drive to breathe plays an important role in determining whether the patient with CAO will hypoventilate. Thus, it is not the type of lung disease alone that determines a patient's clinical state, but the interaction between the lung disease and the drive to breathe. The pink puffer may be looked on as a "fighter" who maintains a normal Pa_{CO_2} in the face of great mechanical difficulties. The blue bloater, on the other extreme, settles for less work and allows the Pa_{CO_2} to rise.

Table 2.2. Features of the Blue Bloater

Ventilatory drive poor.
Relatively mild or even absent dyspnea.
Cyanotic.
Large sputum volume and recurrent respiratory infections.
Often edematous and in right heart failure (cor pulmonale).
The predominant disease is chronic bronchitis or centrilobular emphysema.
Laboratory investigations
Moderate or severe airflow obstruction.
Modest hyperinflation.
Hypercapnia, hypoxia and polycythemia.
Relatively normal gas transfer (DL_{CO}).
No radiological emphysema.

Early Airways Disease

As mentioned previously, not all people who smoke are destined to develop CAO. Except for those few people with α_1-antitrypsin deficiency, we do not know which patients who smoke are likely to develop CAO. In an attempt to identify the people at risk, attempts are made to diagnose CAO in its early stages.

There is evidence that CAO begins with pathological changes in the small airways, those with an internal diameter less than 2 mm. Since these airways account for only 10 to 20% of total airways resistance, relatively advanced disease may be present without clinical or physiological evidence of overt lung disease. For example, total airflow resistance would only increase by 10 to 20% if half the small airways were obliterated by disease.

As discussed earlier, there are lung function tests such as MMEFR, dynamic compliance, closing volume, and the air and helium flow-volume loop that are sensitive to changes in the small airways at an early stage of disease when the patient is asymptomatic and has a normal FEV_1. This is important information insofar as abnormality of these so-called sensitive tests of lung function may predict the later development of CAO. This suggestion awaits confirmation, but if it turns out that these tests are predictors of CAO, it may be possible to identify subjects at high risk and prevent overt disease by an appropriate intervention such as the cessation of smoking.

There is evidence that early changes in lung function in asymptomatic smokers are reversible on quitting smoking. Conversely, patients with overt CAO and abnormal FEV_1 may have irreversible lung disease.

Approach to Therapy and Management of CAO

The optimal management of CAO will depend on a clear understanding of the anatomical distribution, the nature of the pathological lesion, and the physiological consequences of the disease process (Figure 2.26). Adopting this approach, the physician may be in a position to recognize the reversible components of airflow obstruction in any given patient. It is likely that destruction of alveolar walls such as occurs in emphysema will not respond to therapy, whereas inflammatory changes in the bronchial wall might.

The patient must stop smoking, since cigarette smoking is the major contributing factor in the development and progression of CAO. It is rare that people who are nonsmokers develop overt CAO. There is evidence that quitting smoking early in the course of disease may be attended by reversibility of the disease process. In the latter stages of disease, the rate of deterioration may be slightly reduced by cessation of smoking.

Efforts are directed at *reducing airflow resistance.* Since emphysematous changes are irreversible, therapy and management are aimed at the bronchitis component.

Bronchodilators (see p. 154) are employed to release any airway smooth

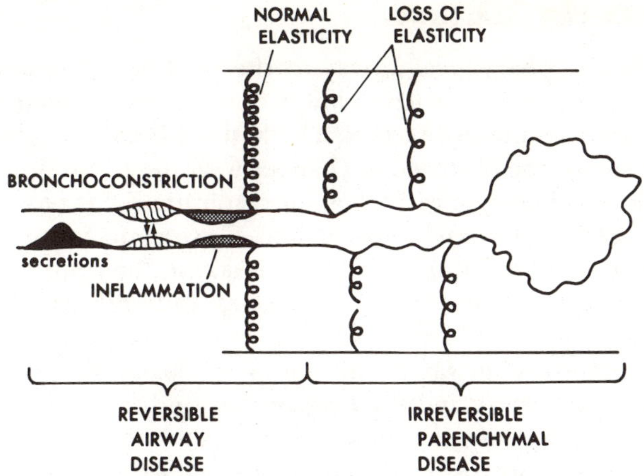

Figure 2.26. Schematic of the mechanisms of disease in CAO. Destructive lesions of the alveoli are likely to be irreversible, while inflammatory changes, bronchoconstriction, and secretions in the airway lumen can be benefited by appropriate chemotherapy and physiotherapy aimed at reducing production and facilitating expectoration of sputum.

muscle spasm that may be present. Antibiotics are used to control infections with increased airway secretions and bronchial wall inflammation. Corticosteroids that are nonspecific anti-inflammatory agents are always worth a carefully controlled trial in selected patients with severe disease.

Physiotherapy has a time-honored place in the management of CAO. Nevertheless, improvement while in a pulmonary rehabilitation program often appears to correlate better with psychological than with physiological parameters. Postural drainage and physiotherapeutic measures aimed at facilitating sputum expectoration may help in some patients. There is evidence that pursed-lip breathing is beneficial, as it slows the respiratory frequency, increases the tidal volume, and has been shown to improve gas exchange.

Since significant hypoxia occurs in the more advanced stages of CAO, it may be necessary to institute *supplementary oxygen* at this stage. Careful evaluation of the arterial oxygen tensions at rest, on exercise, and at night while sleeping must be available when deciding on oxygen enrichment of inspired air. Patients may develop severe oxygen desaturation particularly while they are dreaming. The minimum oxygen enrichment sufficient to raise Sa_{O_2} to about 90% should be established and employed. This objective may be achieved with oxygen therapy via nasal prongs at a 2 to 3 L/min flow rate. In some patients, there is worthwhile symptomatic improvement, increased exercise tolerance, and postponement of total disability and cor pulmonale.

All sedative drugs must be avoided because of possible respiratory center depression and precipitation of acute respiratory failure.

UPPER AIRWAY OBSTRUCTION

Obstruction in the pharyngeal airway or the trachea has important physiological differences from obstruction lower down in the respiratory tract. The differences are related to two factors. The first is whether the diameter of the airway at the site of the obstruction changes with the respiratory cycle. If the obstruction does not change with phase of respiration, it is a *fixed* obstruction; if it does change, it is a *variable* obstruction. The second factor is the location of the lesion. As will be discussed below, a lesion in the upper airway outside the thorax, an *extrathoracic obstruction,* behaves quite differently from an *intrathoracic obstruction.*

The diameter of the airway at the site of an obstruction is related to the pressure inside the airway and the pressure around the airway. With a fixed obstruction, the airway at the site of the obstruction is too stiff to change its dimensions as these pressures change. Thus, with this type of lesion, most commonly caused by scar formation, obstruction will be evident on inspiration and expiration.

If the obstruction is variable, the diameter of the airway will increase when the pressure in the airway exceeds the pressure around the airway. However, when the pressure in the airway is less than the pressure around the airway, the diameter of the airway will decrease, thus increasing the obstruction. When a lesion is intrathoracic, the pressure around the airway is pleural pressure; when it is extrathoracic, the pressure is simply the pressure surrounding the neck, atmospheric pressure.

Extrathoracic Variable Obstruction

The most common causes of such obstruction are paralyzed vocal cords, inflammation, enlarged lymph nodes, fat deposits, and tumors. During inspiration, the pressure in the airway is negative compared to the atmospheric pressure around the airway. This tends to decrease the diameter of the airway. During expiration, the pressure in the airway is positive compared to atmospheric pressure, thus reducing the obstruction (Figure 2.27). The increase in upper airway obstruction with inspiration explains the important finding of *stridor,* a crowing sound during inspiration in severe upper airway obstruction.

Patients with extrathoracic obstruction may have worsening of the obstruction during sleep and may develop *obstructive sleep apnea* (Chapter 6).

Intrathoracic Variable Obstruction

Tumors are the most common cause of intrathoracic variable obstruction. During expiration, the pleural pressure will exceed the intra-airway pressure, worsening the obstruction. During inspiration, the airway pressure is greater than the pleural pressure, lessening the obstruction (Figure 2.28).

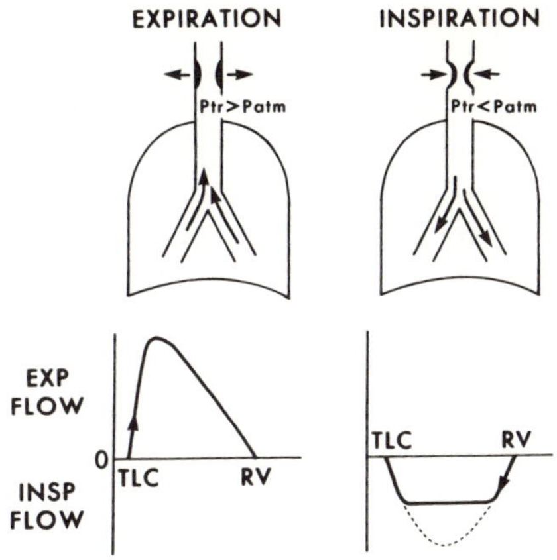

Figure 2.27. Variable extrathoracic obstruction. During forced expiration, the intratracheal pressure (Ptr) exceeds the pressure around the airway (Patm = atmospheric pressure), resulting in a decrease of the obstruction. During forced inspiration, when the pressure around the airway exceeds the intratracheal pressure, the obstruction is increased, hence the plateau on inspiration on the flow-volume curve. The dotted line is the normal curve.

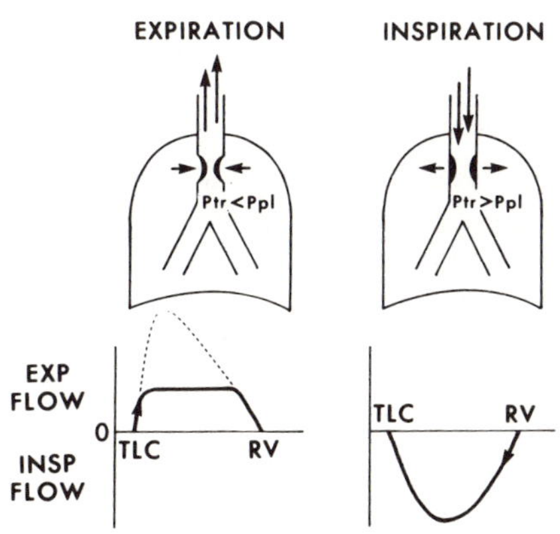

Figure 2.28. Variable intrathoracic obstruction. During forced expiration, the pressure acting around the airway (Ppl = pleural pressure) may be greater than the intratracheal pressure (Ptr), increasing the obstruction and causing a plateau during expiration on the flow-volume curve. During forced inspiration, the intratracheal pressure is greater than the pleural pressure, thus decreasing the obstruction, and the inspiratory curve may be normal. The dotted line is the normal curve.

Diagnosis of Upper Airway Obstruction

Flow-volume curves are used to document upper airway obstruction. Both expiratory and inspiratory curves are done. Inspiratory curves are done because with extrathoracic obstruction the problem is with inspiration. When obstruction is severe, a plateau is seen on the flow-volume loop. With a fixed obstruction, a plateau is present in expiration and inspiration; with an extrathoracic variable obstruction, the plateau is seen during inspiration; with intrathoracic variable obstruction, it is seen during expiration.

ASTHMA

Airflow obstruction caused by reversible airway smooth muscle constriction is discussed in Chapter 8.

BIBLIOGRAPHY

Fletcher C, Peto R, Tinker C, et al: The natural history of chronic bronchitis and emphysema: Eight-year study of early chronic obstructive lung disease in working men in London. Oxford, Oxford University Press, 1976.

Hutcheon M, Griffin P, Levison H, et al: Volume of isoflow: A new test in detection of mild abnormalities of lung mechanics. *Am Rev Resp Dis* 110:458, 1974.

Kryger M, Bode F, Antic R, et al: Diagnosis of obstruction of the upper and central airways. *Am J Med* 61:85, 1976.

Macklem PT: Disease in small airways. *Basics of RD*, vol 4 (no 5), 1976.

Matthay RA (ed): Symposium on obstructive lung diseases. *Med Clin North Am* 65:3, May, 1981.

McFadden ER, Kiker R, Holmes B, et al: Small airway disease: An assessment of the tests of peripheral airway function. *Am J Med* 57:171, 1974.

Morris JF, Koski A, Johnson LC: Spirometric standards for healthy nonsmoking adults. *Am Rev Resp Dis* 103:57, 1971.

Petty TL (ed): Chronic Obstructive Pulmonary Disease. *Lung Biology in Health and Disease*, vol 9. New York, Marcel Dekker, 1977.

Rodarte JR, Hyatt RE: Respiratory Mechanics. *Basics of RD,* vol 4 (no 4), 1976.

Thurlbeck WM: Chronic Airflow Obstruction in Lung Disease. *Major Problems in Pathology*, vol 5. Philadelphia, Saunders, 1976.

3

Lung Restriction

C.P.W. Warren

When the lungs are inflated, fresh air is sucked into them replenishing the oxygen taken up from the alveolar gas. Inflation is accomplished by contraction of the respiratory muscles, the diaphragm and external intercostal muscles. These enlarge the thoracic cage surrounding the lungs. Inflation of the respiratory system may be hindered by disorders of the lung itself or by alterations in the structures surrounding the lungs, the chest wall and diaphragm.

Diseases that reduce lung inflation are classified physiologically as the restrictive disorders. They hamper the movement and reduce the static volumes of the lung through their diminution of the respiratory system's distensibility. Examination of those factors that determine the inflation and distensibility of the respiratory system will enable the student to understand more easily what goes wrong in the restrictive disorders. This chapter describes the resting volume and the distensibility of the normal lungs before examining the consequences of reduced distensibility on the lung's function. Since over two hundred diseases are now known to have the potential to restrict the lungs, a résumé of their frequency, their major clinical features, and their pathology is given at the end of the chapter.

THE NORMAL LUNG

Normal Resting Lung Volume

Inspiration is an active process requiring contraction of the inspiratory muscles. Expiration is a passive process, since the respiratory muscles are relaxed and the energy necessary to empty the lungs is produced from that stored in the expanded elastic lungs. At the end of expiration, all the respiratory muscles are relaxed.

The volume of the air in the lungs when the respiratory system is at rest, that is, when there is no airflow and all the respiratory muscles are relaxed, is called the *functional residual capacity* (FRC). This is the volume of the lungs at the end of a normal expiration. The size of the FRC is determined by the interaction of two structures, the lungs and the thoracic cage. Both these structures are elastic; their tissues have the property that causes them to return to their resting shape after they have been deformed by a force. When removed from the chest, the lungs will empty of air; thus, the natural size of the lungs is even smaller than that of the relaxed respiratory system. On the other hand, the natural size of the thoracic cage is larger than that of the relaxed respiratory system. The final size of the respiratory system at FRC is determined by the balance of the pressure due to the lung's tendency to collapse, the elastic recoil of the lung (Pst_L), and the pressure due to the thoracic cage's tendency to expand, the outward elastic recoil (Pst_{TC}) of the chest wall (Figure 3.1). In life, the lungs and the thoracic cage are bound together by the film of pleural fluid. That this is an effective link is well known to any student who has tried to separate two microscope slides joined by a film of water; the slides slide on each other but cannot be pulled apart. If the pleural film is broken, as with a pneumothorax (a leak of air from the lung into the pleural space), then the lung empties because of its elastic recoil and the chest wall moves outward.

The volume of the lungs is made up of the tissue of the lungs, the blood within the lungs, and the volume of gas in the alveoli and airways. It is the volume of the gas in the lungs (and only 4% is in the airways) that is considered to be the measure of lung volume. The volume of the lungs may be reduced by disorders of the lungs or the structures surrounding the lungs, the pleural space, or the chest wall.

Normal Breathing

Inspiration is the result of contraction of the respiratory muscles enlarging the thoracic cage. The distending pressure (pressure = force per unit area) generated by the muscles is dissipated in overcoming:

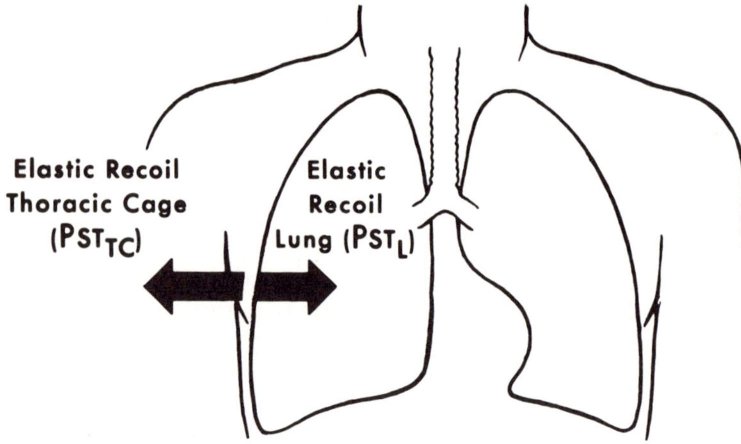

Figure 3.1. The lung volume at functional residual capacity (FRC). Pst_{TC} = elastic recoil of the thoracic cage. Pst_L = elastic recoil of the lung.

Elasticity

- The elasticity of the lungs and thoracic cage.

Resistance

- The frictional resistance of the airways to air flowing through them.
- The frictional resistance of the tissues of the lung and thoracic cage. This is the resistance to displacement of lung, rib cage, abdominal contents, etc.
- The inertia of the system (negligible).

The total pulmonary frictional resistance consists of that of the airways (80%) and that of the tissues (20%). The frictional resistance of the respiratory system is a factor only during movement of the system. The disorders of frictional resistance are covered in Chapter 2. In many of the disorders that increase the elastic recoil of the lungs, there will be increases in tissue frictional resistance as well, but it is rarely sufficient to limit respiratory excursions. For this reason, it will not be considered further.

The normal inspiration (tidal volume) during quiet breathing is 300 to 500 ml of air. The volume of air that enters the lungs will depend on the distending pressure produced by the respiratory muscles and the distensibility of the respiratory system. The pressure that overcomes the elastic recoil of the lungs is stored in the increased elastic recoil of the stretched lung. When the respiratory muscles relax, then the increased elastic recoil of the enlarged lung overcomes the chest wall causing the lungs to empty to functional residual capacity.

Compliance of the Respiratory System

The distensibility of the respiratory system is called *compliance,* which is the volume change produced by a change in the distending pressure.

$$\text{Compliance (C)} = \frac{\text{Change in volume } (\Delta V)}{\text{Change in pressure } (\Delta P)}$$

Since the respiratory system is elastic, the change in distending pressure is stored as elastic recoil. At any lung volume, when airflow is zero the elastic recoil is equal and opposite to the distending pressure that is expanding the lung.

$$\text{Compliance} = \frac{\text{Change in volume } (\Delta V)}{\text{Change in elastic recoil pressure } (\Delta Pst_L)}$$

When the compliance of the respiratory system is low (the system being stiff or less distensible), then a greater distending pressure is needed to enlarge it to the same volume as one with normal compliance. Conversely, the elastic recoil in the lung of low compliance is greater than that of a normal lung at the same volume.

In order to understand the compliance of the respiratory system fully, it is preferable at first to consider the compliance of its two parts, the lungs and the thoracic cage, separately.

Compliance of the Lungs

As mentioned before, when the lungs are removed from the body, their elastic recoil will empty them completely except for some gas trapped behind closed airways. If the lungs are then inflated by an above atmospheric pressure applied to the airway, or the lungs are surrounded by a subatmospheric pressure, then the change of volume that occurs as a result of that pressure can be measured. The relationship between the change in volume and the change in *transpulmonary pressure* (distending pressure) producing inflation gives the lung's compliance.

The pressure-volume curve of a lung during inflation is shown in Figure 3.2. As transpulmonary pressure increases, the volume increases steadily until, at a certain point, increasing the pressure further produces progressively less and less enlargement. When inflation pressure can no longer fill the lung, the elastic recoil of the lung is maximum. This property of the lung is familiar to anyone who has blown up a balloon, and such a balloon is also shown diagrammatically in the figure.

When the pressure-volume relationship of an object such as a rubber balloon is obtained, then the curve during inflation is the same as on deflation, and this is the same whether the balloon is filled with air or water. These observations are not seen when the experiment is done with the lungs. In 1929, von Neergaard performed this experiment on fresh excised lungs and found that the pressure necessary to inflate a lung filled with water was about half that needed to inflate a lung filled with air. The elastic properties of the tissues of the lung would not be altered by inflation with water, so he deduced that the interface between the surface film lining the lung and the air was an important contributor to the elastic properties of the lung. The alveoli of the lung act as millions of little bubbles, and when inflated their surface enlarges.

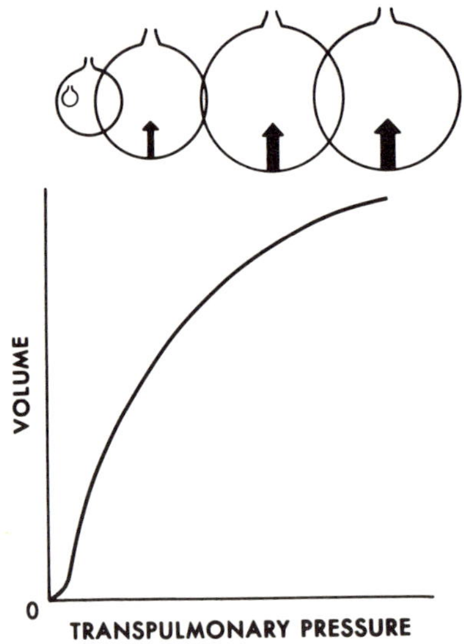

Figure 3.2. The relationship of the volume of the excised lungs to distending pressure. Above the graph is shown the size of a balloon that behaves in a similar way during inflation; the size and direction of the arrows is indicative of the elastic recoil of the balloon.

Release of the distending pressure allows the surface tension of the alveoli to shrink them. This phenomenon is the result of the surface tension forces of a liquid-air interface and is familiar to bubble blowers; the surface of a bubble shrinks to the smallest possible area.

The properties of the alveolar air-surface interface were found to be even more complex (Chapter 13). The surface tension of the lungs is higher at large lung volumes than small volumes, and at a given lung volume the surface tension is greater during inspiration than expiration. This phenomenon, *hysteresis,* is the property of the special surface active material, *surfactant,* which coats the alveoli. Surfactant has been extracted from the lungs, and when a film of this fluid is stretched its surface tension increases, and when compressed it decreases. Because surface tension decreases as lung volume shrinks, the alveoli are prevented from completely collapsing during expiration. Surfactant is a complex material consisting of the lipid lecithin (especially dipalmatyl lecithin) and protein.

The pressure-volume curve of the lung in life is different during inspiration than expiration (Figure 3.3) as a result of this remarkable property of surfactant. By tradition, the pressure-volume curve of the lung is recorded during expiration, since that is when the effect of the surfactant's surface tension recoil is minimum.

Compliance of the Thoracic Cage

The thoracic cage is a semirigid container, which can both diminish and expand in size to some extent; the limits of expansion are not met in life. The

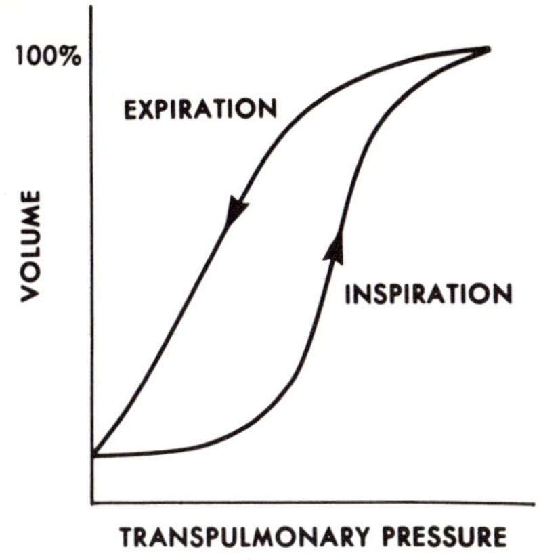

Figure 3.3. The relationship of the volume of the fresh-excised lung in air during inflation and deflation. The phenomenon of hysteresis is apparent from the divergence of the curves.

thoracic cage does not behave like a balloon but rather like a thick-walled rubber bulb that when compressed springs back to normal shape sucking in air. The changes in volume of such a bulb, the pressure-volume curve of the thoracic cage during deflation, and inflation are shown in Figure 3.4. The properties of the thoracic cage are determined by its component parts. First, there is the skeleton of the thoracic spine, ribs, and sternum, which are hinged

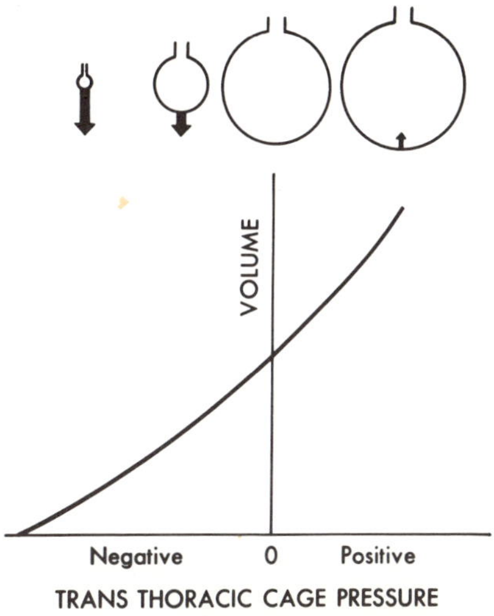

Figure 3.4 The relationship of the volume of the thoracic cage to compressing and distending pressure. Above the graph is shown the size of a rubber bulb that behaves in a similar way; the size and direction of the arrows is indicative of the elastic recoil of the bulb. At low volumes, the thoracic cage has a high elastic recoil that is tending to increase volume.

so that the cage can expand forward and laterally. Attached to the skeleton are the respiratory muscles, which move the bones. The diaphragm, which moves downward, also acts as a floor to the cage; its movement can be affected by the contents of the abdominal cavity and the state of the abdominal wall. The tone of the respiratory muscles affects the rigidity of the chest. Finally, changes in the connective tissue, adipose tissue, and skin may have an influence on the chest wall's expansion.

Compliance of the Intact Respiratory System

In life, the lungs and thoracic cage move in harmony, and the pressure-volume curve of the respiratory system is the sum of the curves of its parts. The pressure-volume curve consists of the sum of the pressure needed to expand the lung and to expand the chest wall at that volume. For any volume $P_{RS} = P_L + P_{TC}$. This is shown in Figure 3.5.

Measurement of Compliance

The Respiratory System

The pressure-volume (PV) curve of the respiratory system is determined clinically by measuring the pressure distending the system at several volumes during expiration. The measurements are made when no flow is occurring,

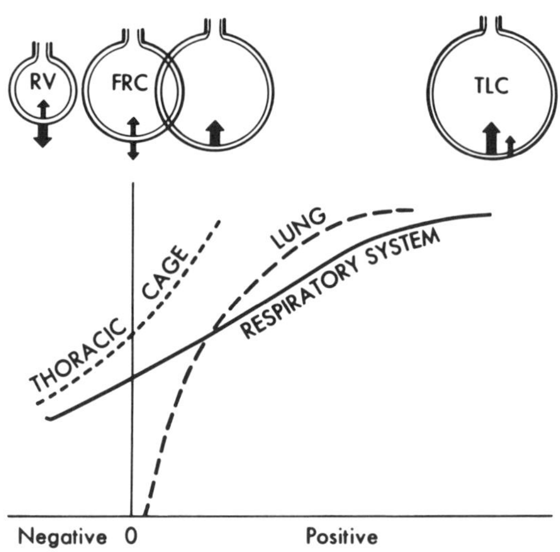

Figure 3.5. The relationship of the volume of the excised lung, thoracic cage, and intact respiratory system to various pressures. Above the graphs are shown the size of a combined balloon inside a bulb that behaves in a similar way to the intact respiratory system; the size and direction of the arrows are indicative of the elastic recoils of the bulb and balloon. At FRC, the lung is tending to decrease its volume, while the thoracic cage is tending to increase its volume. FRC is determined by the balance of these tendencies.

hence we are obtaining static measurements that are not affected by airflow resistance. The person being studied breathes to a lung volume and then fully relaxes all respiratory muscles as much as possible against a closed mouthpiece (Figure 3.6).

We can measure the volume accurately. But what is the pressure distending the respiratory system? It is the pressure across the respiratory system; on one side is alveolar pressure P_{ALV}; on the other side is the pressure on the surface of the chest, atmospheric pressure, which is referenced as zero. When there is no airflow, alveolar pressure equals mouth (or airway opening) pressure, P_{AO}. Thus, the distending pressure is $P_{AO} - 0 = P_{AO}$. To calculate compliance, the change in volume is divided by the change in P_{AO} over the linear portion of the pressure-volume curve near FRC.

The Lungs

The measurement of the PV curve of the lungs is measured in a similar manner to that described above (Figure 3.7). The pressure acting across the lung, the transpulmonary pressure P_L, is pleural pressure on one side and alveolar pressure on the other. Since during no flow, alveolar pressure equals pressure at the mouth, then transpulmonary pressure equals mouth pressure minus pleural pressure:

$$P_L = P_{AO} - P_{PL}$$

In clinical studies, pleural pressure is not measured directly. It has been found that esophageal pressure reflects pleural pressure over most lung volumes. Esophageal pressure is not an exact measurement of pleural pressure,

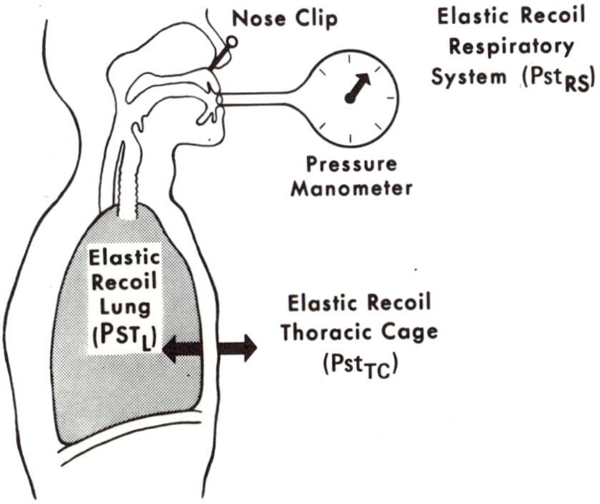

Figure 3.6. The measurement of the compliance of the respiratory system. Pst_{RS} = elastic recoil of the respiratory system; Pst_L = elastic recoil of the lungs; Pst_{TC} = elastic recoil of the thoracic cage. A manometer at the mouth measures airway-opening pressure.

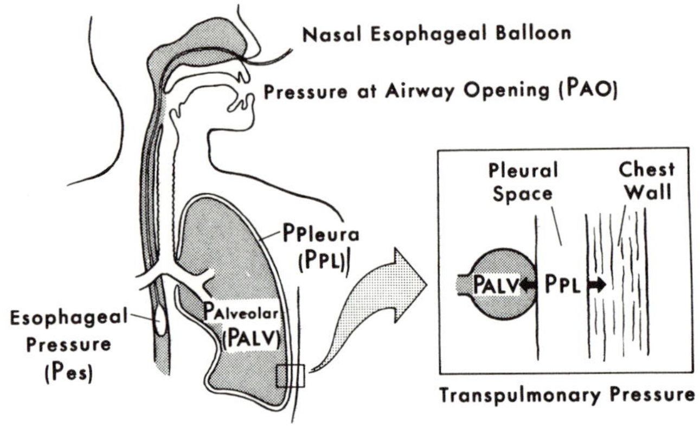

Figure 3.7. The measurements of the compliance of the lungs. P_{es} = esophageal pressure, which is used to measure P_{PL}, the pleural pressure. P_{AO} = pressure at the open mouth that, when the glottis is open and no airflow, equals P_{ALV}, the alveolar pressure.

but it faithfully follows changes in pleural pressure. The person being studied swallows a small balloon into the lower esophagus and the changes in pressure in the balloon are used to measure changes in pleural pressure.

A curve is plotted of the lung volume and the transpulmonary pressure associated with it during expiration from total lung capacity. A measure of compliance can be made by calculations from the linear portion of the PV curve (usually the curve above FRC):

$$\frac{\Delta \text{ Volume}}{\Delta \ (P_{AO} - P_{PL})}$$

The Chest Wall

We can calculate chest wall compliance in a similar way by dividing the volume change by the pressure acting across the chest wall, pleural pressure on one side, minus atmospheric pressure (zero) on the other. Alternately, by measuring the compliance of the respiratory system and the compliance of the lungs, the compliance of the chest wall can be calculated from the equation:

$$\frac{1}{\text{Total compliance}} = \frac{1}{\text{lung compliance}} + \frac{1}{\text{thoracic cage compliance}}$$

THE PHYSIOLOGICAL EFFECTS OF REDUCED COMPLIANCE

Disorders of the Lung

Lung Volumes

Although increases in lung tissue, blood volume, or lung fluid will encroach on the gas space of the lung, the loss will be small compared to the effects produced by concomitant changes in the lung's compliance. Such disorders

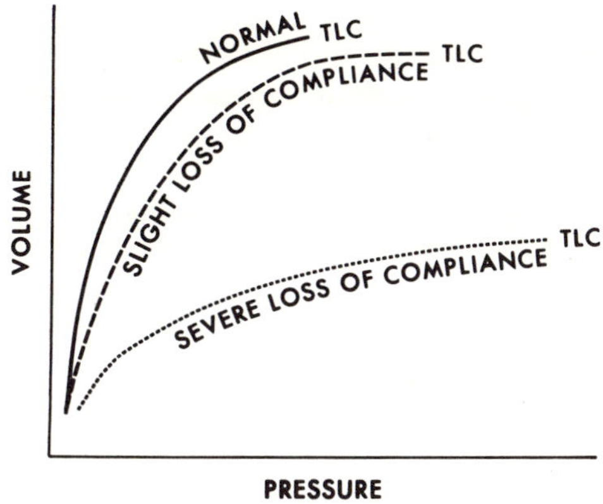

Figure 3.8. The relationship of transpulmonary pressure and lung volume in patients with normal, slight, and severe loss of compliance.

change the composition of the lung tissue and increase the elastic recoil of the lung. This increased inward recoil of the lung will overcome the outward recoil of the chest wall and sway the equilibrium position inward; functional residual capacity is reduced. Total lung capacity will also be lowered. Residual volume may be decreased, but since it reflects primarily airways closure, it may not change. Finally, the whole pressure-volume curve is shifted down and to the right. The changes in the pressure-volume curve are illustrated in Figure 3.8. It should be noted that a person with low compliance generates higher pressure at TLC than a person with normal lungs. This is because the force a muscle can generate increases with fiber length, and fibers of inspiratory muscles shorten with increases in lung volume. Thus, with low lung volumes the inspiratory muscles, being longer, are at a greater mechanical advantage and can generate a greater distending pressure.

Ventilation

The supply of fresh air to the lungs is determined by the frequency and depth of respiration. When compliance is reduced, the respiratory muscles will have to strengthen their contraction to maintain tidal volume, thus increasing the work of breathing. The respiratory system minimizes the increase in work by decreasing the tidal volume and increasing breathing frequency. In fact, most patients with reduced compliance tend to *hyperventilate*. That this is not due to hypoxemia has been demonstrated, since it continues despite correction of hypoxemia. Moreover, it has been found that if the afferent vagus nerve is blocked in the neck of such patients, hyperventilation and the accompanying sensation of dyspnea may be relieved. The hyperventilation and dyspnea arise from the impulses of receptors in the lungs (discussed in Chapter 6).

Patients with reduced compliance of the thoracic cage do not have increased stimulation of lung reflexes and so hyperventilation is not found; in fact, hypoventilation is common with disorders such as kyphoscoliosis.

Airflow

The flow of air entering the lungs is determined solely by inspiratory effort overcoming the airflow resistance and the elasticity of the respiratory system. Thus, increases of elasticity will tend to reduce inspiratory airflow for a given effort; this effect is not significant clinically.

The flow of air leaving the lungs depends primarily on the elastic recoil of the lungs and the degree of resistance to airflow in the airways. The elastic recoil of the thoracic cage and the effort of the expiratory muscles have only a slight effect. The increased elastic recoil of the lungs will increase airflow from the alveoli and, since disorders that reduce pulmonary compliance rarely affect the airways, resistance to the airflow is not increased.

At first sight, measurements of maximum expiratory flow from the lungs, discussed in more detail in Chapter 2, such as forced expiratory volume at one second (FEV_1), maximum midexpiratory flow rate (MMF), or flow at 50% of vital capacity (FEF 50%) are apparently reduced. Although the vital capacity is reduced, the proportion of the vital capacity expired in the first second (FEV_1/FVC) is actually increased above the normal 70 to 80%; the flows are "supernormal." If the flow-volume curve is compared to the predicted curve at the same absolute lung volume (Figure 3.9), then it can be seen that flows are actually increased.

Gas Exchange

Arterial hypoxemia, which is common in subjects with restricted lung movement, could be produced by four mechanisms; alveolar hypoventilation, true shunting, ventilation-perfusion mismatching, and impaired diffusion of oxygen. These mechanisms are discussed in greater detail in Chapter 9.

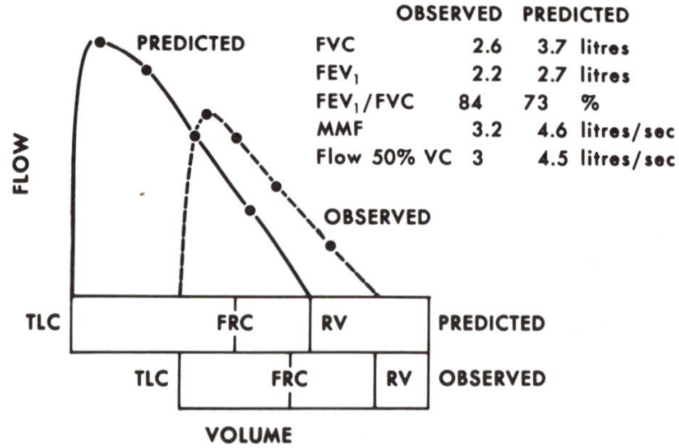

Figure 3.9. The absolute lung volumes and forced expiratory flow-volume curve of the normal (predicted) person and those observed in the patient with reduced lung compliance. Lung volumes are indicated by the horizontal rectangles under the loops.

Alveolar Hypoventilation

It has already been pointed out that the breathing pattern in most patients with reduced lung compliance is rapid and shallow, and minute ventilation is high. It is not surprising, therefore, that the arterial P_{CO_2} is low. Alveolar hypoventilation is thus not the explanation for their arterial hypoxemia. Does alveolar hypoventilation ever occur? Certainly. As mentioned before, it does occur with reduced compliance of the thoracic cage, when compliance becomes so low that the respiratory muscles can no longer generate the pressure necessary to inflate the lungs sufficiently. Alveolar hypoventilation in patients with low compliance identifies a severe disorder and is often a terminal event.

True Shunting

True shunting is mentioned only to dismiss it as a cause of hypoxemia in these disorders. Even with severe pulmonary fibrosis, there is no significant destruction of alveoli without an accompanying loss of the vasculature of that area.

Ventilation-Perfusion Mismatching

Gas Mixing. The mixing of fresh air with alveolar gas is remarkably uniform in the human lungs. The distribution of the gas to the alveoli is determined by the time constant of the lung unit (e.g., a lobe, an acinus, an alveolus) under consideration. The time constant is the product of the resistance of the airways leading to that lung unit and the compliance of the unit. Units with lowered time constants (low compliance in restrictive disorders) fill up less easily than those with normal time constants. If all units in the lung have equal increments in their time constant, then ventilation will still be uniformly distributed. In most chest and lung disorders with reduced compliance, the changes in compliance of lung units are patchy and time constants vary between units. Gas mixing in these disorders is usually nonuniform, but is not as disturbed as with airflow obstruction.

Alveolar Gas-Pulmonary Capillary Matching. The maintenance of normal gas exchange by the lungs is most dependent on the close contact of pulmonary capillaries with alveolar gas. It is not a continuous contact, since the capillaries are spread as a network over the alveoli (Figure 3.10). The capillaries and alveoli are separated only by the alveolar epithelial lining, the fused basement membranes of alveolus and capillary, and the capillary endothelium (Figure 3.11). If the alveoli adjacent to the capillaries are poorly ventilated, then there may be insufficient oxygen in the alveolar gas to saturate the hemoglobin in that area; these are low $\dot{V}/\dot{Q}$ regions. In other areas though ventilation and perfusion may be normal, or even if regions are better ventilated than perfused (high $\dot{V}/\dot{Q}$ units), the hypoxemia that results from the low $\dot{V}/\dot{Q}$ units cannot be corrected. Disturbances in ventilation-perfusion distribution are common in disorders that reduce both lung and thoracic cage compliance. This mismatching is related more to the nature and distribution of the disor-

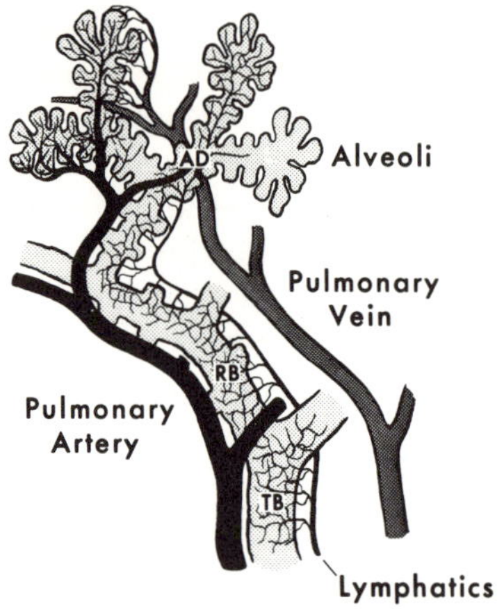

Figure 3.10. A diagram drawing of part of a pulmonary acinus, showing the pulmonary capillaries spread as a network over the alveoli. The pulmonary arteries, pulmonary veins, and lymphatic vessels are apparent. The small airways are shown. (TB = terminal bronchiole. RB = respiratory bronchiole. AD = alveolar duct).

der affecting compliance than to the overall reduction in compliance. These changes of $\dot{V}/\dot{Q}$ combined with changes in distribution of the ventilation combine to produce hypoxemia.

Impaired Diffusion of Oxygen

With each inspiration, fresh air flows through the airways down to the terminal bronchioles where it comes to a halt. From here the inspired oxygen

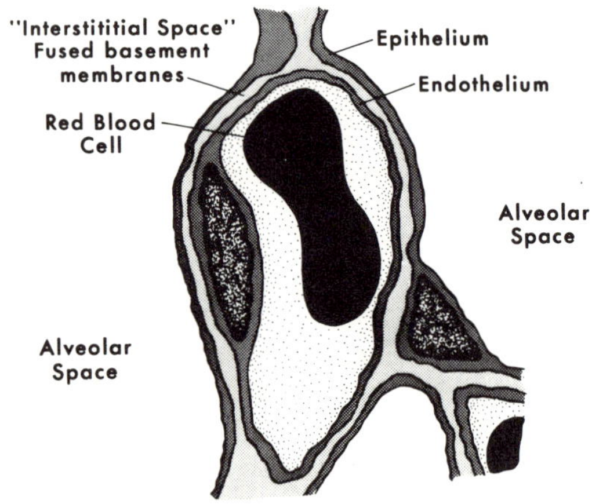

Figure 3.11. A diagram of the alveolar wall taken from an electron microphotograph of the normal lung. Note the fusion of epithelial and endothelial basement membranes.

moves by diffusion down a concentration gradient into the alveoli and then through the alveolar-capillary membrane to the desaturated red blood cells entering the lung from the right heart.

The two factors that may be of importance in limiting the diffusion of oxygen in the restrictive disorders are the volume of the lungs and the distance to be traveled by the gas. The reduction in lung volume that occurs when compliance is low, particularly if alveoli are destroyed by the disease's pathology, will reduce the alveolar surface and impair diffusion. The pulmonary disorders that reduce pulmonary compliance are also associated with widening of the alveolar-capillary distance due to cellular infiltration and deposition of fibrous tissue between the alveolar lumen and capillary endothelium (Figure 3.12). For many years, the result of this increased distance for diffusion of oxygen was thought to be responsible for the hypoxemia of these disorders, and the term "alveolar-capillary block" was coined.

Although there are reasons why O_2 diffusion should be impaired in these disorders, it has been found that *diffusion of oxygen is not hampered sufficiently to explain the hypoxemia observed*. The hypoxemia in these disorders is, as in most other lung disorders, mainly due to ventilation-perfusion mismatching. That is, oxygen may diffuse out from the alveolar gas but not meet a perfused capillary on the other side of the membrane, or conversely, red cells may flow past poorly ventilated alveoli whose alveolar gas is not well replenished with oxygen. The hypoxemia is better called a disorder of oxygen transfer than one of diffusion. It has been estimated that hypoxemia in disorders of restricted lung movement can be attributed 20% at most to poor diffusion and 80% or more to ventilation-perfusion mismatching.

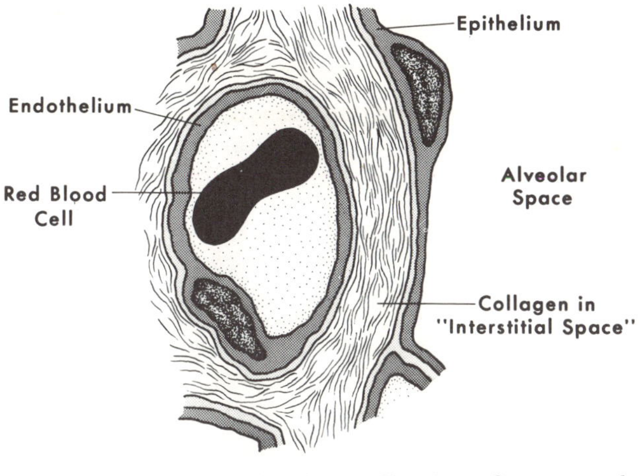

Figure 3.12. A diagram of the alveolar wall taken from an electron microphotograph of a lung from a patient with a form of fibrosing alveolitis. The collagen has been laid down between the basement membranes of the epithelial and endothelial cells.

Carbon Dioxide Excretion

Carbon dioxide excretion is discussed in more detail in Chapter 10. It has already been pointed out that most subjects with a low lung compliance tend to hyperventilate, because lung reflexes produce a rapid shallow breathing pattern. Carbon dioxide washout from the alveolar gas is good, and arterial P_{CO_2} tends to be low as a result. Only in low chest wall compliance and advanced disorders with very low lung compliance is overall ventilation reduced sufficiently for CO_2 to be retained.

Exercise (See p. 195)

Few of the disorders reducing compliance of the respiratory system produce hypoxemia at rest until they are well advanced. Oxygen uptake may be less efficient, but the system meets the demands put upon it. However, during exercise the demands may not be met, and hypoxemia may become apparent or even profound. The hypoxemia is the result of the impaired oxygen transfer in the lungs. On exercise, the cardiac output is increased considerably, and normally such an increase in flow would be accommodated by the recuitment of more pulmonary capillaries. But in the disorders in which lung compliance is reduced, there occurs a partial obliteration of the capillary bed. With an increased cardiac output, and with more blood flowing through insufficient capillaries, there is a reduced transit time for red cells through the lungs; there is insufficient time for oxygen to combine with hemoglobin. An analogy would be the problem of a mechanic bolting nuts on a car assembly line who is faced with having to reach for nuts while the cars are passing more quickly—some bolts will not be tightened.

Disorders of the Pleura

The accumulation of air or fluid in the pleural space will break the adhesion of the lung to the chest wall causing the lung to empty because of its own elastic recoil. This effect will be compounded by the pressure of the air or fluid in the thoracic cavity. These disorders are reviewed in Chapter 7.

Disorders of the Thoracic Cage

The compliance of the respiratory system will be reduced by changes in the shape of the thoracic skeleton (e.g., kyphoscoliosis), by reduction in the elastic recoil of the thoracic cage (e.g., neuromuscular paralysis, obesity), or by changes external to the thoracic cage (e.g., abdominal ascites) that elevate the diaphragm.

The effect of reduced compliance of the chest wall has been studied in normal subjects whose chests have been strapped with rubber tubing. In this situation, the total lung capacity, functional residual capacity, and vital capacity are reduced. The subjects respond to the situation by breathing shallowly and rapidly. There is no change in resistance to airflow in the lungs. Gas distribution becomes nonuniform and arterial oxygen tension falls; this is the result of atelectasis of small units of alveoli.

DISEASES PRODUCING RESTRICTED LUNG MOVEMENT

The main damage of the many lung diseases restricting lung movement occurs beyond the terminal bronchioles and affects mainly the alveoli. The thread that binds these disorders together is that all of them may restrict lung volume with reduction of compliance. The etiology of these diseases is varied and often unknown; their pathogenetic mechanism is usually unclear, and the classification of their pathology can be controversial. These disorders may be grouped under several headings: in this book restrictive lung disease, in another infiltrative lung disorders, in a third interstitial lung disease, and in a fourth the diffuse pulmonary alveolar fibroses. The student of these disorders must use a thesaurus to track them down when consulting the literature. There have been several attempts to classify these disorders and at the moment the best is probably by etiology.

Etiological Classification of Restrictive Lung Disorders

Etiology	*Examples*
Infectious	Viral infections
Neoplastic	Lymphangitis carcinomatosis
Vascular	Mitral stenosis
Inhaled dusts	
Inorganic	Silicosis
Organic	Farmer's lung
Ingested toxins	Busulphan, paraquat
Unknown	
Without any systemic disease	Fibrosing alveolitis
With systemic disease	Rheumatoid lung

Since many of the diseases producing restriction are of unknown etiology, this classification must remain somewhat unsatisfactory for the moment.

The Frequency of the Restrictive Lung Diseases

The prevalence of these restrictive lung diseases in the general population is unknown. The relative frequency distribution of the diseases may be judged by the results of lung biopsies from a large number of patients in an American hospital (Table 3.1). But lung biopsy results cannot be used to judge the frequency of the diseases, since less than half of the patients are biopsied. For instance, such a series will not include asymptomatic people and those with clinically obvious diagnoses. Table 3.2 shows the clinical experience of the

Table 3.1. The Diagnoses Made by Open-Lung Biopsy in Diffuse Pulmonary Disease

Diagnoses that can be made only by lung biopsy:	
Interstitial fibrosis (fibrosing alveolitis)	14
Subacute interstitial pneumonitis	2
Goodpasture's syndrome	2
Idiopathic "pulmonary" hemosiderosis	1
Eosinophilic granuloma	7
Pulmonary alveolar proteinosis	7
Pulmonary arteriolitis	1
Desquamative histiocytic interstitial pneumonitis	1
Diagnoses that may require lung biopsy for confirmation:	
Sarcoidosis	14
Chronic beryllium disease	13
Chemical pneumonitis	1
Pneumoconioses	17
Carcinomatosis	7
Lymphoma	2
Diseases that ordinarily do not need lung biopsy:	
Tuberculosis	4
Fungal infections	2
Cystic disease of the lungs	2
Rheumatoid lung disease	1
Radiation fibrosis	1
Pulmonary emboli	2
No diagnostic help from lung biopsy	5

SOURCE: Adapted from Gaensler EA, Moister MVB, and Hamm J: *N Engl J Med* 270:1319–1331, 1964, with permission.

author in a general teaching hospital over six years and probably reflects the general frequency of the disorders. Most subjects did not have a biopsy.

The Common Pathology of the Restrictive Lung Diseases

The common characteristic of all these restrictive lung diseases is acinar infiltration by fluid and cells in varying amounts and types. Many of the diseases may heal by fibrosis, which further impairs the function of the acinus. Examination of the structure of the acinus reveals the basis for the functional changes already discussed in this chapter; the alveoli, blood vessels, and the lymphatics are intimately intertwined. Interposition of cells, fluids, or fibrotic tissue disrupts their functional structure. In many organs, such as the liver, there is a definite interstitium; in the pulmonary acinus there is no particular interstitium—rather the alveolar cells and the pulmonary capillaries are so close that their basement membranes appear to be fused (Figure 3.11). But in the diseases included in this section, the interstitial space reappears since the basement membranes are often separated by infiltration of the interstitial

Table 3.2. The Diagnoses Made on Clinical Criteria, Transbronchial and Open Lung Biopsy, or Autopsy of Diseases that May Produce Restrictive Lung Disorders over a 6-Year Period in St. Boniface General Hospital, Winnipeg, Canada

Disease	*Number*	*Total (%)*
Sarcoid	32	29
Fibrosing alveolitis	17	16
Collagen diseases	8	7
Pneumoconioses	6	5
Allergic alveolitis	12	11
Carcinomatosis	5	5
Infections	7	6
Drug reactions	4	4
Mitral stenosis	2	2
Goodpasture's syndrome	2	2
Idiopathic pulmonary hemosiderosis	1	1
Radiation fibrosis	1	1
Nonspecific fibrosis	12	11
Total	109	

space (Figure 3.12). It is this interference of the close bond between alveolus and capillary that can make these diseases so disruptive of gas exchange.

The pathological changes in the restrictive lung diseases can be extensive but not produce any symptoms or disturbance in lung function. This is particularly true in sarcoid. Disturbance in lung function is dependent on the properties of the infiltrate. For instance, in fibrosing alveolitis the low compliance does not seem to be due to the presence of more collagen in the lung, but rather to a change in the type of collagen. In carcinomatosis of the lymphatic system of the lung, the cancer grows along the lymph vessels and produces a rigid skeleton to the lung resulting in very stiff lungs. On the other hand, carcinomatosis of the lung produced by scattered islands of tumor deposited in the blood vessels may have little effect on function until the infiltrate is large. Infiltrates of upper lobes, for example, ankylosing spondylitis, interfere less with lung function than infiltration of the lower lobes where the lung's major gas exchange occurs.

All these disorders may result in extensive fibrosis of the lungs, thus totally destroying them. At this stage, the diseases are virtually indistinguishable in their clinical appearance, radiology, lung function, and pathology. At this stage, retraction of fibrous tissue may distend and damage the small airways of the lung giving a honeycomb appearance of the lung and even causing areas of emphysema.

The Clinical Features Common to the Restrictive Lung Diseases

Many patients with restrictive lung diseases are asymptomatic and have no signs.

Symptoms. The most common symptom of these diseases is dyspnea on exercise, and as the disease advances this will also occur at rest. A dry cough is sometimes present. Phlegm production, hemoptysis, and chest pain are not common features. In advanced disease, cor pulmonale and right heart failure will appear.

Signs

- Cyanosis. Central cyanosis may be apparent on exercise and eventually also present at rest.
- Respiration. The patient will tend to breathe rapidly and shallowly.
- Clubbing. Clubbing of the fingernails is associated with all the advanced stages of restrictive lung diseases. Clubbing is commonly found at the early stages of asbestosis and fibrosing alveolitis.
- Examination of the thorax usually reveals few changes by inspection, palpation, or percussion. The characteristic sign on auscultation are crackles (crepitations), which appear late in inspiration; these are thought to be due to bronchioles, normally closed by surrounding infiltrates, popping open on inflation.

Some Clinical Features Distinguishing the Restrictive Lung Diseases

Family History. Some restrictive diseases are inherited, for example, fibrosing alveolitis (rarely) and neurofibromatosis, and so appear in the family tree.

Associated Diseases

- Infectious. Many lung infections have healed by extensive fibrosis, but this is rare. It is seen most often after tuberculosis.
- Congenital. Lung infiltrates are seen occasionally in neurofibromatosis, tuberous sclerosis, and the histiocytoses, for example, Hand-Schüller-Christian disease.
- Collagen disease. Restrictive lung disorders can be seen in scleroderma, rheumatoid arthritis, systemic lupus erythematosus, Sjögren's syndrome, dermatomyositis, and the vasculitides.
- Carcinomatosis. Metastatic cancer may spread in the lung by the blood or lymphatic vessels and rarely by the airways of the lung. Lymphoma may sometimes infiltrate the lungs.

Environment. Some inhaled material may produce restrictive lung diseases. Dusts that may produce these are listed under *inorganic* Table 3.3 and *organic*

Table 3.3. The Inorganic Dusts that May Produce Restrictive Lung Disease

Silica	Talc
Asbestos	Hematite
Coal dust	Aluminum ores and powder
Beryllium	Iron oxide

Table 3.4. Toxic gases such as cadmium fumes, ozone, and oxides of nitrogen may also damage the acinus and lead to fibrosis.

Radiation to the lung will cause local lung infiltration.

Ingested Materials. The herbicide, paraquat, or such drugs as busulphan, bleomycin, nitrofurantoin, and salazopyrine may produce lung infiltration.

The Evaluation of Restrictive Lung Disease

The patient in whom restrictive lung disease is suspected is best evaluated by a careful history in which clues to etiological agents or associated disorders are sought. Physical examination may also reveal important signs, for example, clubbing, coal dust tattooing of the skin, neurofibromatoses, arthritis, and involvement of other organs (skin, spleen, eye) in sarcoid.

Radiology (see Figure 3.13). The radiograph in the early stages of the restrictive lung disease can be normal. The change that reveals its presence is diffuse shadowing, which is usually either a reticular pattern, scattered nodules, or a combination of both. In more advanced disease, shrinkage of the lungs is apparent and eventually honeycombing develops. Most restrictive lung diseases involve the lower lobes preferentially, but sarcoidosis may be most apparent adjacent to the hila, whereas silicosis, ankylosing spondylitis, and chronic allergic alveolitis involve the upper lobes. Hilar node enlargement is characteristic of sarcoidosis.

Immunology. The immunological changes, for example, increased globulins and autoantibodies, associated with the collagen diseases are usually found when the lung is involved. But nonspecific antibodies are found in unrelated restrictive lung diseases; serum rheumatoid and antinuclear factors are quite

Table 3.4. The Organic Dusts that May Produce Restrictive Lung Disease

Material	*Disease*	*Cause*
Moldy hay	Farmer's lung	Thermophilic actinomyces
Bird droppings	Bird-owner's lung	Bird serum
Humidifier water	Humidifier fever	? Thermophilic actinomyces
Mushroom compost	Mushroom-worker's lung	? Thermophilic actinomyces
Sugar cane	Bagassosis	? Thermophilic actinomyces

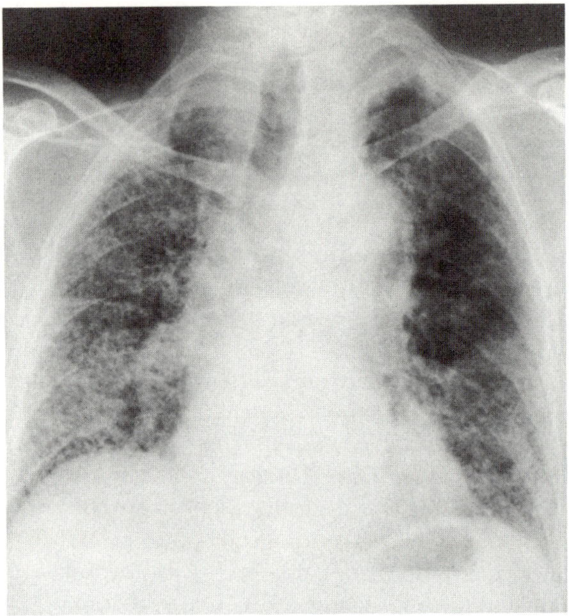

Figure 3.13. A chest radiograph of a patient with advanced fibrosing alveolitis. Severe dyspnea. TLC 77% predicted, VC 61%, FEV_1/FVC 75%, single breath CO transfer 30% predicted, rest Pa_{O_2} 45 mmHg, Pa_{CO_2} 28 mmHg.

frequently found in fibrosing alveolitis, silicosis, and asbestosis. Circulating immune complexes have been detected in fibrosing alveolitis and eosinophilic granuloma.

In allergic alveolitis, specific antibodies against the causative antigen are usually present.

Diagnosis. The diagnosis of the restrictive lung disease may not be revealed by the measures described so far. In that case, a biopsy of the lung may reveal a characteristic appearance so that the disease can be identified; however, in the advanced stages the changes are usually those of nonspecific fibrosis. The biopsy is the only way to confirm the diagnosis in fibrosing alveolitis.

Prognosis. The natural history of these diseases is extremely variable. As long as the patient has no symptoms and normal lung function, the patient can be optimistic.

Therapy. If an etiological agent can be identified, then it must be avoided in the future. If the restrictive lung disease is a feature of a general disease, then it should be treated as part of that.

In such lung diseases as fibrosing alveolitis and sarcoid, the mainstay of treatment is steroids. These probably suppress the inflammatory process and may reduce healing by fibrosis. A therapeutic trial of steroids for 1 to 2 months is worth trying in most of the diseases when abnormal function is present; there may be an amelioration in these disorders.

SUMMARY OF THE MORE COMMON RESTRICTIVE DISEASES

Sarcoid

Sarcoid is a disease characterized by the presence in all of several affected organs or tissues, of epithelioid cell tubercles, without caseation, though some fibrinoid necrosis may be present at the center of a few tubercles. It proceeds either to resolution or to conversion of the epithelioid cell tubercles into avascular acellular hyaline fibrous tissue.

- *Age:* Majority 20 to 40 years. More common in blacks than whites.
- *Sex:* Slightly more common in women than men.
- *Etiology:* Unknown.
- *Clinical:* Usually asymptomatic. Chest x-ray films show hilar glands often enlarged. Sarcoid can involve any organ of the body. In advanced lung involvement dyspnea and cough prominent.
- *Immunological:* Relative lymphocyte anergy.
- *Prognosis:* Good.
- *Treatment:* Steroids for symptoms, abnormal lung function, uveitis, and hypercalcemia.

Fibrosing Alveolitis

Fibrosing alveolitis (interstitial pneumonitis) is a disease (or group of diseases) characterized by inflammation of the alveoli typified by cellular thickening of the alveolar walls with a strong tendencey to fibrosis. The cellular infiltrate includes lymphocytes, plasma cells, and granulocytes. In some cases, there is desquamation of mononuclear cells into the alveolar space. Collagen diseases can be associated with fibrosing alveolitis.

- *Age:* Over 40 years.
- *Sex:* Women and men equally affected.
- *Etiology:* Unknown.
- *Clinical:* Progressively develop dyspnea, sometimes rapidly, sometimes slowly.
- *Immunological:* Serum rheumatoid factor, antinuclear factor, and circulating immune complexes sometimes found.

- *Prognosis:* Usually poor.
- *Treatment:* Those with a cellular lung biopsy and/or circulating immune complexes may respond to corticosteroid therapy.

Inhaled Inorganic Dusts

Workers exposed to inorganic dust (size less than 5 microns) may develop lung fibrosis. The dusts most commonly producing this are listed in Table 3.3. The development of the diseases reflects the quantity of dust inhaled (concentration or duration). Except for asbestosis, the radiological changes of the diseases precede the development of symptoms and abnormal function. In silicosis and coal-worker's pneumoconiosis, progressive massive fibrosis is the hallmark of developing abnormal function.

- *Silicosis:* Predisposes to tuberculosis.
- *Asbestosis:* Usually associated with pleural reaction. Predisposes to lung cancer, especially in smokers.
- *Prognosis:* Usually good unless progressive massive fibrosis supervenes.
- *Treatment:* Prevention by dust control and a medical surveillance program. No specific treatment.

Inhaled Organic Dusts

People exposed to certain organic dusts develop allergic alveolitis, a granulomatous disease of the acinus sometimes leading to fibrosis. The more common causes are listed in Table 3.4. The disease is the result of an immunological reaction to the organic dust and is thought to be mediated through the formation of antigen-antibody complexes or lymphocyte-mediated hypersensitivity. After a sudden heavy exposure to the dust, the sensitized person will develop an acute diffuse pneumonia. With chronic exposure a more insidious illness develops and lung fibrosis results (see p. 158).

- *Immunological:* Serum precipitating antibodies against the dust are usually found. Evidence of immediate and delayed skin reactions to the dust and lymphocyte sensitivity to bird proteins can sometimes be detected.
- *Prognosis:* Usually good except if repeated exposure occurs.
- *Treatment:* Steroids ameliorate the acute illness but probably do not alter the chronic disease. Prevention should be the avoidance of the dust.

OTHER DISEASES ASSOCIATED WITH RESTRICTIVE LUNG DISORDERS

Common Disorders

- *Radiation:* Sufficient radiation to the lungs will produce damage and fibrosis that may respond to corticosteroids.

- *Drugs:* Busulphan and bleomycin produce dose-related lung fibrosis; nitrofurantoin and salazopyrine may produce a hypersensitivity reaction.
- *Toxic Gases:* Cadmium, ozone, ammonia, and oxides of nitrogen can produce severe damage to the terminal bronchioles.
- *Infections:* Widespread infections of the lung may cause a severe restrictive disorder, for example, miliary tuberculosis, viral pneumonia.
- *Carcinoma:* Carcinoma spread by blood or lymphatics may cause restriction. Rarely does cancer spread through the airways (alveolar cell carcinoma). Lymphomas rarely infiltrate the lungs.
- *Collagen Diseases:* Collagen diseases may cause fibrosing alveolitis as well as vasculitis in the lungs.

Rare Disorders

- *Eosinophilic Granuloma:* Age 20 to 40 years. 20% with bone lesions.
- *Tuberous Sclerosis:* Multiple tumors of the connective tissue.
- *Neurofibromatosis:* Typical skin lesions.
- *Idiopathic Pulmonary Hemosiderosis:* Usually in children, hemoptysis associated with iron deficiency anemia
- *Goodpasture's Syndrome:* The disease produces infiltration and bleeding in the lung and glomerulonephritis. Antibodies against the basement membrane of glomeruli and alveoli are present in the serum.

THE CHEST WALL AS A CAUSE OF RESTRICTION

Skeletal Disease

Kyphoscoliosis. Simple kyphosis has little effect on lung function, since diaphragm and rib movement remain uniform. But kyphoscoliosis, in which there is twisting of the spine and hence distortion of the thoracic cage, may interfere with function. Idiopathic kyphoscoliosis is the most common form today and appears during adolescence. In the past, poliomyelitis was the most common cause. In kyphoscoliosis, there is a reduction of total lung capacity and vital capacity, without obstruction to airflow. The disturbed movement of the thoracic cage leads to uneven distribution of ventilation and ventilation-perfusion ratios. Hypoxemia is the result and eventually hypoventilation and cor pulmonale result. The respiratory failure is compounded by a loss of the chemical respiratory drive in these patients.

Ankylosing Spondylitis. Ankylosing spondylitis occurs mainly in men and produces fusion of the vertebral bodies and of the costovertebral joints. Good and uniform diaphragmatic movement is retained. The vital capacity and total lung capacity are slightly reduced. Thoracic wall compliance is low. The effect on ventilation is minor, and blood gases are normal. Uncommonly, ankylosing spondylitis causes fibrous-cystic changes in the upper lungs. This may effect lung function.

Pectus Excavatum. Pectus excavatum is a congenital depression of the sternum. Despite a severe cosmetic disturbance there is little interference in lung function.

Flail Chest. Flail chest occurs after multiple rib fractures and part of the chest wall no longer expands when the respiratory muscles contract. The loss of the rigidity of the ribs means that as inspiration is attempted the chest wall at the site of the fractures is sucked in by the reduced pleural pressure produced by diaphragmatic movement. This can prevent the ribs from healing properly. To stabilize the chest wall, the patient must be mechanically ventilated with positive pressure until the fractures heal.

Neuromuscular Disease

Paralysis of one diaphragm reduces ventilation on that side. Bilateral paralysis leads to loss of total lung capacity and vital capacity. Orthopnea is prominent, since when supine the flaccid diaphragm is displaced headward by the abdominal contents. Reduced chest wall compliance due to loss of muscle tone lowers functional residual capacity. Lower motor neuron lesions of the intercostals hardly matter unless the diaphragm is also affected.

The patient with acute neuromuscular disease, for example, Guillain-Barré syndrome or myasthenia gravis, has reduced peak inspiratory pressure at first and then loses total lung capacity. When the vital capacity is reduced to about 1 liter (in an average man), respiratory failure is imminent and mechanical ventilation should be used.

Skin

It has been suggested that sclerodermatous skin might impair chest wall movements. This effect, if it occurs, would be negligible compared to the lung disease of scleroderma. Severe scarring after burns could impair chest wall movement.

Obesity

Obese patients with normal lungs may develop severe respiratory failure (see p. 113). For many years, this was attributed to the results of impaired chest movement by the excess tissue. These patients may have reduced chemical drive to breathe. More recently upper airway obstruction has been found to occur in these subjects during sleep. Adipose neck tissues may encroach on the relaxed pharynx. In obesity, thoracic cage compliance is reduced; functional residual capacity is reduced but not residual volume or total lung capacity. Ventilation, but not perfusion, of lower lung zones is impaired and leads to chronic hypoxemia. Hypoventilation and cor pulmonale can complicate severe obesity.

BIBLIOGRAPHY

Bates DV, Macklem P, Christie RV: *Respiratory Function in Disease.* Philadelphia, WB Saunders, 1971, p 268.

Crystal RG (Moderator), Fulmer JD, Roberts WC, Moss ML (Discussants): Idiopathic pulmonary fibrosis. NIH Conference. *Ann Int Med* 85:769, 1976.

Gaensler EA, Carrington CB: Open biopsy for chronic diffuse infiltrative lung disease: Clinical roentgenographic and physiological correlations in 502 patients. *Ann Thorac Surg* 30:411, 1980.

Keogh BA, Crystal RG: Pulmonary function testing in interstitial pulmonary disease. *Chest* 78:856, 1980.

Mitchell DN, Scadding JG: Sarcoidosis. *Am Rev Respir Dis* 110:774, 1974.

Murray J: *The Normal Lung.* Philadelphia, WB Saunders, 1976, p 77 and p 151.

Schatz M, Patterson R, Fink J: Immunologic lung disease. *N Engl J Med* 23:1310, 1979.

Turner-Warwick M: A perspective view on widespread pulmonary fibrosis. *Br Med J* 1:371, 1974.

Turner-Warwick M, Burrows D, Johnson A: Cryptogenic fibrosing alveolitis: clinical features and their influence on survival. *Thorax* 35:171, 1980.

Ziskind M, Jones RM, Weill H: Silicosis. *Am Rev Respir Dis* 113:643, 1976.

4

Pulmonary Vascular Disease

Howard S. Goldberg

The pulmonary circulation is designed to allow for exchange of respiratory gases with the environment. A very large surface area between blood and air across an extremely thin tissue barrier allows the lung to perform efficiently. The pulmonary circulation has the important property of being able to increase its surface area for gas exchange as cardiac output increases to match increased tissue oxygen demands. The large cross-sectional area of the pulmonary vascular bed allows the entire cardiac output to flow through the lung at an average pressure of about one-tenth that of the systemic circuit. Furthermore, as cardiac output increases, the pressure in the pulmonary vascular circuit can remain low because of the recruitment of previously unperfused vessels. This serves to lower the resistance to blood flow.

The major clinical problems involving the pulmonary circulation result from disorders in the ability of the pulmonary circulation to function at low pressure. Specifically, these problems are pulmonary hypertension and pulmonary edema. The former leads to derangement in normal cardiovascular function and the latter to hypoxemia.

STRUCTURE AND FUNCTION OF THE PULMONARY CIRCULATION

Anatomical Considerations

Anatomically, the pulmonary circulation is divided into arteries, arterioles, capillaries, venules, and veins. The pulmonary artery is part of a low pressure circulation system. The normal pulmonary artery pressure is 25/8 mmHg compared to 120/70 mmHg for the aorta. Even though the main pulmonary artery has the same intraluminal diameter as the ascending aorta, it has a smaller wall thickness and much less organized elastic laminae. The elastic laminae become regular when the pulmonary artery enters the lung and are present down to vessels of about 1 mm in diameter. Thereafter, elastin gradually disappears as the vessels become purely muscular at about 500 μm. This muscle tissue also gradually diminishes and is absent in vessels less than 30 μm in diameter. These small arterioles form a capillary network within a meshwork of interstitium.

Part of the surface of the capillary vessels has a close structural relationship with the alveolar septum. This surface is so thin that it cannot be separated into its components by light microscopy. The constituents of this surface are capillary endothelial cells and alveolar epithelial cells, with either a fused basement membrane or an extremely thin interstitial space composed of fine elastic fibers, collagen bundles, and an occasional fibroblast (Figure 4.1). The thinness of this surface facilitates the diffusion of gases between the blood and alveolar air. The rest of the capillary surface does not have such a close relationship with the alveoli. Where the barrier is thicker, the basement membranes are not fused and the interstitium contains more collagen, cells, and proteoglycan matrix.

The capillaries drain into amuscular venules. As the venules increase in diameter to 100 μm, muscle and elastin begin to appear. The extrapulmonary portion of the pulmonary veins have a muscular media that is myocardium.

There are few pulmonary artery to pulmonary vein anastomoses, although pulmonary artery to bronchial artery anastomoses are not uncommon. However, the most common type of anastomosis is between the bronchial and pulmonary veins.

Pulmonary lymphatics begin at the level of the respiratory bronchiole and

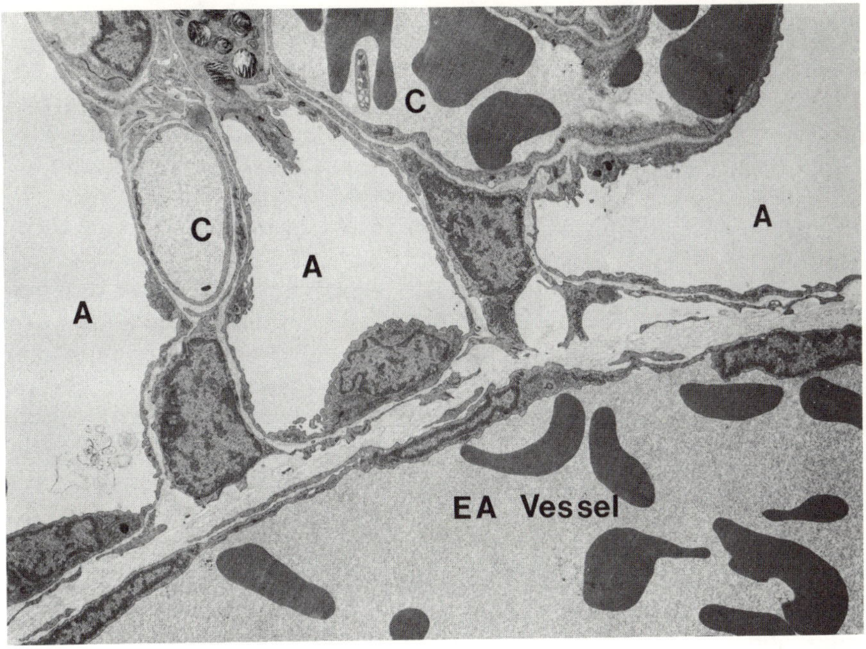

Figure 4.1. The pulmonary microcirculation. A = alveoli. C = capillary. EA = extra-alveolar blood vessel, probably venule. Two capillaries C are shown, one in cross section and one in longitudinal section. Note the thin barrier between capillary blood and alveolar air (magnification ×4000). (Courtesy of Juan Gil and J. McNiff, Hospital of the University of Pennsylvania, Philadelphia, Pennsylvania.)

are quite abundant. Their structure is similar to lymphatics elsewhere in the body.

The pulmonary interstitial space is relatively scanty around the alveolar vessels but may contain fibroblasts and connective tissue fibers. As the vessels in the lung get larger, the interstitium contains more connective tissue, proteoglycans, macrophages, mast cells, and interstitial cells. These interstitial cells contain contractile proteins and may serve a regulating function with regard to blood flow or localization of interstitial fluid. This structural framework may serve the important function of storage of extravascular water and proteins and directing them toward the hilum of the lung and lymphatics.

Pulmonary vasculature has several important metabolic functions. These include the conversion of angiotensin I to angiotensin II and the breakdown of bradykinin at the endothelial surface. The endothelial cells also metabolize serotonin, norepinephrine, and prostaglandins E and F. However, the most important function of the pulmonary circulation is to provide a large surface area for release of carbon dioxide from the body and uptake of oxygen from the air.

Physiological Considerations

Matching of Ventilation and Perfusion

Matching of ventilation to perfusion is important to optimize gas exchange. If there is perfusion to a lung region with no ventilation, the blood does not have an opportunity to exchange gases with the air. The blood undergoes no change in CO_2 or O_2 content. This type of perfusion is called a *right to left shunt.* In the normal lung, this accounts for less than 5% of the total cardiac output.

In other areas of the lung, there may be no perfusion at all, yet ventilation may occur. This is called *dead space ventilation.* Obviously, ventilation of conducting airways is dead space ventilation (anatomic dead space), but ventilation of unperfused alveolar units is also dead space ventilation. The total *physiological dead space ventilation* accounts for less than 30% of the total minute ventilation.

We can express shunt in terms of a ratio of ventilation to perfusion, $\dot{V}/\dot{Q}$. Since there is zero $\dot{V}$, the $\dot{V}/\dot{Q}$ is zero. In similar terms, in physiological dead space, which has zero $\dot{Q}$, $\dot{V}/\dot{Q}$ is infinite.

The normal lung has a $\dot{V}/\dot{Q}$ that lies between these two extremes. Normal alveolar ventilation is about 4,500 ml/min. Normal pulmonary perfusion is about 5,500 ml/min. $\dot{V}/\dot{Q}$ is, therefore, normally about .8.

In the absence of a significant defect in gas diffusion, hypoxemia can occur if $\dot{V}/\dot{Q}$ is reduced. With a $\dot{V}/\dot{Q}$ of zero, increasing the amount of oxygen in alveoli does not improve the O_2 content of the blood leaving the region of shunt. However, in the absence of shunt, blood leaving regions with low $\dot{V}/\dot{Q}$ will have an increase in O_2 content if the alveolar oxygen is increased. The mechanism of these effects are discussed in greater detail in Chapter 9.

Determinants of Pulmonary Blood Flow: Zones 1, 2, and 3

We have not yet considered the pressure-flow relationship in the pulmonary circulation. The understanding of this relationship requires a separation of the pulmonary vasculature into two types of vessels, distinguished by their response to lung inflation.

These vessels are *alveolar vessels* and *extra-alveolar vessels.* Lung inflation compresses alveolar vessels and distends extra-alveolar vessels. This is because lung inflation results from a relative increase in alveolar pressure (the pressure surrounding alveolar vessels) and a relative fall in pleural pressure (the pressure surrounding extra-alveolar vessels).

When the alveolar pressure exceeds the intraluminal pressure of the alveolar vessel, it collapses or closes. It is obvious that no flow can occur through alveolar vessels that are closed. In upright humans, alveolar pressure may exceed pulmonary artery pressure near the top of the lung. If the mean pulmonary artery pressure is 15 cmH_2O at the level of the lung hilum and the lung extends 16 cm above the hilum, then the alveolar pressure at the top of the lung is zero relative to atmospheric pressure and the pulmonary artery

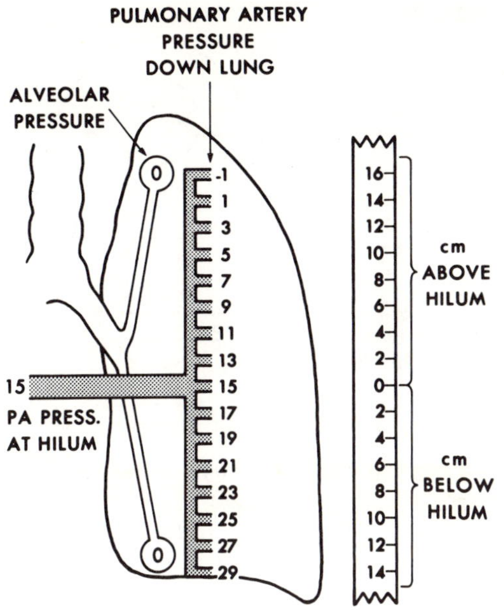

Figure 4.2. The effect of gravity on alveolar and vascular pressures in the lung. Although pulmonary artery pressure is 15 cmH_2O at the hilum, the intravascular pressure decreases by 1 cmH_2O for every cm above the hilum and increases by 1 cmH_2O for every cm below the hilum. Thus, pulmonary artery pressure increases from the top to the bottom of the lung. In contrast, alveolar pressure is not affected by gravity. Thus, in the top of the lung, alveolar pressure exceeds pulmonary artery pressure; thus there is no flow here. This is zone 1.

pressure is -1 cmH_2O (Figure 4.2). In this case the alveolar pressure surrounding an alveolar vessel would be greater than the pressure inside the vessel, and it would be closed. The region of the lung where alveolar pressure exceeds pulmonary artery pressure has been called zone 1. There is no blood flow in zone 1 (Figure 4.3).

For each centimeter down the lung, the pulmonary artery pressure increases while the alveolar pressure remains constant. Once pulmonary artery pressure exceeds alveolar pressure, blood flow through alveolar vessels occurs. Further down the lung the difference between pulmonary artery pressure and alveolar pressure increases and blood flow increases proportionally. This is zone 2.

At some point further down the lung, pulmonary venous pressure will exceed alveolar pressure. From this point down, flow is proportional to the difference between pulmonary artery pressure and pulmonary venous pressure. This is zone 3.

The differences between the zones can be compared to an aqueduct system (Figure 4.4). Water is carried from a height equivalent to the pulmonary

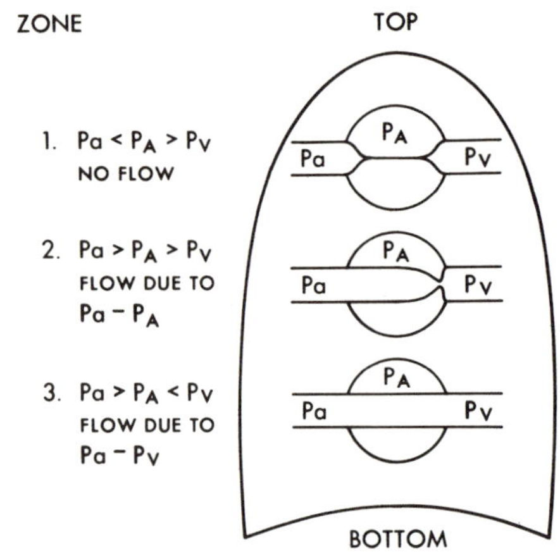

Figure 4.3. The three zones of the lung. The blood flow in the zones is determined by the interrelationship of alveolar, arterial, and venous pressures. (Adapted, with permission, Hughes JMB, Glazier JB, Maloney JE and West JB: Effect of lung volume on the distribution of pulmonary blood flow in man. *Respiration Physiology* 4:58–72, 1968.)

arterial pressure (Pa), down to another height equivalent to the alveolar pressure (PA). Where PA is higher than Pa there is no flow; this is zone 1. In zone 2 flow is determined by the difference between Pa and PA. As long as the height of the draining stream equivalent to the venous pressure (Pv) is below alveolar pressure, the height of Pv has absolutely no effect on the water draining into the stream. When the height of the stream (Pv) exceeds the height of the

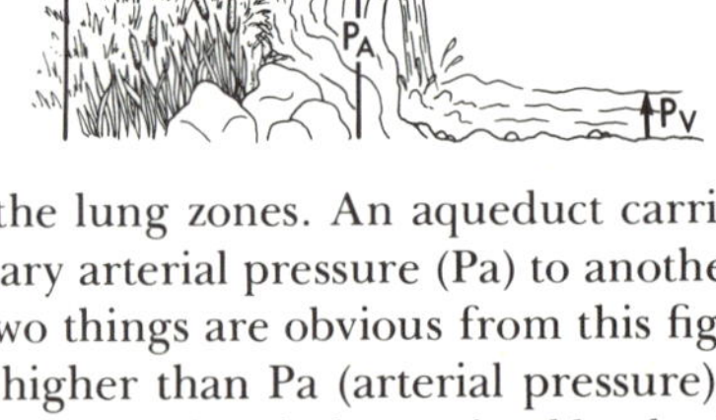

Figure 4.4. Analogy of the lung zones. An aqueduct carries water from one height equivalent to the pulmonary arterial pressure (Pa) to another height equivalent to the alveolar pressure (PA). Two things are obvious from this figure. The first is that if PA (alveolar pressure) were higher than Pa (arterial pressure), there would be no flow, zone 1. In the present case, zone 2 flow is determined by the difference between Pa and PA. As long as the height of the draining stream (equivalent to venous pressure, Pv) is below alveolar pressure, the height of this stream has absolutely no effect on the water falling into the stream.

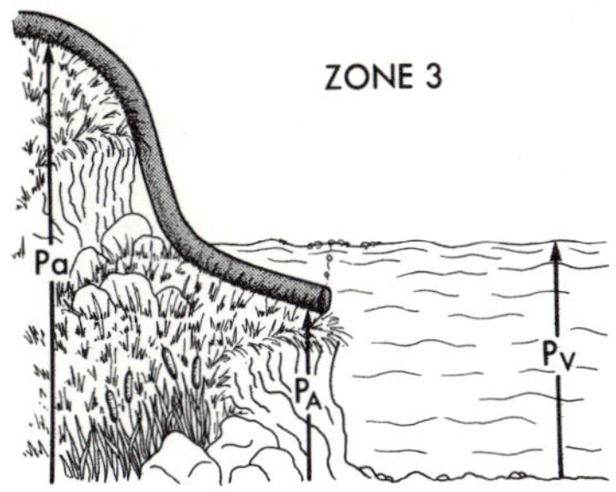

Figure 4.5. Zone 3. The height of the stream (venous pressure) has risen and now exceeds the height of the outlet of the aqueduct (alveolar pressure). Flow is now due to the difference between Pa and Pv.

aqueductal outlet (PA), flow is due to the difference between Pa and Pv (Figure 4.5).

In zone 3 both pulmonary artery pressure and pulmonary venous pressure increase equally going down the lung. Therefore, the gradient for flow does not increase in zone 3 as it does in zone 2. Yet when measured there is an increase in flow down zone 3, although it is less than in zone 2. Since the driving pressure for flow is not changing in zone 3, as it does in zone 2, the resistance to flow down zone 3 must be decreasing. If the resistance to flow down zone 3 is decreasing, then it may also be decreasing down zone 2. So in zone 2 there is an increase in flow due to an increase in driving pressure and perhaps a fall in resistance; while in zone 3 there is an increase in flow due to a fall in resistance without a change in driving pressure. Therefore, a greater change in flow going down zone 2 than in going down zone 3 can be expected. This is the case.

What can account for the alteration in resistance to blood flow in these zones? Where resistance is decreasing, the possibilities are *recruitment of parallel channels* or *distension of channels already receiving flow.* Distension of vessels already receiving flow occurs because of the increase in distending pressure down zones 2 or 3. The recruitment of parallel channels occurs in at least two ways: first, the opening of arterioles with muscular media that were previously closed and second, by distributing the postarteriolar blood flow into a larger capillary network of alveolar vessels. There is evidence that all of these mechanisms occur.

In summary, the perfusion of the lung can be subdivided into zones. Zone 1 occurs when pulmonary alveolar pressure is greater than both pulmonary arterial and pulmonary venous pressure. Zone 2 occurs when pulmonary alveolar pressure is less than pulmonary arterial pressure but greater than pulmonary venous pressure. Zone 3 occurs when pulmonary alveolar pressure is less than both pulmonary arterial and pulmonary venous pressure.

Pulmonary Vascular Resistance

Calculation of pulmonary vascular resistance is often simplified by taking the difference between pulmonary artery pressure and left atrial pressure and then dividing by the flow. This can lead to serious errors if the blood flow is not all in zone 3. The back pressure for flow in zone 2 is the alveolar pressure, not the venous pressure. If left atrial pressure and thus venous pressure is lowered in zone 2, this does not influence flow at all, any more than lowering the level of a stream formed at the base of a waterfall can influence the amount of water going over the falls. At any level in zone 2, the driving pressure is the difference between pulmonary artery pressure and alveolar pressure.

But even if the proper driving pressure is used in determining pulmonary vascular resistance, it should be noted that the pressure-flow relationship in the lung is not linear. Furthermore, it has not been established that in a no flow state the driving pressure is zero. In other words, even with some positive pressure, arterioles in the pulmonary vascular bed may be closed, just as in the systemic vasculature.

The importance of this is most evident when interpreting the effects of drugs or other interventions. If pulmonary blood flow is decreased, it will appear as if there is an active increase in pulmonary vascular resistance. This effect may be no different than the normal pressure-flow relationship in the lung. Therefore, caution must be used when interpreting apparent changes in pulmonary vascular resistance.

Regulation of the Pulmonary Circulation

The pulmonary circulation is not simply a series of passive tubes. The circulation can be regulated. This is accomplished by local vasoconstriction. Unlike the systemic circulation, which generally dilates in the presence of hypoxia and hypercapnia, the pulmonary circulation constricts. In addition, when blood flow to the lungs is increased (as during exercise), recruitment of vessels occurs. That is, flow occurs in parallel channels that were "empty." This has the effect of increasing the size of the vascular bed. This latter mechanism can keep the pressure low in spite of marked increases in flow.

In low $\dot{V}/\dot{Q}$ units, the alveolar oxygen tension becomes reduced. This reduction in alveolar oxygen tension can lead to pulmonary vasoconstriction, by a mechanism that is not yet understood.

It is clear that the entire "reflex arc" for hypoxic vasoconstriction is in the lung itself. This response can be elicited in the lung when it is removed from the body. The stimulus appears to be low O_2 concentration in the vicinity of small branches of the pulmonary artery. The most important source of this hypoxia is a reduced Po_2 in airspaces adjacent to these vessels, although a low Po_2 in the blood in the vessel itself can also cause constriction. Whether the constriction involves local neural reflex arcs or humoral agents such as histamine is unclear. It could be that hypoxia simply induces metabolic alterations within the smooth muscle cell itself and that these metabolic changes cause the muscle to contract.

Hypercapnia and acidosis, which also independently cause pulmonary vasoconstriction, tend to augment the effect of hypoxic vasoconstriction. Thus, patients with hypoxia and hypercapnia tend to have more severe pulmonary hypertension than patients with hypoxia alone. Figure 9.24 shows the effect of hypoxemia on pulmonary artery pressure in patients with lung disease.

This response of the circulation to abnormal gas tension has some theoretical advantages. In lung disease, there may be regional differences in lung function. Those areas that are poorly ventilated have a lessened influence on total gas exchange if the fractional blood flow to the poorly ventilated region is reduced. The pulmonary vasoconstriction occurring in hypoxic regions would increase the resistance to blood flow and would then have the desired effect of reducing the regional fraction of the pulmonary blood flow. That is, flow would be increased in less hypoxic regions.

This effect becomes less beneficial as more and more lung regions become poorly ventilated. If too many regions undergo hypoxic pulmonary vasoconstriction, the pulmonary artery pressure necessary to have a normal cardiac output may rise to higher levels. This can then lead to higher pressure in the right heart. If the right heart pressures rise sufficiently, signs of right heart failure such as ankle edema, large tender liver, prominent neck veins that don't empty with inspiration, or even anasarca may develop. Under such a circumstance, the patient may also show electrocardiographic signs of right heart enlargement or strain. When this sequence of events is seen in the patient, a diagnosis of *cor pulmonale* can be made.

At high altitude, where the partial pressure of oxygen is reduced, even people with normal lungs may undergo hypoxic pulmonary vasoconstriction and suffer the sequelae of pulmonary hypertension.

Although this effect has been regarded as uniformly bad, it should be noted that with the increase in pulmonary artery pressure a more uniform distribution of pulmonary blood flow occurs. This tends to lessen the $\dot{V}/\dot{Q}$ in excessively high $\dot{V}/\dot{Q}$ areas and tends to normalize $\dot{V}/\dot{Q}$ for the entire lung, with a resultant improvement in arterial oxygen tension.

If pulmonary hypertension is long-standing, anatomic changes in the pulmonary arteries and veins can occur. These changes are primarily characterized by medial hypertrophy.

The pulmonary circulation responds to a wide variety of exogenous and endogenous compounds (Table 4.1). Endogenous agents such as angiotensin II, serotonin, and prostaglandin $F_2\alpha$ cause constriction of the pulmonary circulation. Acetylcholine can dilate the pulmonary circulation.

α-Adrenergic agents such as norepinephrine cause constriction, whereas β-adrenergic agents such as isoproterenol produce vasodilation. Blockade of α-receptors and β-receptors produces the following results. β-Blockade enhances the constrictor response, while α-blockade reduces the constrictor response.

Other pharmacological agents such as the methylxanthines, the nitrates, and the smooth muscle dilator hydralazine can reduce vasoconstriction. However, the clinical experience of using agents that reduce pulmonary vasocon-

Table 4.1 Agents Acting on the Pulmonary Circulation

Constrictors	*Dilators*
Hypoxia	β-Adrenergic agents
Hypercapnia	Nitrates
α-Adrenergic agents	Hydralazine
Serotonin	Acetylcholine
Angiotensin II	
Prostaglandin $F_2\alpha$	

striction in treating pulmonary hypertension has been disappointing. Only hydralazine appears to be effective, and this is only true in some patients.

Congenital heart disease, mitral stenosis, and other forms of acquired heart diseases can also lead to pulmonary hypertension. A discussion of these ailments is outside the scope of this chapter.

PULMONARY HYPERTENSION

Pulmonary Hypertension Secondary to Lung Disease

As discussed above, hypoxia and hypercapnia cause pulmonary vasoconstriction. Thus, disorders such as chronic airflow obstruction, which cause hypoxemia and sometimes hypercapnia, can lead to pulmonary hypertension and cor pulmonale. Disorders in which hypoventilation is prominent (obesity-hypoventilation, idiopathic hypoventilation, kyphoscoliosis) also can lead to pulmonary hypertension.

In restrictive lung diseases, the fibrotic disorder may actually engulf and obliterate vessels. This form of pulmonary hypertension occurs during the late stages of pulmonary fibrosis.

In patients who develop severe hypoxemia during sleep, those with sleep apnea and those with chronic airflow obstruction, there occurs a marked rise in pulmonary artery pressure during sleep.

Pulmonary Embolism

A sequela of pulmonary embolic disease is pulmonary hypertension. Since all materials in the systemic venous blood will reach the pulmonary circulation, it follows that such materials can occlude pulmonary vessels. The most common form of embolism is clot, thromboembolism. Other materials that can embolize and occlude the circulation include amniotic fluid, tumor masses, air, and catheters. The fat embolism syndrome may develop following a variety of metabolic and traumatic insults to the body. The pathogenesis of this condition is unknown, but it may be related to the toxic rather than the occluding effect of the offending agents thought to be free fatty acids.

The most common source of the clots in pulmonary thromboembolism is from deep vein thrombosis of the lower extremity. There are several factors that predispose to the development of venous thrombosis. These include immobility, pregnancy, heart failure, obesity, oral contraceptives, and malignancies. Surgical patients who are kept immobile for long periods on the operating theater table are at increased risk to develop venous thrombosis.

If an embolus is large enough to occlude 50% or more of the main pulmonary artery or one of its two main branches, an acute increase in pulmonary vascular resistance may occur that is potentially life threatening. With a greatly increased pulmonary vascular resistance, the pressure in the right heart necessary to generate a normal cardiac output may exceed the capabilities of the right ventricle. Heart failure or shock secondary to decreased cardiac output ensues.

The major problem of pulmonary embolism is hemodynamic. Other effects relate to change in $\dot{V}/\dot{Q}$. An embolized area getting no blood flow is in essence dead space. With time, an area that has been embolized may lose surfactant and atelectasis can occur. Release of hormonal agents, especially from platelets, leads to bronchoconstriction and additional vasoconstriction. These effects add to the deleterious effects of the embolus itself.

Rarely, pulmonary thromboembolism causes necrosis or infarction of lung tissue. This event is not as common as expected because lung tissue receives its own oxygen supply from the bronchial circulation and directly from alveoli.

Although hypoxemia is a usual concomitant to pulmonary embolus, it need not occur. When hypoxemia is seen, it is usually a result of increased perfusion to poorly ventilated areas (i.e., low $\dot{V}/\dot{Q}$). If a patent foramen ovale or atrial septal defect is present, pulmonary hypertension could lead to an atrial right to left shunt causing a reduction in arterial oxygen tension. If cardiac output is reduced, there may be a reduction in the venous O_2. With a lowered venous O_2, any venous admixture effect, through shunts or low $\dot{V}/\dot{Q}$ areas, will further reduce the arterial oxygen tension.

Pulmonary embolus is, therefore, a dangerous acute stress to anyone, but in a compromised patient it is potentially lethal.

Some patients have many episodes of pulmonary embolism. Patients with multiple pulmonary emboli may develop chronic pulmonary hypertension resembling primary pulmonary hypertension, which is described below.

The most common feature of thromboembolism is acute shortness of breath. Pleuritic chest pain, often a localized "stitch in the side," and hemoptysis indicate that atelectasis or infarction has occurred. Severe crushing retrosternal chest pain may also occur.

The laboratory methods available to diagnose thromboembolism include the perfusion lung scan, which demonstrates the pulmonary circulation. The combination of a defect on lung scan in the presence of a normal chest x-ray film is very suggestive of this diagnosis (Figure 4.6). Injection of dye into the pulmonary artery, pulmonary angiography, is a more specific method of diagnosing embolism.

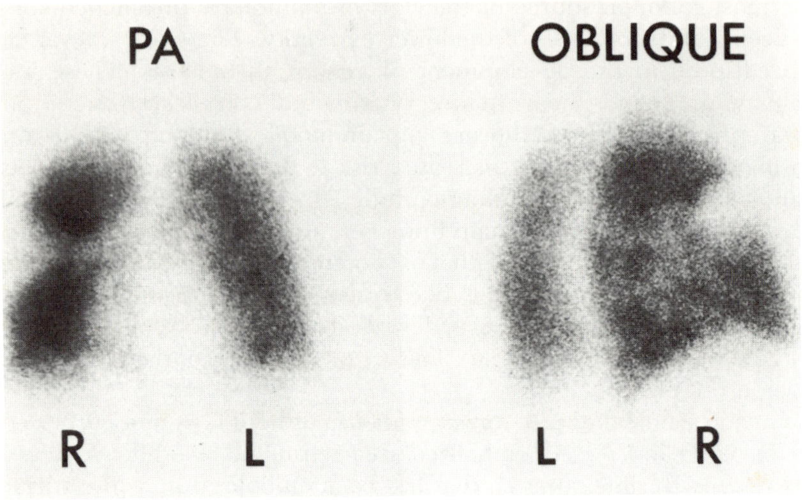

Figure 4.6. Lung perfusion scans in pulmonary thromboembolism. The pulmonary circulation is labeled with a radioisotope that can be photographed using a gamma camera. A defect is seen in the anterior segment of the right upper lobe. This scan is that of a woman who developed deep venous thrombosis and then dyspnea and pleuritic chest pain.

Heparin, an anticoagulant, is used to treat patients with thromboembolic disease. Recently, enzymes that dissolve clots, urokinase and streptokinase, have been used to treat emboli. The role of the enzymes is still unknown.

Primary Pulmonary Hypertension

Primary pulmonary hypertension (PPH) is an often lethal form of chronic pulmonary hypertension. The etiology of the disease is not identifiable. The disease is characterized anatomically by intimal proliferation with concentric laminar intimal fibrosis, fibrinoid necrosis, pulmonary arterial dilatation, and so-called plexiform lesions in addition to medial hypertrophy.

It is likely that this disorder can be caused by many factors. The disorder has also been found to be more common in people with autoimmune disorders (polymyositis, rheumatoid arthritis, scleroderma, and dermatomyositis), particularly if they also have Raynaud's phenomenon of the digits, another vascular disorder. PPH is primarily a disease of young women (women : men = 2 : 1) and may have its onset during pregnancy.

These patients demonstrate abnormal ventilation, gas exchange, and limitation in cardiac output. Characteristically PPH patients hyperventilate at rest and markedly during exercise. The cause of the hyperventilation is not adequately explained by hypoxemia. It has been postulated that activation of lung reflexes (see Chapter 6) causes the hyperventilation.

In spite of hyperventilation, these patients are at least slightly hypoxemic;

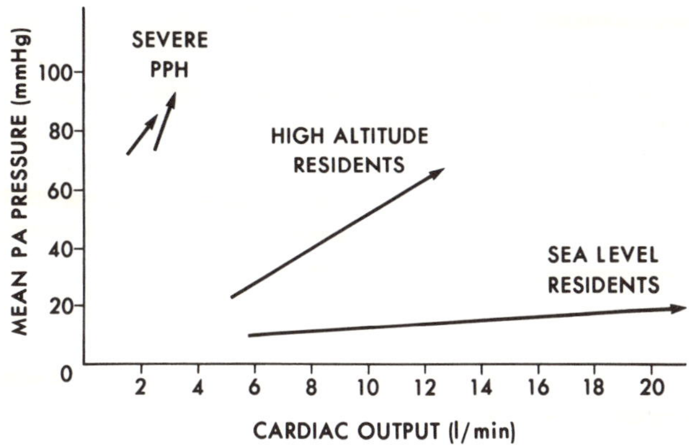

Figure 4.7. Relationship of cardiac output and pulmonary artery (PA) pressure. In normals, at sea level, an increase in cardiac output due to exercise is associated with very little or no change in pulmonary artery pressure. Residents of high altitude, who have mild pulmonary hypertension, have a moderate increase in PA pressure when cardiac output is increased. In contrast, patients with primary pulmonary hypertension (PPH) have a low cardiac output and a very high PA pressure at rest. The slightest increase in exercise causes marked increases in PA pressure. Hence, the marked exercise limitation of these patients. (Adapted, with permission, from Voelkel N. and Reeves JT: Primary Pulmonary Hypertension, in *Pulmonary Vascular Diseases*. New York, Marcel Dekker, Inc. 1979.)

thus they have an elevated (A − a) P_{O_2} gradient. The cause of the hypoxemia is most likely $\dot{V}/\dot{Q}$ mismatching.

Patients with PPH have marked limitations in their cardiac output. In attempting to increase flow through the constricted circulation, there occurs a marked increase in pulmonary artery pressure. This is in marked contrast to normals, who can increase cardiac output fourfold without significantly increasing pulmonary artery pressure (Figure 4.7). Since exercise requires an increased cardiac output, not surprisingly, exercise is very limited in these patients, and the earliest symptom is shortness of breath on exercise. In fact, during exercise pulmonary artery pressure may rise to levels high enough to cause retrosternal pain, which is similar to angina pectoris.

In spite of the fact that many pharmacological agents can reduce pulmonary artery pressure in the laboratory, the clinical use of these has by and large been disappointing. Patients usually die 2 to 4 years after the onset of symptoms. Recently, vascular dilators such as hydralazine and diazoxide have been used with some success in a small number of patients.

Effect of Pulmonary Hypertension on the Circulation

The major effects of pulmonary hypertension are on the cardiovascular system. Since the right heart is pumping against a greater load, the pressure within the right ventricle rises. This leads to right ventricular hypertrophy.

Right atrial pressure (Pra) also increases in order to allow filling of the right ventricle to a higher pressure during diastole.

This increase in Pra has a major effect on venous return and, therefore, cardiac output. The pressure gradient between the circulatory pressure driving blood back to the heart and the Pra narrows as the Pra increases. In order to maintain a normal gradient, the mean circulatory pressure must increase. As this pressure increases, systemic venular and capillary pressures may increase sufficiently to cause edema to form. This effect is most prevalent in the more dependent portions of the body and is clinically manifested in its early stages as pedal edema.

With increased pressures on the right side of the heart, pressures in the left side of the heart may also rise. Most often increases in left sided pressures result from disease of the left ventricle. However, with increases in right sided pressures, the rise in left heart pressure may be a consequence of the mechanical linkage or interdependence of the two sides of the heart. These mechanical linkages are provided by shared muscle fibers, the interatrial and interventricular septa, and the pericardium.

Unfortunately, the consequences of this pressure increase are not related to the cause. If the pressure in the left atrium, pulmonary veins, and pulmonary microvasculature rise sufficiently, pulmonary edema can result.

PULMONARY EDEMA

The factors governing the passage of fluid from capillary to alveolus are contained in an equation derived from Starling. The relationship expressed in this equation shows that the rate of fluid movement across the vessels into the lung is directly proportional to the pressure gradient across the vascular membrane and to the ability of the vascular membrane to allow fluid movement. The pressure gradient is made up of two parts: one, the hydrostatic pressure gradient across the membrane and two, the pressure equivalent of a concentration gradient across the membrane.

This relationship is algebraically expressed as:

$$\dot{Q}f = Kf\,[(Piv - Pis) + \sigma\,(\pi is - \pi iv)]$$

$\dot{Q}f$ is the rate of fluid movement from the vessels into alveoli in ml/min. Kf expresses the ability of the vascular membrane to allow fluid movement; it is an index of permeability or leakiness. It is related to the physical properties of the membrane and the surface area of membrane available for fluid transport. Piv is the intravascular pressure in the vessels that can leak. Pis reflects the interstitial hydrostatic pressure. $\pi$is and πiv are the osmotic pressures of the interstitial space and intravascular space respectively. σ is called the reflection coefficient. It is really a correction factor for the fact that the vascular membrane allows some protein to leak across. Under ordinary circumstances, the pulmonary lymphatics probably serve to remove the small amounts of fluid that enter into the pulmonary interstitium. When the system is severely stressed, for example, when Piv increases, the lymphatics become inadequate to clear the extravascular fluid. The fluid then begins to collect in the interstitium.

From the above equation, it is clear that fluid flow into the airspaces can be caused by several types of abnormality. Alterations in permeability, hydrostatic pressure, and osmotic pressure can all theoretically cause pulmonary edema.

Increased Hydrostatic Pressure

Increases in pulmonary capillary pressure (Piv) cause pulmonary edema. The most common cause of this occurrence is left heart failure or mitral valvular disease. These increase left atrial pressure and thus pulmonary venous pressure and hence capillary pressure. This is also called *high pressure pulmonary edema*.

The interstitium around the microvascular bed normally is very noncompliant like the interstitium elsewhere in the body. Therefore, small changes in fluid volume cause large increases in interstitial hydrostatic pressure. This increase in pressure (Pis) serves to reduce the hydrostatic gradient for further fluid transudation. Additionally, since the fluid volume is increasing, the protein concentration and hence π is, the osmotic pressure, decreases. This also tends to oppose further movement of fluid into the interstitium.

As fluid continues to move into the interstitium from the vasculature, it begins to move toward the hilum and becomes visible on a histological section as periarteriolar and peribronchiolar cuffs. As more and more fluid moves into the interstitium, more cuffing around the larger airways and blood vessels occurs as fluid tracks toward the hilum. This accounts for the so-called butterfly or bat wing appearance seen in x-ray films of those people with modest amounts of pulmonary edema.

Increased Membrane Permeability

So far, the discussion has focused on edema caused by an increase in hydrostatic driving pressure. Obviously, if Kf increased, that is, if the vascular membrane became more leaky, then even with normal pressures the same sequence of events could occur. Diffuse injury to the alveolar capillary membrane increases permeability and causes leakage of fluid into alveoli. This topic is reviewed in Chapter 5. This type of edema is called *low pressure pulmonary edema.*

Reduced Osmotic Pressure

Although a marked reduction in plasma protein can substantially reduce osmotic pressure, this alone seldom causes pulmonary edema. However, the combination of increasing hydrostatic pressure and reduced osmotic pressure will increase the rate of edema formation acutely.

Interactions in Pulmonary Edema

There is clearly an interaction in the variables that can cause edema formation (Figure 4.8). When increased permeability is present, a small increase in

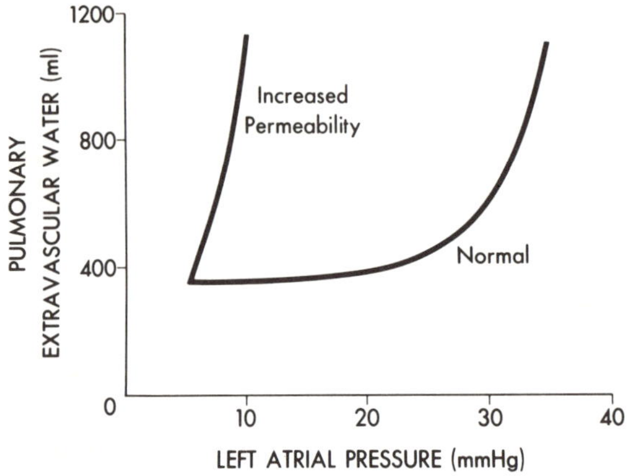

Figure 4.8. The effect of left atrial pressure on pulmonary edema formation. When the alveolar-capillary membrane is normal (the right curve), increasing left atrial pressure up to about 20 mmHg has little effect on the rate of edema formation. When the membrane is abnormally permeable, increased edema formation occurs with much lower left atrial pressure. (Adapted, with permission, Hopewell P, Murray JF: Adult Respiratory Distress Syndrome, in Shibel EM, Moser KM (eds): *Respiratory Emergencies.* St. Louis, the C.V. Mosby Company, 1977, p 101.)

hydrostatic pressure, even in the low range, can dramatically increase edema formation. Thus, a hydrostatic pressure that is "safe" with an intact alveolar-capillary membrane can have disastrous effects when increased permeability is present.

Treatment of Pulmonary Edema

If enough fluid accumulates in the interstitium under sufficient pressure, fluid can then move from the interstitium across the relatively tight alveolar wall into the alveoli. This has profound effects on gas exchange and lung elastic properties. The fluid-filled air spaces do not participate in gas exchange but may still receive blood flow. These units now become shunts. The shunt fraction may become so significant that even with 100% oxygen, it may be impossible to maintain Pa_{O_2} above 50 mmHg.

One modality of treatment is to reduce capillary hydrostatic pressure. As shown in Figure 4.8, this should help even when capillary pressure is normal. This can be accomplished by reducing intravascular volume either by limiting the patient's fluid intake or by using diuretic agents. Another approach is to use agents that reduce the afterload of the left heart. This results in a fall in Piv and hence hydrostatic pressure.

In the presence of increased permeability, it is unclear whether increasing plasma osmotic pressure has an effect. Any plasma proteins administered to the patient may simply leak through the permeable alveolar-capillary membrane.

To effectively oxygenate a patient, maneuvers to increase FRC and reduce shunt are employed. These are discussed more fully in Chapter 11. One modality that is almost always used is positive expiratory pressure above atmospheric pressure (PEEP). With PEEP there is an increase in FRC and intrathoracic pressure.

Effect of PEEP on Cardiac Output

The effect of increasing intrathoracic pressure is to increase the pressure around the heart. If the same volume in the right atrium is maintained, the pressure within the right atrium is not changed relative to the new intrathoracic pressure around the heart. It does, however, increase right atrial pressure relative to the pressure surrounding the rest of the body. The pressure gradient for return of blood to the heart is reduced, venous return decreases, and cardiac output falls. In many patients, vascular reflexes can overcome this effect; but in those patients who are unable reflexly to increase venous return, the consequent fall in cardiac output may become clinically significant.

Thoracic reflexes or cardiac responses to increased intrathoracic pressure may play a role in decreasing left heart function. These effects, if they exist, are probably minor. The major cause for the decrease in cardiac output in patients on PEEP is the decrease in venous return.

BIBLIOGRAPHY

Bergofsky EH: Active control of the normal pulmonary circulation, in Moser KM (ed): *Pulmonary Vascular Diseases.* New York, Marcel Dekker, 1979, p 233.

Hughes JNB: Pulmonary circulation and fluid balance, in Guyton JG (ed): *International Review of Physiology, Respiratory Physiology II*, vol 14. Baltimore, University Park Press, 1977, p 135.

Hurley JV: Current views on the mechanisms of pulmonary edema. *J Pathology* 125:59, 1978.

Matthay RA, Wood LDH (eds): Seminar: Cardiovascular function in respiratory failure. *Am J Cardiol* 47:683, 1981.

Moser KM: Pulmonary vascular obstruction due to embolism and thrombosis, in Moser KM (ed): *Pulmonary Vascular Diseases.* New York, Marcel Dekker, 1979, p 341.

Parker JC, Guyton AC, Taylor AE: Pulmonary transcapillary exchange and pulmonary edema, in Guyton AC, Young BB (eds): *International Review of Physiology, Cardiovascular Physiology III*, vol 18, Baltimore, University Park Press, 1979, p 261.

Voelkel N, Reeves JT: Primary pulmonary hypertension, in Moser KM (ed): *Pulmonary Vascular Diseases.* New York, Marcel Dekker, 1979, p 573.

West JB: Regional differences in the lung. *Chest* 74:426, 1978.

5

Adult Respiratory Distress Syndrome

Thomas L. Petty

The adult respiratory distress syndrome (ARDS) is the final common pathway of a variety of unrelated but massive insults to the lung that injure its gas-exchanging interface. This often fatal syndrome is characterized by severe dyspnea, hypoxemia, and diffuse bilateral pulmonary infiltrations following lung injury occurring in persons who were previously healthy. The clinical presentation, pathophysiology, current understanding of the pathogenesis of the disorder, and an approach to systematic physiologically oriented management are briefly reviewed in this chapter.

Historical Perspective

Certainly, the adult respiratory distress syndrome is not new to medicine; it is only that it is now recognized as an important clinical state and is better understood and better managed. Previous descriptions along with numerous clinical reports and reviews of the underlying pathology resulted in numerous terms: congestive atelectasis, traumatic wet lung, postperfusion lung, "white lung," and "Da Nang lung" crept into the medical literature and the lay press.

Table 5.1. Clinical Terms Often Synonymous with ARDS

Acute alveolar failure
Acute respiratory failure[a]
Adult hyaline membrane disease
Blast lung
Capillary leak syndrome
Congestive atelectasis
Da Nang lung
Postcardiopulmonary bypass perfusion lung (pump lung)
Respirator lung
Shock lung
Stiff lung syndrome
Traumatic wet lung
Whiteout lung or white lung syndrome

[a]Versus acute ventilatory failure

Table 5.1 lists many of the previous designations, all of which refer to the adult syndrome of acute diffuse lung injury. None are especially accurate or descriptive of all of the pathways to the development of ARDS.

The author and members of his department first described ARDS as a clinical syndrome in 1967. Twelve patients were reported as exhibiting a syndrome that was believed "remarkably similar to the infantile respiratory distress syndrome." Mechanical ventilatory support with a technique of trapping air within the lung against a pressure, later called positive end expiratory pressure (PEEP), was used to treat some of these patients. Five patients survived. Autopsy findings of the seven who died revealed striking alveolar atelectasis, engorgement of capillaries, and hyaline membrane formation.

Shortly after, in 1968, a conference on the pulmonary effects of nonthoracic trauma was conducted by the Committee on Trauma of the Division of Medical Sciences, National Academy of Sciences—National Research Council. It became apparent that shock, multiple long bone trauma and, in patients resuscitated with large volumes of fluid, there often developed a pulmonary picture that bore a monotonous regularity and striking similarity to the original description of the adult respiratory distress syndrome. Many of the presenters were clinicians who had cared for combat casualties in Vietnam. It was believed that a large number of cases coming to the attention of physicians were due to huge numbers of combat casualties cared for by "alert, informed physicians whose minds have been sensitized to detect the unusual and the unexplained." The excellent battlefield resuscitation and prompt evacuation to surgical care facilities allowed people who previously would have died to reach medical attention.

The mechanism(s) of the acute lung injury, which was clearly the common denominator present in all cases presented at this conference, was, and remains, unknown. Speculations offered as possibilities were toxic factors or vasoactive substances, the pulmonary effects of fat embolization, lung ischemia, surfactant abnormalities, hemodynamic factors, and exogenous factors such as overtransfusion of fluids.

Over the years, controversy over the appropriateness of the ARDS designation arose and as our understanding of the process began to unfold, it became likely that the conceptual parallelism between the adult respiratory distress syndrome and that suffered by the newborn infant may have been inappropriate. Specifically, the central role of surfactant abnormality in the adult is not established, and experimental evidence suggests that a surfactant abnormality is not a primary event but rather a late complication of acute diffuse lung injury, compared to the infantile respiratory distress syndrome where surfactant abnormality is the primary cause. Whether the lumping together of all forms of injury under the syndrome is wise today can be debated. The term *ARDS* does create a conceptual framework on which to base therapy and further serves as a stimulus to better understand the basic mechanisms of injury caused by a variety of acute diverse pulmonary insults.

The remainder of the chapter presents the current understanding of ARDS, beginning with a clearer clinical definition, current understanding of pathogenesis, and then pathophysiology. The contemporary approach to management will be briefly reviewed.

Definition

It is extremely important to adhere to the original definition of the adult respiratory distress syndrome, summarized briefly in Table 5.2. ARDS is best

Table 5.2. Criteria for Diagnosis of the Adult Respiratory Distress Syndrome (ARDS)

Clinical history of catastrophic event:
Pulmonary or
Nonpulmonary (e.g., shock, multisystem trauma)
but exclude:
Chronic pulmonary disease
Left ventricular failure
Must have clinical respiratory distress:
Tachypnea > 20 breaths/minute
Labored breathing
Central cyanosis when breathing air
with chest radiograph showing:
Diffuse pulmonary infiltrates
and physiological measurements of:
$Pa_{O_2} < 50$ mmHg (6.6 kPa) when $FI_{O_2} > .6$
Total respiratory compliance < 50 cc/cm H_2O (usually 20 to 30)
Increased shunt fraction and deadspace ventilation

recognized in patients with no previous underlying lung disease who have suffered a sudden catastrophic, often multiorgan system insult, which has led to dyspnea, labored breathing, and noncardiogenic pulmonary edema with associated abnormalities of lung mechanics and gas exchange. In defining this syndrome, it is important to exclude primary left ventricular failure, subacute and chronic infiltrative lung disease, and other forms of respiratory insufficiency such as those associated with chronic airflow limitation.

Pathophysiology and Pathogenesis

The respiratory distress syndrome is caused by diffuse damage to the gas-exchanging surface—the alveolar-capillary membrane. Damage to either the alveolar or capillary side of this membrane can cause ARDS.

Diffuse alveolar injury, that is, injury to the alveolar-lining cell (type I alveolar cell), results from contact of these cells with a toxic substance. Inhalation of toxic gases, hydrocarbons, or gastric acid can cause such damage.

Diffuse capillary endothelial injury is probably the most common mechanism causing ARDS, but the precise pathogenesis remains unknown. It has been postulated that humoral agents, toxins, components of the coagulation system, activation of the complement system, and excessive sympathetic activity may individually or collectively play a role. Lung injury by infusion of oleic acid, endotoxin, salicylates, narcotics, and central nervous system insults are among the most common methods used to produce ARDS in experimental animal studies designed to explain acute diffuse lung injury in people. However, so far no model of acute lung injury accurately reflects all facets of the human syndrome.

Whether the primary lesion is alveolar or vascular, an increase in vascular permeability occurs. The mechanisms keeping fluid in these capillaries may thus fail and fluid may leak into the interstitial space and may flood into the alveoli (see Chapter 4) causing pulmonary edema.

A pathological examination in the acute stage shows fluid and red blood cells in the interstitial space and in the alveoli. Later hyaline membranes are seen, which are made up of proteins, mainly fibrinogen, that have leaked into alveoli.

The response of the lung to injury is limited. The type I alveolar cells do not replicate. The type II cells, which are the producers of surfactant, can replicate and differentiate into type I cells. Thus, hyperplasia of type II cells may be prominent. In addition, the repair reaction in the interstitial space may result in fibrosis.

Lungs become noncompliant (stiff) in ARDS. This is caused by fluid accumulation in the interstitial space and alveoli. Another mechanism that may be responsible is the inactivation of surfactant by edema fluid, leading to an increase in surface tension that can lead to alveolar instability and collapse. The noncompliant lungs have greater recoil, a greater "tendency to collapse." Since functional residual capacity is determined by the balance of forces

Table 5.3. Pathophysiology of ARDS

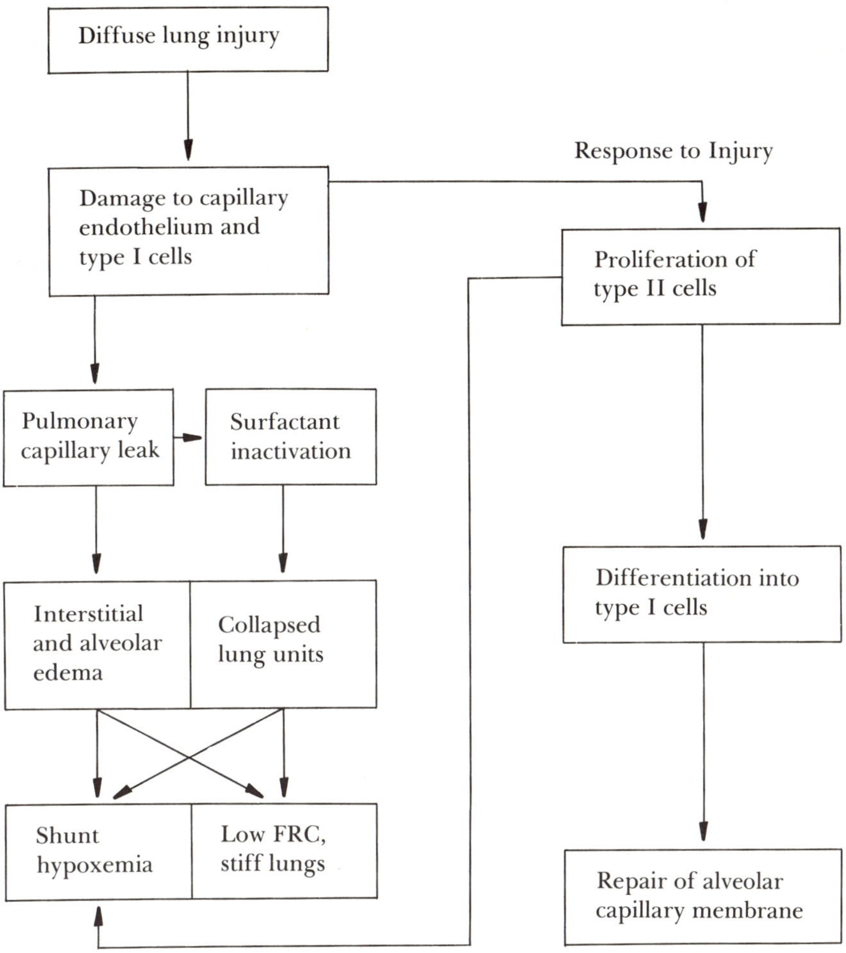

caused by the chest wall recoiling outward and the lungs recoiling inward, the increased recoil of the lungs in ARDS causes a low functional residual capacity (Table 5.3).

Recent research into the pathogenesis of ARDS has focused again on surfactant abnormalities. This reflects the continued comparison with the respiratory distress syndrome of the newborn in which deficient surfactant plays a central role. There are certainly many similarities between the infantile respiratory distress syndrome (IRDS) and ARDS:

Similar abnormalities in lung mechanics and gas transport.

- Indistinguishable pathological features of congestive atelectasis, alveolar debris, and hyaline membrane formation.
- A comparable approach to supportive therapy.

This analogy remains one of the major reasons why the term ARDS was coined to designate this syndrome.

Unlike premature infants with IRDS, previously healthy patients with ARDS must have had normal surfactant function before the acute lung injury occurred. Since surfactant loss may promote alveolar collapse, which in turn may encourage the sequestration of alveolar edema, this could lead to further inactivation of surfactant function, so that a vicious circle might be set up. Thus, surfactant abnormalities found in ARDS may influence the secondary pathogenesis of the syndrome. If a convenient means of monitoring surfactant function and/or chemistry could be established, this might serve as a marker of injury and/or recovery. It is also conceivable that surfactant function could be restored pharmacologically or artificially by infusion or nebulization.

Hypoxemia is a cardinal feature of ARDS. The hypoxemia can be difficult to treat. *The major cause of hypoxemia in ARDS is shunting*—continued perfusion of alveoli that are filled with fluid or collapsed and thus not ventilating. Hypoxemia caused by shunt is relatively resistant to oxygen therapy (see p. 179).

Because hypoxemia stimulates ventilation, and because the lung disease stimulates receptors that cause rapid shallow breathing (see p. 115), hyperventilation is common in ARDS. Hypercapnia is not usually the major problem.

Clinical Setting

Many etiological factors lead to this clinical picture of ARDS including major insults such as:

- Shock from any cause.
- Multisystem trauma.
- Overwhelming infection.
- Overdoses of drugs, etc., likely to damage the pulmonary circulation.
- Inhaled toxic substances.
- Infectious alveolar insults, including bacterial and nonbacterial pneumonia.

Table 5.4 lists the clinical states most commonly resulting in ARDS, but most often these clinical events occur without the complication of ARDS.

Developing Clinical Features

ARDS usually occurs in previously healthy people. Characteristically there is a latent period between the insult and the development of the full-blown clinical picture, which is usually 18 to 24 hours (with extremes of 12 to 48 hours).

Table 5.4. Clinical States Associated with ARDS

Shock
Septic
Hemorrhagic
Cardiogenic
Anaphylactic
Trauma
Direct pulmonary contusion
Nonpulmonary, multisystem
Infection
Viral pneumonia
Bacterial pneumonia: staphylococcal or streptococcal
Miliary tuberculosis
Legionnaire's pneumonia
Disseminated intravascular coagulation
Fat emboli
Amniotic fluid emboli
Aspiration: especially of highly acid gastric contents (pH < 2.5)
Near drowning
Inhaled toxic agents
Smoke
Phosgene
Oxides of nitrogen
Pancreatitis
Oxygen toxicity
Narcotic drug abuse
Heroin
Methadone
Propoxyphene
Radiation pneumonitis
Drugs
Ethchlorvynol
Salicylates

After this interval tachypnea, labored breathing, air hunger, and cyanosis are observed, and arterial blood gas analysis confirms hypoxemia. The abnormalities in lung mechanics and oxygen transfer are readily estimated once the patient is intubated and receiving mechanical ventilatory support. It is likely that monitoring the respiratory rate and simple bedside measurements of respiratory mechanics during ventilatory support or of indices of gas transfer will yield important clues to the impending development of the fully established syndrome.

Three important clinical indices that could be continuously monitored in those patients thought to be at risk are:

- A fall in total respiratory compliance ($\Delta V/\Delta P$ in cc/cmH_2O) as shown by an increase in the pressure to inflate the stiff lungs at their maximal tidal volume.
- Tachypnea—often causing the patient to fight the respirator.
- An increase in the concentration of inspired oxygen ($F_{I_{O_2}}$) or tension ($P_{I_{O_2}}$) necessary to maintain an adequate arterial P_{O_2}.

The chest radiograph shows diffuse, bilateral, usually symmetrical interstitial and alveolar infiltrations, characteristically sparing the costophrenic angles (Figures 5.1 and 5.2).

Management

Today the management of ARDS is empirical and supportive. Mechanical ventilatory support is essential, and this requires:

- A definitive airway—an endotracheal tube placed through either the nose or the mouth, or a tracheostomy.
- A volume-cycled ventilator that allows exquisite control of the inspired oxygen concentration and modification of pressure wave forms, as well as sufficient power to provide high levels of mechanical work.

The tidal volume is usually set at 10 to 12 cc/kg of body weight at first, with a patient-initiated respiratory rate. This may be a relatively rapid rate, chosen

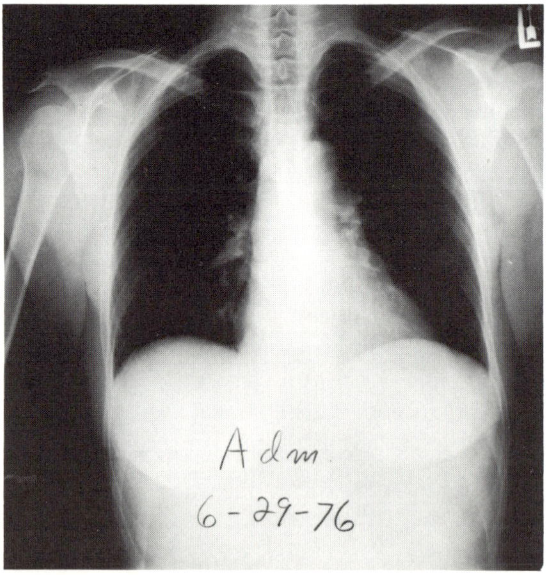

Figure 5.1. Admission chest x-ray of a 48-year-old woman suffering acute hemorrhagic shock from massive peptic ulcer bleeding.

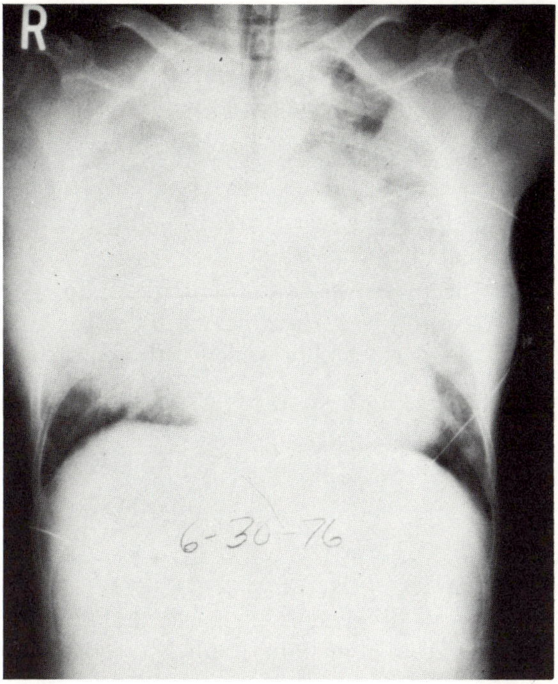

Figure 5.2. Chest x-ray appearance following resuscitation with 44 units of whole blood and corrective surgery. Although the cardiac silhouette appears enlarged, pulmonary venous pressure measured by Swan-Ganz catheter was normal. The patient recovered.

by the patient's respiratory center due to reflexes received from stretch receptors of the stiff (noncompliant) lungs.

PEEP

The use of positive end expiratory pressure (PEEP) has continued to receive considerable attention. This technique maintains an end expiratory pressure of 5 to 15 cm of water by imposing a threshold resistor during exhalation. PEEP keeps open lung units that are otherwise likely to collapse and be unavailable for gas transfer. These lung units may be "unstable" or collapsed due to surfactant abnormalities. PEEP raises functional residual capacity and improves arterial oxygenation by opening up nonventilating units, effectively reducing shunt, and thus allowing mechanical ventilation with a lower inspired oxygen concentration ($F_{I_{O_2}}$). Reducing the $F_{I_{O_2}}$ may prevent or delay oxygen-induced pulmonary damage (described on p. 228) that may take place after 24 to 48 hours of ventilation with an $F_{I_{O_2}}$ of over 0.6 or after only 12 to 24 hours with an $F_{I_{O_2}}$ of 1.0. The benefit of PEEP is counterbalanced by the potential disadvantages of reducing cardiac output and the risk of further damage to the lungs by the excessive intra-alveolar pressure (barotrauma). These two considerations are seldom problems in the case of markedly impaired pulmonary compliance, when conventional levels of PEEP (5 to 15 cm of water) are used. Although some advocate higher levels of PEEP, these are reasons for caution:

- There is no good experimental evidence to support this risky maneuver.
- Recent evidence suggests an increased accumulation of lung water at higher levels of PEEP in isolated perfused lungs.
- Higher levels of PEEP may impair left ventricular function, adding a circulatory burden that would be highly undesirable in the face of the increase in pulmonary capillary permeability, which is the hallmark of ARDS.

Whether or not PEEP actually improves survival has also recently been questioned in a retrospective analysis, but unfortunately this study included patients with all forms of acute respiratory failure and not only patients with well-defined ARDS.

Pharmacological Therapy

Pharmacological therapy is discussed only briefly and in principle. Almost all investigators agree that antibiotics should only be used for specific identified infections. The author has not found that so-called prophylactic antibiotics reduce bacterial colonization or invasion, and the uncontrolled use of antibiotics has not been shown to reduce the burden of sepsis, which often results from infection with relatively resistant Gram-negative bacilli.

Inotropic agents, such as dopamine, which increase cardiac output, would seem appropriate in the face of a failing circulation. Theoretically, a combination of inotropic agents and drugs to promote peripheral vasodilatation, such as nitroprusside, would allow adequate tissue perfusion and oxygen delivery, even with a low left ventricular filling pressure. This approach might lower pulmonary microvascular pressure and, despite increased capillary permeability, could reduce capillary leak. These considerations at present remain theoretical but are the subject of intense investigation in some centers.

The use of corticosteroid drugs remains controversial. Corticosteroids given early in acute lung injury can reduce transcapillary fluid flux, may combat the damage to the capillary endothelium resulting from complement fragments such as C5a, and promote membrane "stability." Against corticosteroid therapy is the potentially harmful effect on the function of the lung macrophages, which play a major role in lung defense against bacterial infection. Whether or not corticosteroids can improve surfactant elaboration in ARDS, as they appear to do in immature lungs, is highly debatable, but we must suppose that steroids may accomplish this in certain patients. The author currently uses methylprednisolone sodium succinate in pharmacological doses, 30 mg/kg body weight for 24 to 48 hours, in an attempt to capitalize on the potential beneficial effects discussed above, yet aiming to minimize side-effects such as bacterial colonization that theoretically should occur after the first 24 to 48 hours. So far, no controlled study has been conducted to either support or challenge the use of corticosteroids in ARDS, but their use is widespread in current practice.

Outcome

It is of interest to review the outcome of ARDS in 100 recent consecutive cases selected from one of our five hospitals, over a period of just over 5 years. Patients were selected consecutively by the author and his colleagues using the definition in Table 5.2. The etiological factors underlying these cases were analyzed and classified as major (common) and minor (uncommon) causes (Table 5.5). Although in some patients only a single etiological factor was present, in the majority there was a combination of causes: a total of 57 different combinations of etiological factors was found in this group of patients. This is why it is *impossible* to categorize patients with ARDS in terms of a single lung insult; in most patients not one, but many factors operate.

Only 44 of these 100 patients survived, which is similar to other large series, though no other well-defined consecutive study of this type has been reported. The outcome in these 100 consecutive patients, analyzed in terms of

Table 5.5. Etiological Factors Associated with the Adult Respiratory Distress Syndrome in 100 Consecutive Patients

Factors	*Single Cause*	*Multiple Cause Combination*[a]	*Total %*
Common	23 Patients	66 Patients	
Sepsis	9	16	25
Shock	2	22	24
Trauma	2	21	23
Fluid overload	2	19	21
Aspiration	2	13	15
Major viral pneumonia	6	4	10
Disseminated intravascular coagulation syndrome	0	8	8
Fat embolism	0	7	7
Uncommon	7 patients	4 patients	
Drug overdose	2		
Drowning	2		
Pulmonary embolism and transplant	0	2	
Hemorrhage and transplant	0	2	
Air embolus	1		
Pancreatitis	1		
Inhaled irritant	1		

[a]57 different combinations were found in the 100 patients

the eight major etiological factors, suggests that sepsis and shock are most clearly associated with a poor prognosis. Overall, the outcome must depend not only on the type of the original injury but also on the effectiveness of the initial respiratory support and the avoidance of such subsequent complications as oxygen toxicity, sepsis, and barotrauma. Initial respiratory support is usually successful, so that it is within the narrow area of avoiding complications that an additional margin of success might be achieved:

- Using the lowest possible oxygen fraction (preferably $F_{I_{O_2}} < .4$).
- Using meticulously clean techniques to avoid infecting the patient's unprotected airway.
- Keeping a careful watch for infection by daily clinical assessment, paying particular attention to fever, leucocytosis, new pulmonary infiltrates, and culture of tracheobronchial secretions.
- Avoiding excessive levels of PEEP or ventilation with an unnecessarily high level of tidal volume to prevent barotrauma, which can result in pneumothorax and/or pneumomediastinum, with subsequent septic complications.

Sequelae

Patients can be weaned from mechanical ventilation when they no longer require either PEEP or an $F_{I_{O_2}} > .4$, and when they can provide the necessary effort for breathing without fatigue. Patients in a group followed for more than 7 years have shown progressive improvement, except for one patient who had a substantial degree of underlying chronic airflow limitation before ARDS was diagnosed. It is surprising that radiographically apparent intersti-

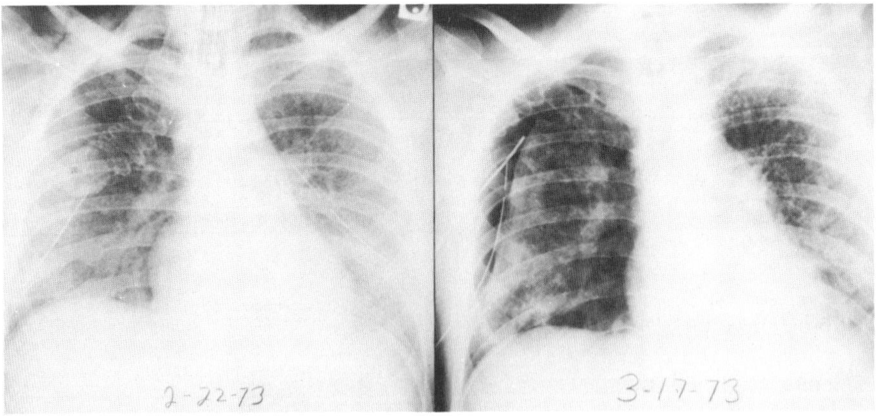

Figure 5.3. Paired chest x-rays from a 25-year-old man suffering ARDS, associated with septic shock and self-induced drug administration. Note bilateral chest tubes to manage pneumothorax. The following two figures demonstrate changes in the same patient.

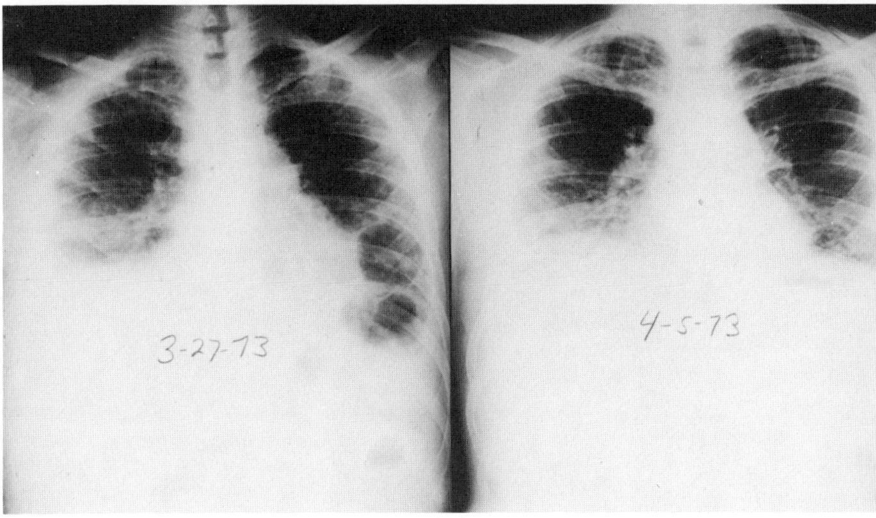

Figure 5.4. Improvement in chest x-ray over time with the evidence of bilateral basilar infiltration suggesting pulmonary fibrosis.

tial fibrosis does not progress; in fact, the reverse is true. Figures 5.3 to 5.5 show x-ray resolution over a period of time in one of the cases in this follow-up series.

This series of patients demonstrated a progressive improvement in forced vital capacity (FVC), total lung capacity (TLC), and single breath carbon monoxide transfer over a period of months or years. Thus, although in the early stages of recovery a patient may have moderate to severe respiratory insufficiency, further improvement in overall lung mechanics and gas transfer can be expected.

The probable explanation for the progressive improvement in gas transfer is that although type I cells die after injury, this is followed by a proliferation of type II cells, which then line the alveolar spaces. These metabolically active cells may, of course, create an impediment to gas transfer. Later, however, the type II cells differentiate into type I cells, thus perhaps "reconstituting" the alveolar epithelium. This is most likely to occur if the basement membrane is intact.

The Future of ARDS

There remain many unanswered questions and challenges. We urgently need to find a circulating marker to ARDS in order to identify those patients who are likely to develop the syndrome. If markers can be found that relate to pathogenesis, perhaps pharmacological blockers can be developed. Experimental models are also needed for controlled studies designed to offer better pharmacological approaches to the problem. For example, can the

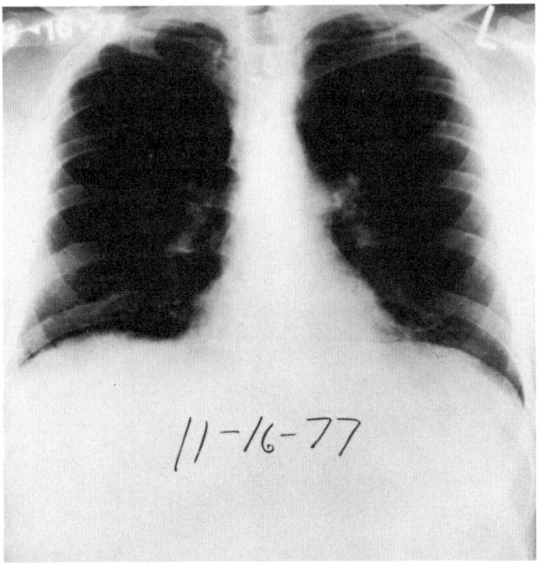

Figure 5.5. Chest x-ray from same patient more than four and a half years after onset of ARDS, showing marked roentgenographic clearing. Improvement in forced vital capacity, FEV_1, diffusing capacity, and rest and exercise blood gases occurred during recovery.

lung be encouraged to tolerate high inspired oxygen concentration for longer periods of time? Can early pulmonary fibrosis be avoided? Can lung surfactant production be stimulated? Most important, can septic complications be avoided or better treated? All of these challenging questions remain for the clinical investigator of the future. In the meantime, supportive therapy and empirical approaches that have been established during the past 14 years should continue to be applied in a systematic and physiologically oriented way, for experience has shown that they can save 50% of the patients suffering from ARDS in many hospitals throughout the world today.

BIBLIOGRAPHY

Ashbaugh DG, Bigelow DB, Petty TL, et al: Acute respiratory distress in adults. *Lancet* 2:319, 1967.

Bachojen M, Weibel ER: Basic patterns of tissue repair in human lungs following nonspecific injury. *Chest* 65:145, 1974.

Petty TL, Hudson LD: Acute pulmonary injury and repair. *Chest* 65:15, 1974.

Lakshminarayan S, Stanford RE, Petty TL: Prognosis after recovery from adult respiratory distress syndrome. *Am Rev Resp Dis* 113:7, 1976.

Toung TJK, Suharia P, Mitzner WA, et al: The beneficial and harmful effects of positive end expiratory pressure. *Surg Gynecol Obstet* 147:518, 1978.

Wood LH, Prewitt RM: Cardiovascular management in acute hypoxemic respiratory failure. *Am J Cardiol* 47:963, 1981.

6

Abnormal Control of Breathing

Meir H. Kryger

BEHAVIORAL FACTORS: INFORMATION ABOUT THE STATE OF THE CEREBRAL CORTEX
Wakefulness
Sleep
  Sleep apnea
Limits to Breathholding

BREATHING PATTERNS
  Breathing patterns with little variation in tidal volume and frequency
  Breathing patterns with irregular tidal volume and frequency
Dyspnea

To breathe we need a *pacemaker* (Figure 6.1) or a *respiratory center* located in the medulla, which sends impulses via the spinal cord to the respiratory muscles. Unlike heart muscle, which has the capacity to generate its own rhythmic contractions, the respiratory muscles rely on the medullary respiratory center. There are neurons in the medulla that fire mainly during inspiration and others that do so mainly during expiration. It is a complex interaction of inspiratory and expiratory neurons that causes the rhythmic output of the pacemaker. Contraction of the respiratory muscles causes the pressure changes that lead to fresh air entering the lungs.

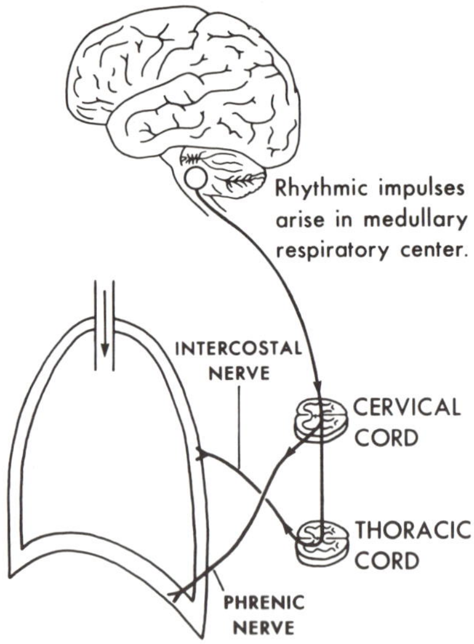

Figure 6.1. Interaction between inspiratory and expiratory neurons in the respiratory center results in rhythmic impulses that travel down to the cervical and thoracic spinal cord, the origins of the intercostal and phrenic nerves, which innervate the respiratory muscles.

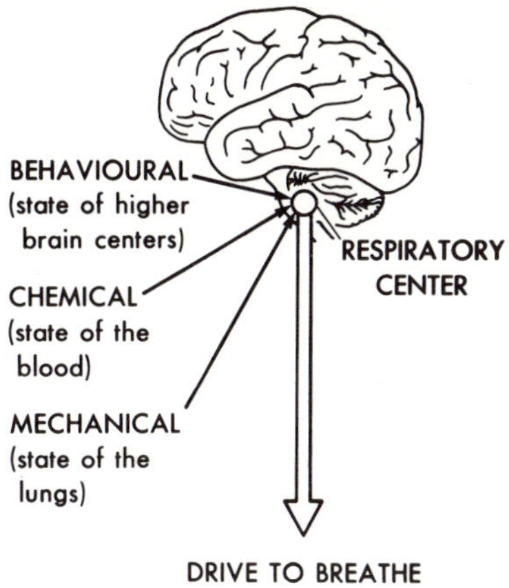

Figure 6.2. For breathing to be appropriate to changing conditions, three types of information modify the output of the respiratory center.

The system as described above is incomplete. Such a system does not know how much to breathe. In order for breathing to be appropriate to changing conditions and to maintain normal blood gas tensions, the output of the respiratory pacemaker must change with changing ventilatory requirements. Three types of information modify or modulate breathing: chemical, mechanical, and behavioral (Figure 6.2). The modulated output of the respiratory center can be thought of as the *drive to breathe.* If the respiratory center is deprived of its modulating inputs, rhythmic breathing becomes very slow. Adequate ventilation is critically dependent on adequate afferent information.

CHEMICAL CONTROL OF BREATHING: INFORMATION ABOUT THE STATE OF THE BLOOD

Carbon Dioxide

An elevation in arterial CO_2 tension (Pa_{CO_2}) results in a brisk increase in ventilation (Figure 6.3). Changes in Pa_{CO_2} are detected by chemoreceptors located in the medulla close to the respiratory pacemaker and by chemoreceptors located in the carotid body. The medullary chemoreceptor is bathed in cerebrospinal fluid. The chemoreceptors most likely respond directly to $[H^+]$; carbon dioxide is a diffusing acid capable of rapidly altering intracellular and cerebrospinal fluid (CSF) pH. About $\frac{1}{3}$ of the hypercapnic response is mediated by the carotid body, and $\frac{2}{3}$ of the response is mediated by the medullary chemoreceptor. The carotid body responds very rapidly to changes in Pa_{CO_2}; the response of the medullary chemoreceptor is slower but more sustained.

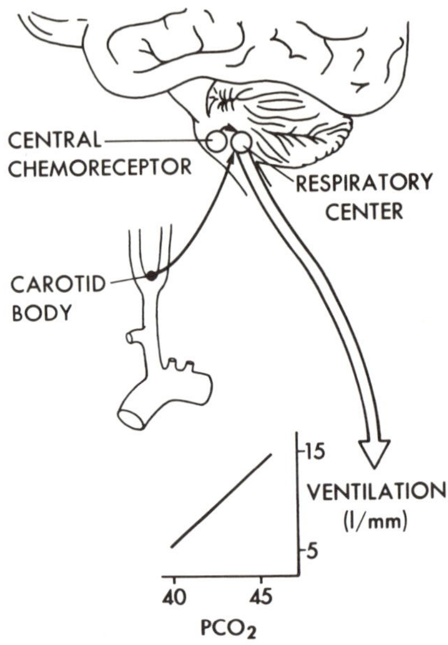

Figure 6.3. Hypercapnic drive to breathe. Changes in carbon dioxide tension are detected in the central chemoreceptor located in the medulla and the peripheral chemoreceptor in the carotid body. Increase in P_{CO_2} causes an increased output from the respiratory center, resulting in increased ventilation.

The cerebrospinal fluid, which bathes the medullary chemoreceptor, is separated from blood by the blood-brain barrier, which is freely permeable to CO_2 but not to H^+ or HCO_3^-. Thus, an elevation in Pa_{CO_2} causes an equal rise in CSF P_{CO_2}. Since CSF contains little protein buffer compared to blood, and since CSF $[HCO_3^-]$ does not change rapidly, the elevation in Pa_{CO_2} causes a greater change in CSF $[H^+]$ and pH than in blood.

CO_2 Airway Receptors

An increase in ventilation occurs when people breathe air containing a small amount of CO_2. This may occur in the absence of an increase in arterial P_{CO_2}. This response is probably mediated by receptors in the large airways that sense CO_2. Airway CO_2 receptors have been extensively studied in birds and dogs; in response to changes in airway P_{CO_2} the vagus nerve has been found to be carrying impulses to the medulla. Although the response can be demonstrated in humans, its role is entirely unknown.

How CO_2 Response Is Measured

The subject rebreathes from a bag containing oxygen-enriched air. This causes parallel increases in CO_2 in the bag, alveoli, blood, and CSF. In normal people, ventilation will increase by 2 to 3 liters per minute for every 1 mmHg increase in P_{CO_2}.

Oxygen

In response to hypoxemia, ventilation increases briskly only when Po_2 is less than 60 mmHg. Because of the shape of the oxyhemoglobin dissociation curve, the oxygen content of arterial blood does not drop significantly until Po_2 is less than 60 mmHg. It is therefore not surprising that ventilation does not increase unless Po_2 is below this level. Above this Po_2, increasing ventilation, with its reduction in Pco_2 and increase in Po_2, would therefore not actually increase the oxygen content of arterial blood and thus would not be a useful physiological response.

Hypoxemia in humans is sensed in the carotid body. Resection of the carotid body totally abolishes ventilatory response to hypoxemia. The tissue in the carotid body that is the sensor is nervous tissue, which sends impulses via the IX cranial nerve to the medulla. The respiratory center integrates this information; the output of the respiratory center is modified by the impulses from the carotid body. In the carotid body, impulses from the sensor are modulated by dopamine neurotransmitter released by glomus cells that are also found in the carotid body and by the sympathetic and parasympathetic nervous systems.

Although it would seem from what was said above that the oxygen sensor specifically senses changes in the oxygen *content* of blood, this is not so. Oxygen content is reduced in anemia and carbon monoxide poisoning, which do not cause an increase in impulses from the carotid body. Studies in people with abnormal oxyhemoglobin dissociation verify that ventilation usually responds to *partial pressure* of oxygen (Po_2) and not to the oxygen content of arterial blood.

Since hypoxemia and hypercapnia are both sensed by the carotid body, it might be expected that the removal of the carotid body would have deleterious effects on breathing. This is not so when lungs are normal, because $\frac{2}{3}$ of the hypercapnic response is mediated by the central medullary chemoreceptor and the hypoxemic drive is not important until Po_2 drops below 60 mmHg. However, when hypoxemia caused by lung disease or high altitude is present, absence of the carotid body can result in life-threatening hypoxemia, since hypoxic ventilatory response will be absent. In addition, during sleep, as will be discussed below, there normally occurs a blunting of the CO_2 drive but not of the hypoxic drive. Carotid body resection would, therefore, permit more severe hypoxemia to occur during sleep in hypoxemic persons.

How Hypoxic Response Is Measured

Inspired oxygen pressure is gradually reduced by adding nitrogen to a bag from which a person is breathing. Ventilation is then plotted as a function of alveolar Po_2, which is measured at the mouth, or as a function of arterial oxygen saturation (Sa_{O_2}), which is measured with an ear oximeter.

Synergism of Chemical Drives

Although, as was mentioned above, when Po_2 is greater than 60 mmHg, ventilation does not normally change much with changing Po_2, this is not so

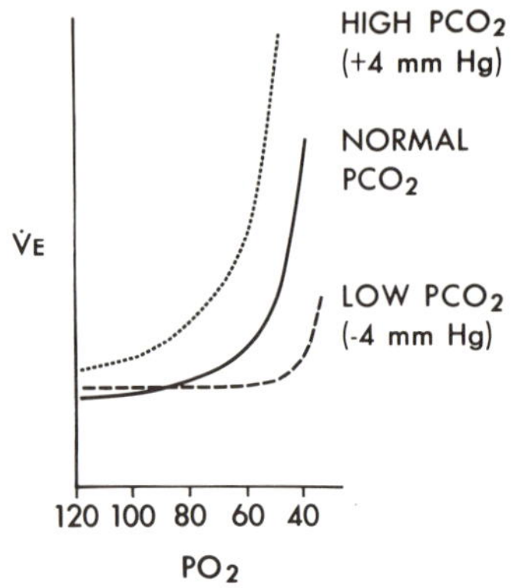

Figure 6.4. Synergism of the chemical drives can be demonstrated by the changes in hypoxic drive with different levels of Pco_2. Levels of Po_2 that normally stimulate breathing slightly (for example $Po_2 = 60$) can markedly increase ventilation when Pco_2 is high. Conversely, low Pco_2 depresses hypoxic drive. Po_2 is in mmHg.

when hypercapnia is present. Hypoxic response is markedly increased when Pco_2 is elevated; levels of Po_2 that do not normally stimulate breathing can stimulate breathing when hypercapnia is present (Figure 6.4). Similarly, hypercapnic drive is markedly increased when hypoxemia is present. The importance of this is that the body has a powerful response available to defend against asphyxia and hypoventilation, which result in hypercapnia and hypoxemia. Conversely, hypocapnia that occurs during hyperventilation blunts hypoxemic ventilatory response.

The Nature of Ventilatory Response

An increase in ventilation can be accomplished by one of two ways: by breathing more deeply (increasing tidal volume) or by breathing more rapidly (increasing frequency). In the presence of chemical stimulation to breathe, the initial response is to increase tidal volume with little or no change in breathing frequency. Only with a marked increase in ventilation does an increase in breathing frequency occur.

Factors Influencing Chemical Drives to Breathe

Genetic Factors. In some people, blunted chemical drives are inherited. Patients with idiopathic hypoventilation (see below), who have depressed chemical hypoxic and hypercapnic drives to breathe, may have other family members with depressed drives. Endurance athletes who often have depressed chemical drives frequently have other (nonathletic) family members with depressed drive. Identical twins have virtually identical hypoxic (but not hypercapnic) drives. In addition, familial depression of hypoxic drive may explain depressed chemical drive to breathe when there is lung disease (see below).

Metabolism. Ventilation changes parallel metabolic demand. In exercise, the relationship of ventilation to CO_2 production remains remarkably constant. Increase in hypoxic drive occurs when metabolic rate increases, by as yet unknown mechanisms in exercise, hyperthermia, and hyperthyroidism. In hyperthyroidism, dyspnea on exercise is common, and this may be due to the increased hypoxic drive of these patients.

In starvation and hypothyroidism, which are associated with a reduction in metabolic rate, there occurs a marked reduction in ventilatory responsiveness to chemical stimuli. Hypoventilation in hypothyroidism may be so severe as to cause coma.

Metabolic Acidosis and Alkalosis. In the presence of chemical stimulation to breathe, as occurs with metabolic acidosis, the initial response is to increase tidal volume with little or no change in breathing frequency. In patients with diabetic ketoacidosis, who demonstrate a slow sighing breathing pattern (Kussmaul respiration), the marked hyperventilation is not suspected because the respiratory rate is counted; the increased depth of breathing is often unnoticed.

With acute *metabolic acidosis,* the H^+ in the blood is buffered by HCO_3^- in the blood and H^+ ions do not easily cross the blood-brain barrier. As a result, $[H^+]$ is higher and $[HCO_3^-]$ is lower in the blood than in the brain extracellular fluid. When the carotid body stimulates breathing as a response to the high blood $[H^+]$, blood P_{CO_2} drops; because CO_2 diffuses freely, CSF P_{CO_2} also drops. Since $[HCO_3^-]$ is higher in the CSF, this will cause a CSF alkalosis that inhibits breathing and partly offsets the stimulation from the carotid body. After several hours, CSF $[HCO_3^-]$ drops and CSF pH approaches normal. Because the peripheral and central chemoreceptors "see" different $[H^+]$, respiratory compensation does not restore blood $[H^+]$ to normal. This is discussed in greater detail in Chapter 12.

In severe *metabolic alkalosis,* as occurs with acid loss from the body (protracted vomiting), there is inhibition of both hypoxic ventilatory response and hypercapnic ventilatory response, and hypoventilation may occur. This reflects in part the synergism of the chemical drives and that the CO_2 response is mediated by $[H^+]$, which is low in metabolic alkalosis. In fact, because of these interactions, in metabolic alkalosis the response of the respiratory system is very unpredictable, ranging from no change in ventilation to severe hypoventilation.

Hypoxemia

Hypoxemia itself can blunt hypoxemic drive. Severe hypoxemia blunts hypoxemic drive more quickly than mild hypoxemia.

Severe Hypoxemia. P_{O_2} below 35 mmHg, besides stimulating the carotid body, actually can depress brain function because neural tissue requires a constant supply of oxygen. Thus, severe hypoxemia will interfere with the function of the respiratory control system and depress breathing. Such depression, which is reversible, occurs within minutes of the onset of the hypoxemia.

Mild Hypoxemia. Po_2 greater than about 35 mmHg results in a blunted hypoxic drive that has its onset within *months, years, or even decades.* It is likely that with this degree of hypoxemia the carotid body continues to fire impulses to the medulla; however, some central mechanism excludes this input or does not respond to it and hypoxemic drive becomes blunted. This type of blunting occurs in patients with chronic airflow obstruction and in children with right to left cardiac shunts. In the latter condition, the blunting may involve a "learning" process. Increasing ventilation will not improve Po_2 when hypoxemia is due to shunt, and the respiratory control system may "learn" that hyperventilation is not improving hypoxemia and thus stop hyperventilating. Another explanation for this blunting is that there may develop receptor adaptation, that is, loss of response due to adaptation of the O_2 sensor in the carotid body. In children with right to left cardiac shunts, the hypoxic drive may return to normal after corrective surgery.

Po_2 between 50 to 65 mmHg occurs in people living at altitudes between 3,000 and 4,000 meters. This degree of hypoxemia will result in blunting of hypoxic drive, which is demonstrable only after *decades.* Newborns and children up to 10 years of age at high altitude have normal hypoxic drives, but people who have lived at high altitude more than 20 years will begin to demonstrate blunting of hypoxemic drive. In such people, the blunting appears to be irreversible and hypoxemic drive will not return when hypoxemia is corrected by moving to sea level.

Diseases Causing Hypoventilation when Lungs and Chest Wall Are Normal

When a neurological or muscular disorder affects the respiratory control system, reduction in ventilatory response to chemical stimulation and hypoventilation may occur (Figure 6.5).

In the Arnold-Chiari malformation, the nerves carrying impulses to the medulla or the medulla itself are damaged. In inflammatory disorders or infections involving the medulla (such as bulbar poliomyelitis or viral encephalitis) there may be dysfunction of the medullary chemoreceptor or of the respiratory pacemaker. Patients with such disorders have an irregular breathing pattern and often hypoventilate during wakefulness. In spite of hypoxemia and hypercapnia, which are powerful stimuli of ventilation and dyspnea, these patients hypoventilate and do not usually complain of shortness of breath. These patients characteristically can *voluntarily* hyperventilate, proving that the neural pathways involved in breathing that bypass the respiratory pacemaker are normal and that the lungs are normal. During sleep, hypoventilation worsens and sleep apnea (see below) may occur. If there is no direct evidence of neurological disease in the face of hypoventilation with normal lung function, the patient is said to have *idiopathic hypoventilation,* also

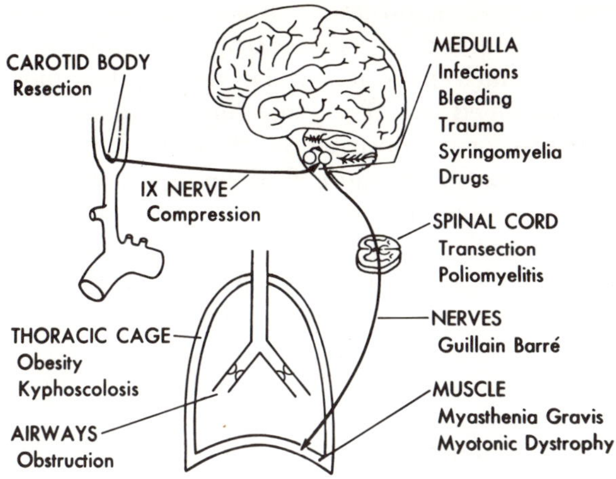

Figure 6.5. Causes of abnormal drive to breathe. Abnormal drive to breathe may occur if a disease directly involves portions of the respiratory control system, in which case respiratory failure may occur when lungs and thoracic cage are normal. Abnormalities of the airways and thoracic cage (chest wall) can also be associated with reduction in chemical drive to breathe.

called primary alveolar hypoventilation and Ondine's curse. However, it is most likely that most of such patients have an abnormality in the medulla. Since the output from the respiratory pacemaker to the respiratory muscles are abnormal, these patients can be treated by an artificial electronic pacemaker that rhythmically stimulates the phrenic nerves.

Generalized paralysis of muscle can cause hypoventilation, since the respiratory muscles may also be paralyzed. Hypoventilation is the major life-threatening complication of high cervical cord transection, myasthenia gravis, and the Guillian-Barré syndrome.

Diseases of the Lung or Chest Wall Causing Hypoventilation

Chronic Airflow Obstruction

When the lungs are normal, ventilation is a good indicator of the output of the respiratory control system i.e. the drive to breathe. When lungs are abnormal, ventilation may no longer accurately reflect the drive to breathe. Obstruction to airflow may depress *ventilatory response* to hypercapnia and hypoxemia; it must be understood that in this setting the actual drive to breathe may be low, normal, or above normal. The person with airway obstruction may be trying very hard to breathe but cannot because of the severity of the lung disease. This can be demonstrated by obtaining a measure of the effort to breathe instead of measuring ventilation. Tests that have been used include the measurement of the work of breathing, the electrical activity of the respiratory muscles, and the pressure generated by the respiratory muscles during inspiration. In this latter measurement, *mouth occlusion pressure* ($P_{0.1}$), mouth pressure is measured with the mouthpiece briefly occluded while the subject is breathing in. Using such tests it can be shown that most people with obstructed airways indeed are trying harder to breathe. They are trying harder to compensate for the obstruction. When such people hypoventilate, they do so because they *cannot* breathe hard enough to overcome the obstruction (Figure 6.6). Some patients with chronic obstructive lung disease who hypoventilate have sufficient lung function to be able to ventilate normally; these patients can be demonstrated to have a true reduction in drive to breathe. These patients *will not* breathe hard enough to overcome the obstruction.

Among patients with chronic airflow obstruction two clinical types may be observed, the pink puffer and the blue bloater (see also Chapter 2).

The pink puffer is well oxygenated (pink) and dyspneic (puffing). He compensates for the airway obstruction by trying to breathe harder and thus maintains normal ventilation. He has few complications of hypoxemia.

The blue bloater is poorly oxygenated (blue) and has peripheral edema ("bloated"), which is a complication of hypoxemia. He has a decreased drive to breathe, which in some cases is inherited, and does not compensate for the airway obstruction by trying to breathe harder. He hypoventilates. In spite of

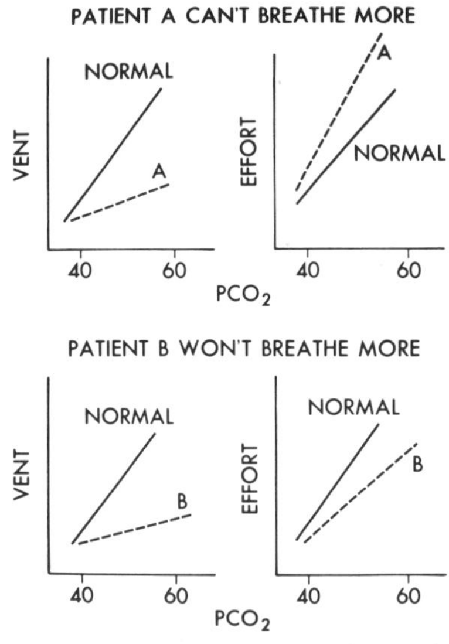

Figure 6.6. Two patients A and B have airway obstruction; both have depressed ventilatory response to hypercapnia compared to a normal subject. In subject A, effort to breathe is in fact much greater than normal; he is trying harder to breathe. When such a patient hypoventilates, it is because he *can't breathe*. In subject B, effort to breathe is reduced; this patient can try harder. When such a patient hypoventilates, it is because he *won't breathe* harder.

severe hypoxemia and hypercapnia, he does not usually complain of shortness of breath. Hypoxemia results in an increase in erythropoietin production and hence red blood cell production that leads to polycythemia. In the presence of alveolar hypoxia, there is constriction of pulmonary arterioles that causes pulmonary artery hypertension and leads to an increase in afterload of the right ventricle. Eventually the ventricle fails, and this results in an increase in right ventricular end diastolic, right atrial, and systemic venous pressures. This increase in venous pressure causes edema in the lower extremities by mechanisms described in Chapter 4.

Although airway obstruction itself can depress chemical drives to breathe, in addition there is wide *genetic variability* in the drives to breathe. On developing chronic airway obstruction, a person who inherited normal drives will become a pink puffer. A person who inherited depressed drives will become a blue bloater. The vast majority of patients fall somewhere between the pink puffer and blue bloater clinical types.

CO_2 Narcosis

Patients with chronic hypercapnia appear to be dependent on hypoxemic drive to breathe and have virtually absent hypercapnic drive. When such patients are given oxygen to breathe, the major stimulus to breathe (hypoxemia) is relieved and the patients may hypoventilate and develop further CO_2 retention. The rapid rise in P_{CO_2} and $[H^+]$ can cause coma and death. It has recently been shown that in some patients the progressive rise in arterial P_{CO_2} while breathing oxygen is not due to a reduction in ventilation. In these patients, oxygen breathing may worsen $\dot{V}/\dot{Q}$ matching by the mechanisms described on page 186. The deterioration in $\dot{V}/\dot{Q}$ matching together with the blunted chemical drive, can explain the rise in Pa_{CO_2} (see also p. 210).

Extrapulmonary Lung Restriction

When inflation of the lung is restricted by stiff structures surrounding the lung, depression of chemical drives and hypoventilation may occur. In contrast, when inflation of the lung is restricted by stiff lungs due to disease in the interstitial space, hypoventilation is rare because of the activity of lung reflexes (see p. 117).

Obesity-Hypoventilation (Pickwickian) Syndrome

A small number of obese patients who have normal lungs hypoventilate. These patients have depressed chemical drives to breathe. They have the complications of hypoxemia, such as polycythemia, pulmonary arterial hypertension, right ventricular failure, and peripheral edema. The most characteristic feature of these patients is daytime somnolence (sleepiness), which is related to recurrent cessation of breathing during sleep—the sleep apnea syndrome (see p. 118). Joe, the fat boy in *Pickwick Papers*, had this problem, hence the name Pickwickian syndrome.

When extrapulmonary restriction is present, there must be an increased effort to breathe to maintain normal levels of ventilation. In these patients, hypoventilation occurs most likely because of an acquired depression of the chemical drives to breathe. Loss of weight in obesity-hypoventilation may cause the drives to breathe to return to normal and result in clinical cure of the disorder.

Kyphoscoliosis

When deformity of the rib cage is severe, depressed chemical drives and hypoventilation occur and patients develop the complications of hypoxemia. This is the cause of death in severe kyphoscoliosis.

Drugs

Respiratory Depressants

Barbiturates (which are used as hypnotics and sedatives), *narcotic analgesics,* and *general anesthetics* depress breathing. These agents can be shown to depress hypoxemic and hypercapnic drives in normal people (Figure 6.7). As has been mentioned above, with airway obstruction, people try to breathe harder. Another effect of these drugs is that they interfere with this effort response to airway obstruction. Patients at risk from these drugs are those who have already blunted drives to breathe or who have lung disease. Indeed even tiny doses of sedative may cause respiratory arrest and death in patients with lung disease.

Naloxone is a specific narcotic antagonist and dramatically reverses the hypoventilation caused by narcotics.

Respiratory Stimulants

Respiratory stimulants can be divided into two general categories, central nervous system stimulants and progestational agents.

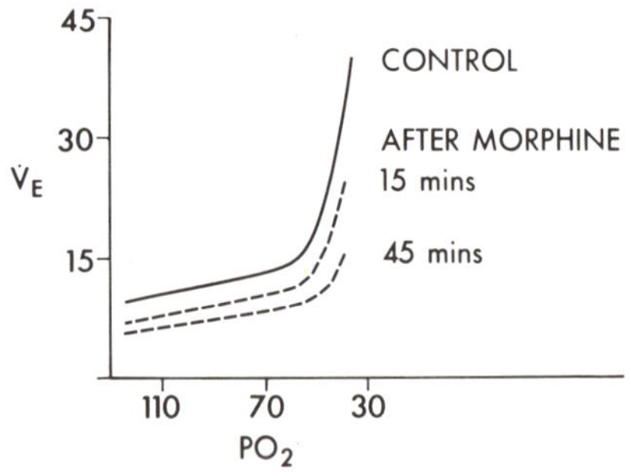

Figure 6.7. Morphine is the most widely used narcotic analgesic. Marked depression of hypoxic drive is present in a normal person 45 minutes after administration. This can cause respiratory arrest and death in patients with lung disease.

Nikethamide, ethamivan, and *doxapram* are general central nervous system stimulants that can enhance respiration and hypercapnic responses in doses below those that cause central excitation or convulsions.

Nikethemide and ethamivan have their effect mainly in the medulla. Doxapram also stimulates the carotid body at doses that are lower than those that cause general nervous system stimulation and, therefore, may be a safer drug than the other two. These agents may increase metabolic rate (oxygen consumption and carbon dioxide production), which offsets some of the beneficial effects of increased ventilation and, therefore, are not particularly useful in patients with lung disease. Doxapram has been used to stimulate breathing depressed by anesthetics. The other drugs are no longer often used because of unwanted effects.

Aminophylline stimulates the central nervous system, acts on the kidney to produce diuresis, stimulates cardiac muscle, and relaxes bronchial smooth muscle. The stimulant effects on the medulla cause an increase in ventilation and an increase in ventilatory response to hypercapnia. The respiratory stimulant effects have been used to treat apnea in infants. Aminophylline is not a powerful respiratory stimulant, and it is used mainly to treat bronchoconstriction (see Chapter 8).

Progesterone. Pregnant women hyperventilate and have a P_{CO_2} that is about 8 to 10 mmHg lower than when they are not pregnant. Hyperventilation also occurs during the luteal phase of the menstrual cycle. Progesterone causes the hyperventilation in both these situations.

Progesterone stimulates breathing centrally without causing any nervous system excitation; so its mechanism of action is different from the central nervous system stimulants. Progesterone causes an increase in hypoxemic and hypercapnic ventilatory response without increasing metabolic rate.

Progesterone has been used successfully in the obesity-hypoventilation syndrome. Experience with this drug indicates that it is likely not to be useful if hypoventilation is caused by structural damage in the medulla.

MECHANICAL CONTROL OF BREATHING: INFORMATION ABOUT THE STATE OF THE LUNG

There are receptors in the lung that respond to inflation, deflation, irritation, and congestion of blood vessels. The impulses from these receptors are carried by the vagus nerve to the medulla. The major effect of these reflexes in humans is to shorten inspiration or to initiate coughing (Figure 6.8). In some people these reflexes induce constriction of airways (see Chapter 8).

Stretch Receptors

Inflation of the lung causes inhibition of inspiration (Hering-Breuer reflex). In animals, this reflex is important and a negative feedback loop may operate to

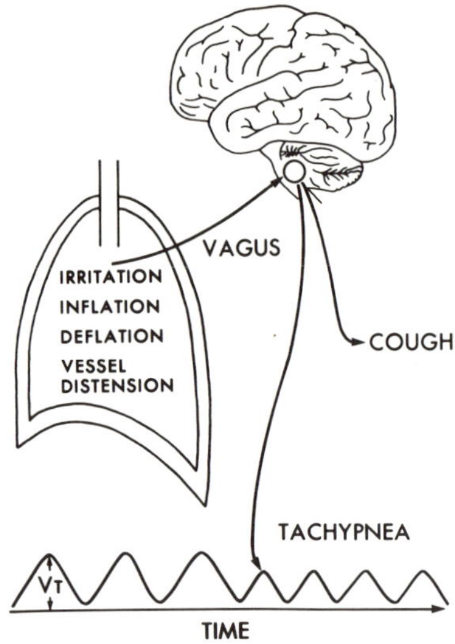

Figure 6.8. Receptors in the lung respond to changes in the state of the lung. Impulses from these receptors travel in the vagus nerve. The response to these impulses is either cough or tachypnea, rapid shallow breathing.

maintain rhythmic breathing. In other words, when the inflation receptors indicate that a certain level of inflation has been reached inspiration ceases. The receptor for this reflex is located in airways and is sensitive to "stretching" of the airways, which occurs with increasing lung volume. In normal people, this reflex is absent or easily overcome by other mechanisms that control breathing. *Deflation* of the lung, as may occur with a pneumothorax, also results in shortened inspiration and in an increased frequency of breathing.

J Receptors

Juxtapulmonary capillary receptors are stimulated by distension of pulmonary capillaries and fluid in the interstitial space of the lung, and they may explain the hyperventilation of pulmonary vascular disease and pulmonary edema.

Irritant Receptors

In the upper airways, receptors responding to mechanical or noxious chemical stimulation initiate *coughing.* Information from these receptors travels via the vagus nerve to the medulla, and a complex series of events is initiated. Inspiration is followed by closure of the glottis (the vocal cords coming together) and vigorous contraction of the expiratory muscles. This results in a marked increase in pleural pressure that narrows the airways and increases alveolar pressure. The opening of the glottis then leads to explosive expiration and material in the narrowed airway is expelled. The narrower the airway about the material the greater the linear velocity of the material during coughing (the "peashooter" effect).

Interstitial Lung Disease

Patients with disease of the interstitial space of the lung hyperventilate. They are usually hypoxemic because of $\dot{V}/\dot{Q}$ mismatching and have intense dyspnea. The dyspnea and hyperventilation are not abolished when oxygen therapy is used to correct the hypoxemia. Therefore, chemical drives do not cause the hyperventilation of these patients.

These patients hyperventilate because of reflexes arising from the lung (most likely initiated by inflation receptors and possibly the J receptors). The stretch receptors can be "stretched" by the large pressure difference between the pleural and airway pressures. These high pressures are necessary to inflate the stiff lungs. Blockade of the reflexes with local anesthesia of the vagus nerves decreases ventilation and relieves dyspnea.

The reflexes result in early termination of inspiration. This leads to a shortened amount of time spent in inspiration, a shorter breathing cycle duration (or an increased breathing frequency), and a smaller tidal volume.

BEHAVIORAL FACTORS: INFORMATION ABOUT THE STATE OF THE CEREBRAL CORTEX

Behavioral factors can override the homeostatic function of the respiratory control system. Talking, singing, laughing, and crying are activities that utilize the respiratory system. People can also voluntarily breathhold or hyperventilate. The neural pathways involved in these activities arise in the cerebral cortex, and some of the efferent pathways entirely bypass the portion of the medulla involved with the automatic control of breathing. In the presence of inflammatory disease in the medulla, as may occur with bulbar poliomyelitis, the respiratory control system may be so abnormal that hypoventilation and death may occur. Yet in such patients, the voluntary neural pathways may be entirely normal and the patients can voluntarily breathe indefinitely.

Most research in the control of breathing in disease has been done in awake patients. Only now is it becoming clear that the most severe physiological derangements occur while patients are sleeping. The level of neurological arousal has a profound effect on breathing.

Wakefulness

Just as there is a respiratory drive related to hypoxemia, hypercapnia, and lung reflexes, there appears to be a respiratory drive related to wakefulness. This may be the most important stimulus to breathe in awake man.

Sleep

The transition from wakefulness to sleep is associated with the loss of the respiratory drive of wakefulness; a reduction in ventilation occurs. During *nondreaming sleep* (also called NREM for nonrapid eye movement), breathing is primarily controlled by chemical drives, which are maintained. Breathing is usually very regular in this state. However, if chemical drive is absent, apnea may occur, since the respiratory drive of wakefulness is also absent.

During *dreaming sleep* (REM sleep), breathing is not primarily controlled by the automatic respiratory control system. In dogs hypercapnic drive is reduced, but hypoxemic drive is present. Breathing is linked more closely to the behavioral characteristics of dreaming than to physiological requirements. Consequently, the breathing pattern during REM is often erratic.

When normal people develop abnormal breathing patterns during sleep, arterial blood gases change little. When people with lung disease who are hypoxemic develop abnormal breathing patterns during sleep, life-threatening hypoxemia may occur. This occurs because a similar drop in Pa_{O_2} will be associated with a much greater drop in Sa_{O_2} when the subject is already hypoxemic (Figure 6.9). Thus, patients with chronic obstructive lung disease often have severe hypoxemia during sleep.

Sleep Apnea

Some patients may stop breathing during sleep, even though the lungs are entirely normal. This is common in patients who have a marked abnormality in chemical control of breathing such as those with the obesity-hypoventilation syndrome (Pickwickian syndrome). During sleep, such patients have recur-

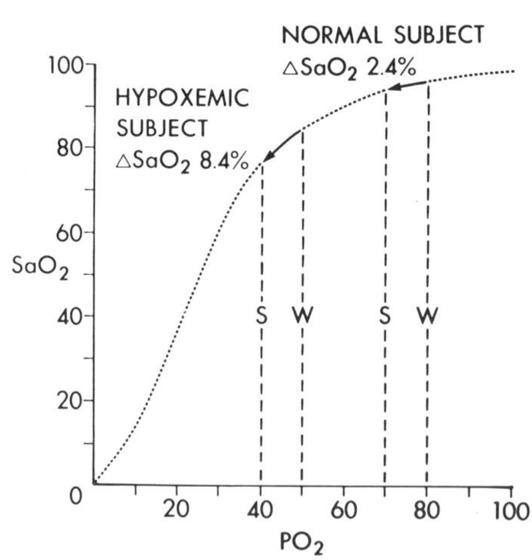

Figure 6.9. A normal subject in the transition from wakefulness (W) to sleep (S) may have a 10 mmHg reduction in Po_2, which results in a small reduction in Sa_{O_2}. Because the Po_2 in a hypoxemic subject is on the steep part of the oxyhemoglobin dissociation curve, the fall in Sa_{O_2} will be three to four times greater for a similar fall in Po_2.

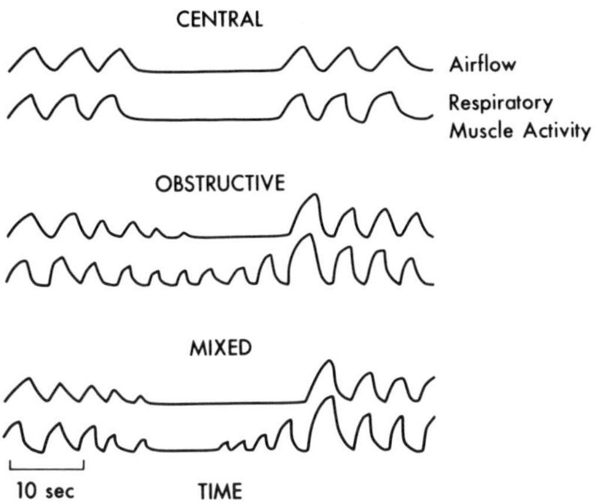

Figure 6.10. Types of sleep apnea: central, absence of muscle activity and airflow; obstructive, absence of airflow in the presence of muscle activity; mixed, central followed by obstructive apnea.

rent episodes of apnea resulting in a periodic breathing pattern. Three types of apnea are observed (Figure 6.10):

- *Central apnea* occurs when breathing stops, because there is a cessation of neural output from the medulla to the respiratory muscles.
- *Obstructive apnea* is characterized by contraction of the respiratory muscles but absent airflow, because of obstruction of the upper airway. This type of obstruction resembles snoring.
- *Mixed apnea* is a central apnea followed by an obstructive apnea.

A major complication of sleep apnea is excessive daytime sleepiness. This occurs because the end of each apneic period (and there are 300 to 500 such periods per night) is associated with a neurological awakening, which can be recorded by electroencephalograph. The patients are sleepy because their sleep is so abnormal. In addition, during obstructed breathing, vagal reflexes are activated that slow the heart rate (bradycardia).

Sleep apnea occurs in people with no apparent abnormalities in their upper airway when they are awake and in patients who have upper airway obstruction, as may occur in children with enlarged tonsils. Such patients are treated by surgical correction of the airway obstruction or by tracheostomy. Sleep apnea is a cause of the sudden infant death syndrome, a poorly understood disease in which apparently healthy infants die in their sleep.

Limits to Breathholding

Breathholding is an excellent example of the interaction of the various modulators of breathing, since breathholding time depends on chemical information, information from the lung and chest wall, and higher cortical centers.

Chemical Information. Breathhold time is prolonged when the chemical drive to breathe is low (high Po_2, low Pco_2) and, conversely, is markedly shortened when the drive to breathe is high (hypoxemia, hypercapnia).

Information About the State of the Lung. Breathhold time is shortened when the lung is in a state of deflation and prolonged when the lung is inflated. Simply breathing a single breath (even if the inspired air is very hypoxic and hypercapnic) can prolong breathhold time proving that information of the state of lung volume, independent of chemical drives, plays a role in determining limits to breathholding.

Higher Cortical Centers. These cortical centers must play an important role since the initiation of breathhold is voluntary. Only when the above factors overcome voluntary control does breathhold cease. This is advantageous, making it impossible for people to kill themselves by simply breathholding.

BREATHING PATTERNS

Examination of the breathing pattern may yield important information about physiological mechanisms.

Breathing Patterns with Little Variation in Tidal Volume and Frequency

Most people breathe regularly (between 10 and 20 times each minute) with little variation in tidal volume or breathing frequency. Every few minutes a deep breath or sigh is taken. Tachypnea most often occurs when lung reflexes mediated by the vagus nerve cause rapid, shallow breathing (Figure 6.11). With chemical stimulation, the initial response is an increase in tidal volume with little change in breathing frequency. The best example of this type of breathing pattern is *Kussmaul's respiration;* this is marked hyperventilation due entirely to a sighinglike, large-tidal volume breathing pattern that occurs with metabolic acidosis.

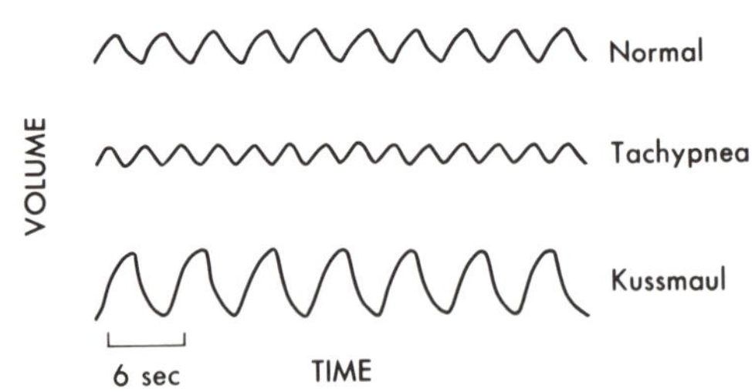

Figure 6.11. Breathing patterns in which breathing frequency and tidal volume are regular. Tachypnea is usually caused by reflexes arising in the lung. The large tidal volume pattern (Kussmaul) usually occurs when intense chemical stimulation (as occurs with metabolic acidosis) is present.

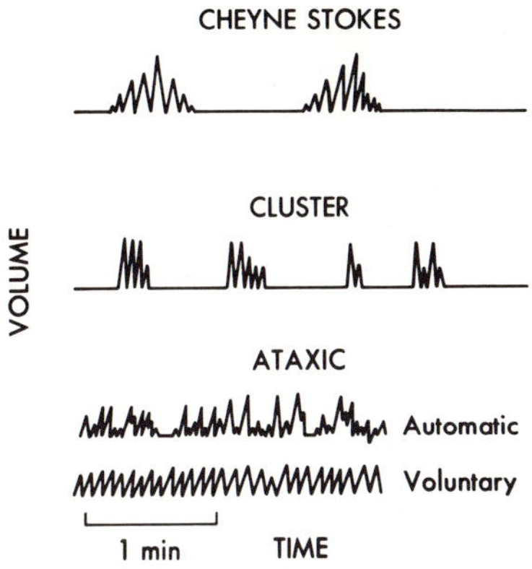

Figure 6.12. Breathing patterns in which breathing frequency and tidal volume are irregular. These breathing patterns usually indicate severe disruption of the respiratory control system and are described in the text.

Breathing Patterns with Irregular Tidal Volume and Frequency

Cheyne-Stokes respiration is a crescendo increase in tidal volume followed by decrescendo decrease in tidal volume and an apneic period (Figure 6.12). This pattern is most commonly observed with *bilateral lesions in cerebral hemispheres.* Hypercapnic drive to breathe is abnormally increased and causes overbreathing that causes P_{CO_2} to drop to levels below which it stimulates breathing. The bilateral cerebral hemispheric lesions lead to a reduction in respiratory drive from the cerebral cortex and apnea occurs until P_{CO_2} rises again to levels that stimulate breathing.

This type of breathing pattern also occurs with slow blood circulation as happens in heart failure. Whereas usually the rapidly responding chemoreceptor, the carotid body, "sees" blood that has just left the lung, with heart failure it "sees" blood that left the lung a while before. Thus, there is a discrepancy in the P_{O_2} and P_{CO_2} of the lung and in the P_{O_2} and P_{CO_2} in the carotid body. If P_{CO_2} in the chemoreceptor is high, it will cause hyperventilation; when P_{CO_2} in the lung becomes normal, the P_{CO_2} in the carotid body is still high and hyperventilation will continue and P_{CO_2} in the lung will continue to drop. By the time P_{CO_2} becomes normal in the carotid body, P_{CO_2} in the lung is very low. Eventually the low P_{CO_2} blood will reach the carotid body and cause apnea and a rise in P_{CO_2}, which causes the cycle to repeat. Therefore, overcorrection and undercorrection of P_{CO_2} occurs.

Cluster breathing (Biot's respiration) is manifested as clusters of irregular breaths alternating with periods of apnea. It is most commonly seen with disease in the pons, which destroys connections between the medullary respiratory center and the higher regions of the nervous system.

In *ataxic breathing* there is complete irregularity of tidal volme and breathing frequency. It is seen in patients with disease of the medullary chemoreceptor or the respiratory center. In spite of severe hypoventilation, dyspnea is absent. These patients can voluntarily hyperventilate.

Dyspnea

Dyspnea, the uncomfortable awareness of trouble in breathing, is related to the drive to breathe and is discussed in Chapter 17.

BIBLIOGRAPHY

Aubier M, Murciano D, Milic-Emili J, et al: Effects of administration of O_2 on ventilation and blood gases in patients with chronic obstructive pulmonary disease during acute respiratory failure. *Am Rev Resp Dis* 122:747, 1980.

Berger AJ, Mitchell RV, Severinghaus JW: Regulation of respiration. Part 1 *N Engl J Med* 297:92, 1977; Part 2 *N Engl J Med* 297:138, 1977, Part 3 *N Engl J Med* 297:194, 1977.

Fleetham JA, Kryger MH: Sleep disorders in chronic airflow obstruction. *Med Clin North Am* 65: No. 3 May, 1981.

Guilleminault C, Dement WC: *Sleep Apnea Syndromes.* New York, Alan R Liss, 1978.

Kryger M, Quesney LF, Holder D, et al: The sleep deprivation syndrome of the obese patient. *Am J Med* 56:531, 1974.

Lyons HA: Centrally acting hormones and respiration. *Pharmacol Ther* [*B*] 2:743, 1976.

Phillipson EA: Regulation of breathing during sleep. *Am Rev Respir Dis* 115:217, 1977.

Read DJC: A clinical method for assessing the ventilatory response to carbon dioxide. *Aust NZ J Med* (supersedes *Australian Annals of Medicine*) 16:20, 1967.

Rebuck AS, Campbell EJM: A clinical method for assessing the ventilatory response to hypoxia. *Am Rev Respir Dis* 109:345, 1974.

Weil JV, Byrne-Quinn E, Sodal I, et al: Hypoxic ventilatory drive in normal man. *J Clin Invest* 49:1061, 1970.

Widdicombe JG: Reflex control of breathing, in Widdicombe JG (ed): *Respiratory Physiology.* MTP International Review of Science, Physiology Series One, vol 2, 1974.

7

The Pleural Space

Meir H. Kryger

The lung is covered by a single layer of mesothelial cells, the visceral pleura; a similar layer, the parietal pleura, covers the inner surface of the chest wall. As lung volume changes, the pleural surfaces slide over each other. The space between the two surfaces is a potential space. Even though the mesothelial surfaces are permeable to liquid and gas, except for a lubricating film, the pleural space is empty. In this chapter, we will consider how the pleural space is kept empty, that is, free of gas and fluid. In diseases of the pleural space, fluid, gas, or cells are present in this usually empty space.

AIR IN THE PLEURAL SPACE: PNEUMOTHORAX

An accumulation of air in the pleural space is called a pneumothorax. Air may enter the pleural space through the chest wall (as occurs with trauma) or by rupture of lung parenchyma. Young people may have blebs in the lung apices, which rupture spontaneously. In some lung disorders such as histiocytosis X, pneumothorax is a common occurrence. A marked increase in alveolar pressure, as can occur in a patient being mechanically ventilated, can rupture lung parenchyma and cause pneumothorax.

In a *tension pneumothorax,* air continues to enter the pleural space, but because of a check valve mechanism it cannot leave. This medical emergency causes a marked increase in pleural pressure, which may actually impede venous return to the heart. In neonates, if there is rupture of lung parenchyma, air may travel in the interstitial space of the lung, toward the hilum, and cause a collection of air in the mediastinum.

The major manifestation of pneumothorax is *sudden* deterioration of cardiorespiratory status. Tachypnea occurs almost immediately, because of the activity of receptors that respond to a reduction in lung volume. This reflex is mediated by the vagus nerve (see Chapter 6).

Pneumothorax will cause an increase in the pressure in veins draining into the right atrium (central venous pressure). Figure 7.1 shows that central venous pressure goes up faster than intrapleural pressure, suggesting that pleural pressure alone does not explain the rise. Two possibilities may explain the finding. First, there may be displacement of the mediastinum, which may kink the vessels that traverse it to empty into the right atrium. Second, it has been shown that a reduction in lung volume results in an increase in pulmonary vascular resistance (Figure 7.2). This is probably due to compression of alveolar vessels, which may lead to an increase in central venous pressure. When central venous pressure is sufficiently elevated, venous return and hence cardiac output are reduced.

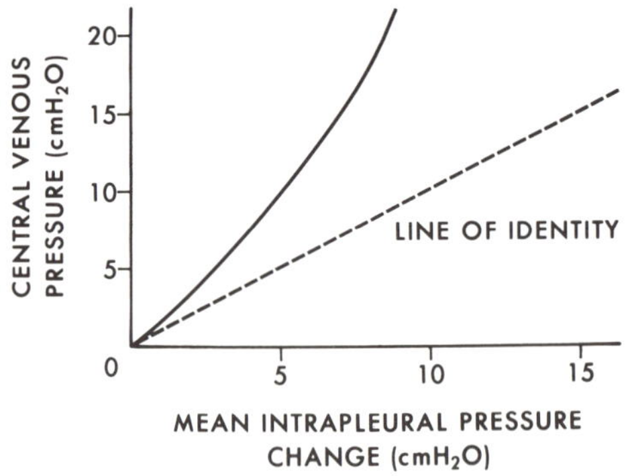

Figure 7.1. The effect of increasing intrapleural pressure in pneumothorax in an experimental animal. If the change in central venous pressure simply reflected intrapleural pressure, the two would change identically (dashed line). In fact, central venous pressure goes up more than pleural pressure.

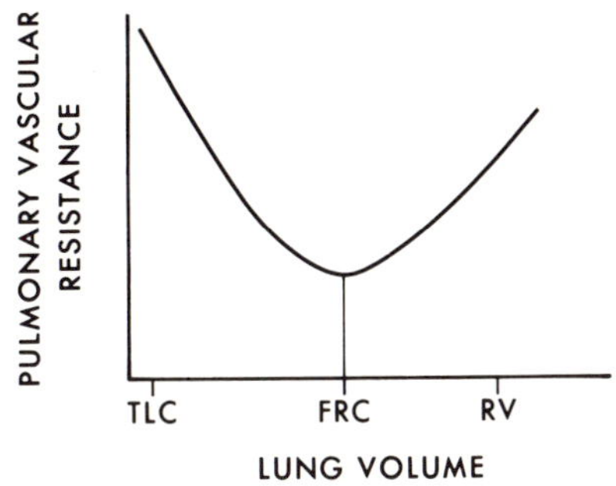

Figure 7.2. Pulmonary vascular resistance increases as lung volume is reduced below normal resting levels (FRC). This may be one reason why central venous pressure rises out of proportion to the increase in pleural pressure in pneumothorax.

Normally the mediastinum is in the midline, because the pleural pressures on either side of the mediastinum are equal. When a pneumothorax is present, pleural pressure on the affected side will exceed pleural pressure on the normal side. The mediastinum will shift to the side of less pleural pressure, the normal side.

When air enters the pleural space, the layers of pleura are separated; the chest wall will spring outward, and the lung will collapse due to its elastic recoil. There is a tendency to grade pneumothorax by using percentages; for example, an x-ray report might say that a 70% pneumothorax is present, which attempts to say that the lung is 70% collapsed. This is extremely misleading; for example, the lung of a patient with emphysema has a loss of recoil and, because of airway closure, may not collapse very much. Thus, a small amount of air in the pleural space of such a patient has the same physiological consequence as a huge amount of pleural air in a normal person (see Figure 7.3).

Hypoxemia occurs acutely in pneumothorax because some perfusion continues to the collapsed hypoventilating lung regions causing $\dot{V}/\dot{Q}$ mismatching. Usually within a day, perfusion is reduced by hypoxic vasoconstriction, and there is improvement in $\dot{V}/\dot{Q}$ and improvement in Pa_{O_2}.

Resorption of Pneumothorax

Eventually a pneumothorax will be resorbed by the mechanisms that keep the pleural space free of gas. When air enters the pleural space, its gas composition will change, because it will tend to equilibrate with the blood-tissue environment that surrounds the pleural space. It has been found that this environment approximates mixed venous blood. The total gas pressure of the air in the pneumothorax is about 713 mmHg (barometric pressure −47). The total gas pressure of mixed venous blood is much less, only about 660 mmHg. This total is the sum of P_{N_2} 574 mmHg, P_{O_2} 40 mmHg, and P_{CO_2} 46 mmHg.

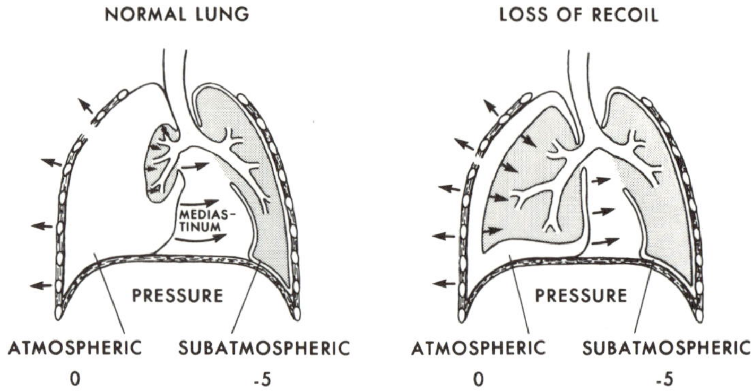

Figure 7.3. Effect of lung recoil on pneumothorax. When atmospheric air communicates with the pleural space, the chest wall springs outward and the lung collapses. The pressure in the pleural space becomes atmospheric, instead of the usual subatmospheric pressure (of about -5 cmH_2O) found in an intact pleural space. A lung with normal recoil will collapse to a very small volume. When loss of recoil is present, the lung will not collapse to as small a volume as a normal lung. The mediastinum will shift to the side of the more negative (lower) pleural pressure.

Because the total gas pressure in the pneumothorax exceeds the mixed venous pressure, gas will be absorbed into the venous blood and the pneumothorax will be resorbed.

Any maneuver that will reduce the total gas pressure in venous blood will increase the total pressure gradient between the pneumothorax and the blood-tissue environment. One way to do this is to breathe oxygen. This will markedly reduce the venous P_{N_2}, but it will have only a small effect on venous P_{O_2} and will markedly increase the total pressure gradient from the pleural air to the blood-tissue environment. This will speed up resorption of the nitrogen (which makes up the major volume of pleural air) in the pneumothorax.

HOW THE PLEURAL SPACE IS KEPT FREE OF FLUID

The parietal and visceral pleural membranes are permeable to liquid. Pleural liquid is formed at the parietal pleura and resorbed by the visceral pleura. The amount of fluid present is determined by the balance between the forces that move fluid into the pleura and those that resorb fluid. Just as in any other part of the body, fluid movement is governed by four variables; these are hydrostatic pressure (HP), colloid osmotic pressure (COP), permeability of blood vessels, and lymphatic drainage. Colloid osmotic pressure is determined by protein content and is about 32 cmH_2O (1 mmHg = 1.36 cmH_2O) in plasma and only about 6 cmH_2O in the pleural liquid, which has low protein content. Remember that fluid goes from an area of high to low hydrostatic pressure but travels from an area of low to high colloid osmotic pressure.

The net force tending to drive fluid from the parietal pleura into the pleural space is:

$$(HPc - HPpl) - (COPc - COPpl)$$

HPc is the mean capillary hydrostatic pressure; HPpl is intrapleural pressure; COPc is plasma colloid osmotic pressure, and COPpl is the colloid osmotic pressure of the pleural fluid.

The parietal pleura, the site of fluid formation, receives its blood supply from systemic vessels, branches of the intercostal arteries. Mean hydrostatic pressure is about 30 cmH_2O in these capillaries. If mean capillary hydrostatic pressure is 30 cmH_2O, pleural pressure is -5 cmH_2O, plasma colloid osmotic pressure is 32 cmH_2O, and pleural liquid osmotic pressure is 6 cmH_2O, then the total pressure driving fluid into the pleural space is:

$$[(30 - (-5)] - (32 - 6)$$

$$= 35 \qquad - 26$$

$= 9$ cmH_2O (Positive number indicates movement into pleural space.)

The visceral pleura receives its blood supply from the lower pressure pulmonary circulation. Except for the lower capillary hydrostatic pressure, all the remaining pressures at the visceral pleura are the same as at the parietal. The lower visceral capillary hydrostatic pressure is the reason that the pleural liquid is absorbed. The net force driving fluid from the pleural space into the visceral pleural capillaries, using the same equation as above except that the visceral capillary hydrostatic pressure is only 11 cmH_2O, is:

$$[(11 - (-5)] - (32 - 6)$$

$$= 16 \qquad - 26$$

$= -10$ cmH_2O (Negative number indicates movement out of pleural space.)

Thus, the pressure driving fluid out of the pleural space exceeds the pressure driving fluid into the pleural space by 1 cmH_2O. In addition, the visceral (resorptive) pleura is more vascularized than the parietal pleura and hence offers less resistance to flow. These factors all favor resorption of fluid (Figure 7.4).

The lymphatics remove protein and cells from the pleural space; maneuvers that increase ventilation increase lymphatic flow, probably because the cycles in pleural pressure occurring during breathing act as an accessory pump.

FLUID IN THE PLEURAL SPACE: PLEURAL EFFUSION

Pleural fluid will accumulate if an imbalance occurs in the mechanisms that tend to keep the pleural space free of fluid. A large pleural effusion restricts lung inflation and causes extrapulmonary lung restriction. Pleural effusion

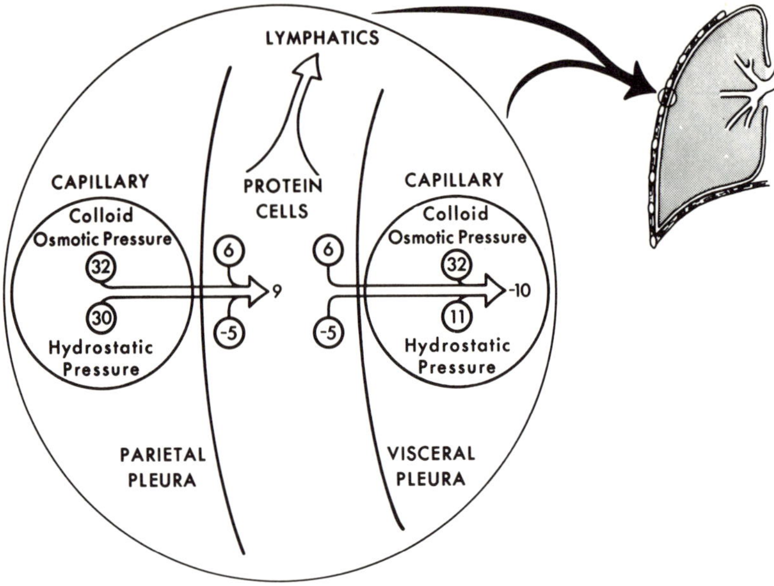

Figure 7.4. Forces keeping the pleural space free of fluid. Fluid is formed at the parietal pleura with a net pressure of 9 cmH_2O and absorbed at the visceral pleura with a pressure of -10 cmH_2O. Thus the pressures resorbing fluid exceed the pressures forming fluid by 1 cmH_2O. The lymphatics remove protein and cells. Numbers refer to pressure cmH_2O.

could be expected when changes occur in capillary permeability, colloid osmotic pressure, hydrostatic pressure, or lymphatic drainage. In general, when the effusion is caused by a reduction in colloid osmotic pressure, or an increase in hydrostatic pressure, the fluid formed is basically an ultrafiltrate of plasma and contains little protein and few cells and is called a *transudate.* When the effusion is caused by an increase in capillary permeability or abnormal lymphatics, the fluid is protein rich and contains many cells and is called an *exudate.*

Capillary Permeability

Capillary permeability is increased when inflammation of the pleura is present. This commonly occurs with infection of the pleural space, which is called empyema, and may occur with infections adjacent to the pleural space including the lung and the subdiaphragmatic region of the abdomen. The increased permeability causes the leakage of protein rich fluid and leukocytes into the pleural fluid. If many cells are present in the pleural fluid, the end products of metabolism of these cells may cause the fluid to be acidic. The increase in protein concentration will increase the pressure driving fluid into the pleural space and reduce the pressure driving fluid out of the pleural space. This can be demonstrated by examining the effect of changing colloid osmotic pressure of pleural fluid from 6 to 12 cmH_2O.

Driving Pressure

Parietal Pleura to Pleural Space	*Pleural Space to Visceral Pleura*
(HPc − HPpl) − (COPc − COPpl)	(HPc − HPpl) − (COPc − COPpl)
[30 − (− 5)] − (32 − 12)	[11 − (− 5)] − (32 − 12)
= 35 − 20	= 16 − 20
= 15 cmH_2O	= − 4 cmH_2O

Thus, the pressure driving fluid into the pleural space exceeds the pressure driving fluid out by 11 cmH_2O (15 − 4 = 11 cmH_2O), and thus fluid will accumulate.

Colloid Osmotic Pressure

Colloid osmotic pressure of serum is reduced when serum proteins are reduced. Decreased albumin production due to liver disease or the urinary protein loss of glomerular disease may both reduce colloid osmotic pressure to levels that will cause pleural effusion. Colloid osmotic pressure may be about 15 cmH_2O (instead of 32 cmH_2O) when serum albumin is reduced to about 1.5 gm%; if all other factors are constant, this will cause pleural fluid accumulation.

Driving Pressure

Parietal Pleura to Pleural Space	*Pleural Space to Visceral Pleura*
(HPc − HPpl) − (COPc − COPpl)	(HPc − HPpl) − (COPc − COPpl)
[30 − (− 5)] − (15 − 6)	[11 − (− 5)] − (15 − 6)
= 35 − 9	= 16 − 9
= 26	= 7

In this situation, fluid will enter the pleural space both at the parietal pleura (with a net driving pressure of 26 cmH_2O) and at the visceral pleura (with a net driving pressure of 7 cmH_2O). Fluid can only be absorbed by the lymphatics when this occurs (Figure 7.5).

Hydrostatic Pressure

Hydrostatic pressure in the capillaries of the parietal and visceral pleura can be increased when venous hypertension due to heart failure is present. Left ventricular failure alone does not result in pleural fluid accumulation, prob-

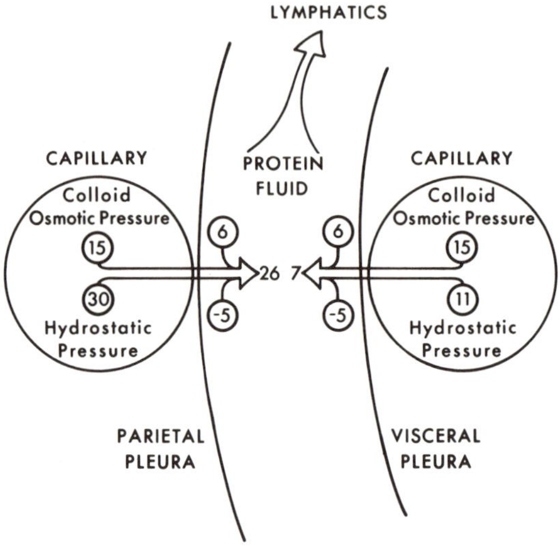

Figure 7.5. Pleural fluid accumulation with reduction of colloid osmotic pressure of blood. When colloid osmotic pressure is reduced from 32 cmH_2O to 15 cmH_2O, fluid is formed both at the parietal and visceral pleural surfaces. The only way fluid can now leave the pleural space is to be taken up by the lymphatics.

ably because the lymphatics can compensate for the reduction in resorption by the visceral pleura. Similarly, systemic venous hypertension due to right ventricular failure alone seldom causes pleural effusion, probably because absorption by the very vascular visceral pleura can keep up with fluid production. On the other hand, biventricular heart failure, by increasing capillary hydrostatic pressure at both surfaces, commonly causes pleural effusion. The increased systemic venous pressure increases fluid formation at the parietal pleura and also decreases lymphatic flow. The latter occurs because lymphatics empty into systemic veins; therefore, venous hypertension will also impede lymphatic flow.

Lymphatic Obstruction

Lymphatic obstruction or increased lymphatic pressure may cause pleural effusion. In patients with portal hypertension and ascites (fluid in the peritoneal cavity), the lymphatics that absorb ascitic fluid traverse the mediastinum, which increases the pressure of the lymphatics that drain the pleural space. Thus, ascites may be associated with pleural effusion. When the major lymphatic channels are obstructed, the effusions may become milky due to the chylomicrons found in lymph fluid originating in the gastrointestinal tract. These are called *chylous* pleural effusions.

Turnover of Pleural Fluid

Once an effusion is present, it may not change much in volume over a short period of time; however, mechanisms that resorb and form pleural fluid are quite active. It has been found that effusions actually have a fairly high turnover of fluid, 30 to 75% of the volume being produced and resorbed per hour.

Diagnosis

The diagnosis of pleural effusion is suggested by the findings of dullness to percussion and reduced breath sounds with usually a shift of the mediastinum to the normal side. Chest x-ray confirms the presence of pleural disease. A small effusion can sometimes be detected only by doing a chest x-ray with the patient lying with the diseased side down, a lateral decubitus x-ray. Attempts to further characterize the effusion can be done by withdrawing a sample of the fluid to do various biochemical tests, microbiological evaluations, and cytological examinations. A biopsy of the pleura can be performed. Occasionally the pleural space is examined visually using a thoracoscope.

Exudate versus Transudate (Table 7.1)
When a patient has a pleural effusion, an attempt is made to characterize it as being caused by increased permeability or reduced lymphatic flow, an exudate, or as being caused by increased hydrostatic pressure or reduced colloid osmotic pressure, a transudate, which is an ultrafiltrate of plasma. Analysis of the pleural fluid is used to determine the mechanism causing effusion. At one

Table 7.1. Diseases with Pleural Effusions

Transudates[a]
Biventricular heart failure
Liver failure
Acute renal failure (fluid overload)
Nephrotic syndrome
Myxedema, sarcoid, peritoneal dialysis
Exudates[b]
Infections (all types)
Pulmonary infarction
Malignancy
Vasculitis (rheumatoid arthritis, lupus erythematosis)
Benign ovarian tumor (Meig's syndrome)
Hepatic abscess, intra-abdominal infection, or pancreatitis
Lymphatic abnormalities

[a] Increased hydrostatic pressure or decreased colloid osmotic pressure.
[b] Increased permeability or increased lymphatic pressure.

time the major test used was the measurement of the protein concentration of the fluid. If more than 3 gm/100 ml protein was present, an exudate was likely; a concentration of less than 3 mg/100 ml suggested a transudate. Recently, the following criteria have been added to document more accurately exudate: pleural fluid to serum protein ratio greater than .5, pleural lactic dehydrogenase (LDH) greater than 200 IU, or pleural fluid to serum LDH ratio exceeding .6. LDH is an enzyme that is easily measured and used as a protein marker. A high pleural fluid white blood cell count suggests inflammation, an exudate. Pleural fluid glucose is reduced in bacterial infection or malignancy, since cells in the pleural fluid in these conditions are metabolically active and utilize glucose. Pleural glucose is also very low in the effusion of rheumatoid arthritis. Infection is also likely when pH of pleural fluid is low, due to accumulation of products of metabolism of cells.

OTHER PLEURAL DISORDERS

Hemothorax. Blood in the pleural space occurs most often with trauma, malignancy, or rupture of a great vessel. Resorption of the blood is often complete, but fibrosis in the pleural space, *fibrothorax,* may occur.

Fibrothorax. Fibrosis of the pleural space occurs as a response to an infection or hemothorax. *Fibrous pleural plaques* commonly occur in persons previously exposed to asbestos.

Neoplasms. Neoplasms arising from the pleural surfaces, mesotheliomas, also occur primarily in persons with asbestos exposure. These tumors, when malignant, can grow extensively and entrap the lung and blood vessels in the mediastinum. Hypertrophic pulmonary osteoarthropathy is common in these patients.

TREATMENT OF PLEURAL DISEASES

Two aspects must be remembered in treating pleural disease. First, the disease may increase pleural pressure and thus compromise lung function. In these sometimes life-threatening situations, the pleural pressure must be reduced usually by draining the pleural space.

Second, the disease causing the effusion must be treated specifically. For example, pleural pyogenic infections must be drained, as must localized infections in other parts of the body. As shown on the list in Table 1, specific treatment is available for most of the causes of pleural effusion.

Unfortunately, at present there is no satisfactory treatment for malignant mesothelioma.

BIBLIOGRAPHY

Agostoni E: Mechanics of the pleural space. *Physiol Rev* 52:57, 1972.

Black LF: The pleural space and pleural fluid. *Mayo Clin Proc* 47:493, 1972.

Black LF: Pleural disease. *Basics of Respiratory Disease* Vol 6, No 5, 1978.

Light RW, MacGregor MC, Luchsinger PC, et al: Pleural Effusions: The diagnostic separation of transudates and exudates. *Ann Intern Med* 77:507, 1972.

Light RW, MacGregor MC, Ball WC, et al: Diagnostic significance of pleural fluid pH and P_{CO_2}. *Chest* 64:591, 1973.

Monin P, Vert P: Pneumothorax. *Clinics in Perinatology* 5(no 2):335, 1978.

8

Immunological Lung Disease and Asthma

W. Kepron

STRUCTURE AND FUNCTION OF THE IMMUNE SYSTEM
T-cells, B-cells, and Macrophages
Cellular and Humoral Immunity
Complement

ALLERGY: ABNORMAL FUNCTION OF THE IMMUNE SYSTEM

ASTHMA
- Prevalence
- Etiology

Pathology
- Smooth muscle hypertrophy
- Mucosal alterations

Bronchial secretions
Pathogenesis of Asthma
- Immunological release of mediators
- Hyperirritability of cholinergic irritant receptor
- Partial beta-adrenergic blockade

Pathophysiologic Alterations in Asthma
- Airflow obstruction
- Lung volumes
- Abnormalities in gas exchange

PHARMACOLOGY OF ASTHMA
Receptors
- Adrenergic receptors
- Cholinergic receptors
- Glucocorticoids and receptors

Therapeutic Agents
- β_2-Receptor agonists
- Phosphodiesterase inhibitors

The immune system protects us from a variety of potentially harmful substances. These substances originate from outside the body (infectious agents, toxins, and foreign particles) and from inside the body (malignant cells). The immune system must first recognize the presence of the harmful substances before mounting an attack. The major defense mechanisms are humoral and cell-mediated immunity. The immune response, when excessive or exaggerated, may actually cause disease. In this chapter, we will review the normal immune system and the effect on the lung of abnormal immune responses. The role of deficient immune responses in the pathogenesis of infections is found in Chapter 15.

STRUCTURE AND FUNCTION OF THE IMMUNE SYSTEM

T-cells, B-cells, and Macrophages

The basic elements of the immune system are the thymus-derived lymphocyte (T-lymphocyte or T-cell), the bursa equivalent lymphocyte (B-lymphocyte or B-cell), and the macrophage. These three cell types arise from a hematogenous stem cell early in the development of the fetus.

The T-lymphocyte begins as a prothymocyte, which migrates to the thymus where under the influence of macrophages it matures into a T-lymphocyte. At the same time, the precursor cells for B-lymphocytes migrate to peripheral lymphoid tissue in liver, spleen, lymph nodes, and lymphoid aggregates within the gastrointestinal tract where maturation and differentiation to B-lymphocytes occur. Structurally and functionally, the two lymphocyte populations remain distinct from one another. The B-lymphocytes possess on their surface immunoglobulin and receptors for both complement and antigen-antibody complexes. These cells elaborate specific immunoglobulins following appropriate activation to perform their main function, humoral immunity. In contrast, T-lymphocytes, which are responsible for cell-mediated immunity, do not possess surface immunoglobulins.

The macrophage is derived from a hematogenous stem cell, the promyelocyte. Following a maturation process in the bone marrow, the cell appears as a circulating monocyte, which eventually populates peripheral tissues. In these tissues, the cells mature further into macrophages, which are capable of participating in various secretory or phagocytic defense functions. The macrophage possesses surface receptors that are able to bind the third component of complement (C_3) or the crystallizable fragment (Fc portion) of immunoglobulin.

Cellular and Humoral Immunity

The development of either cellular or humoral immunity is closely dependent on a close interaction between macrophages and either T-lymphocytes for cell-mediated immunity or B-lymphocytes for humoral immunity. The macrophage initiates the process by acting as both a phagocytic cell and as a secretory cell, capable of elaborating a variety of active agents or mediators. Following contact with a foreign antigen, a macrophage will bind antigen to its cell membrane receptors, then phagocytose, and lyse the antigen. Following lysis, the antigen fragments are reexpressed by the macrophage and once again bound to cell membrane receptors on the macrophage. This process enhances the immunogenicity of the antigen prior to presentation to lymphocytes for the development of the immune responses (see Figure 8.1). Presentation of this bound antigen to T-lymphocytes induces a subset of T-

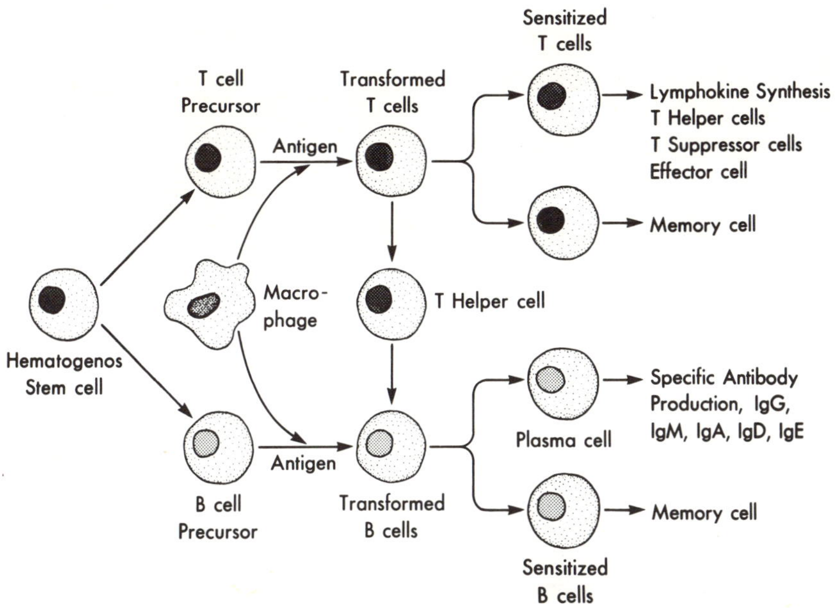

Figure 8.1. Development of the humoral and cellular immune systems. Macrophage processing of antigen occurs prior to presentation to B-lymphocytes and T-lymphocytes, with T-helper lymphocyte facilitation of immunoglobulin production.

lymphocytes, the T-helper cell, which facilitates cooperation between macrophage-bound antigen and B-lymphocytes to produce antibody to the antigen. Then depending on numerous variables, the organism will elaborate specific immunoglobulins of the IgG, IgM, IgA, or IgE class. The T-lymphocytes may produce another subset, the T-effector cells, which are responsible for the cell-mediated immune responses of the organism.

Once the T-lymphocyte is activated to a specific antigen, reexposure to that antigen will induce the release of several proteins called lymphokines that include a macrophage-activating factor (MAF) and a migration inhibitory factor (MIF), which maintains the activated macrophage in the area of antigen exposure. Similarly, activated macrophages secrete several specific lymphocyte-activating factors that act to recruit and activate additional T-lymphocytes or B-lymphocytes at the site of the immune reaction. Thus, an amplification system is established that rapidly facilitates the production of either humoral or cell-mediated immune reactions at the sites of immune reactions. In addition, the T-lymphocyte is also able to promote a direct cytotoxic effect largely through the elaboration of several mediators, which provides protection against various intracellular pathogens, the capacity for allograft rejection and the function of tumor resistance.

Complement

In order for the humoral immune system to function normally in host defense, it is necessary for the complement system to be activated and to participate in the ensuing inflammatory reaction. The complement system is the primary humoral mediator of the antigen-antibody reaction sequence. Once complement is activated, interactions occur between complement, antigen-antibody complexes, and cell membranes to produce a variety of effects. These include cell lysis, recruitment of both humoral and cellular immune mechanisms, release of histamine and lysosomal contents, and inhibition of macrophage, lymphocyte, and polymorphonuclear cell migration.

The individual components of the complement system circulate in the serum as 15 distinct proteins. Activation of the classic complement sequence occurs following antigen-antibody interaction and fixation to cell membrane. Figure 8.2 illustrates the sequence of events that occurs as each serum protein component is activated and, in turn, activates the next precursor in the sequence until the final activation of C_5 through C_9 occurs. Completion of this activation sequence causes cytolysis of the cell or organism. Important by-products of this sequence are the generation of the split products, C_{3a} and C_{5a}, which are anaphylotoxins which can contribute to the generation of an acute anaphylactic reaction via histamine release. Also important is the increase in phagocytosis promoted by C_{3b}, and the chemotactic effect for mononuclear and polymorphonuclear cells promoted by C_{5b}. This "classic pathway" of complement activation is mediated by immunoglobulin of the IgG and IgM class, but may also be activated by DNA, C-reactive protein, and trypsinlike enzymes. An "alternate pathway" of complement activation is recognized with increasing frequency and occurs without the presence of antibody. Although originally described as being activated by properdin, a bacterial protein product released during acute infections, this pathway is now known to be induced by grain dust, moldy hay, cotton dust, and red cedar dust. Both the classic pathway and the alternate pathway (Figure 8.2) produce complement activation through a final common pathway after activation of the third component of complement (C_3). The importance of complement activation is that it mediates lytic destruction of bacteria, viruses, erythrocytes, and platelets. Although some aspects of complement activation are important for host defense mechanisms to operate normally, the resulting inflammatory reactions may have serious detrimental effects on organs should they be involved in a secondary fashion, for example, in acute allergic alveolitis or hypersensitivity pneumonitis (discussed below).

ALLERGY: ABNORMAL FUNCTION OF THE IMMUNE SYSTEM

The major defense mechanisms of the body are mediated by the immune system and are effected by the generation of an inflammatory response at the site of antigen-antibody reactions. Allergy results from the same immunologically mediated inflammatory responses but occurs as antibody is produced against environmental antigens, which are not normally harmful. The reactivity or the hypersensitivity developed by the allergic person is an abnormal reaction by the immune system. This acquired reactivity may be mediated by a variety of different immunological reactions and may involve any organ

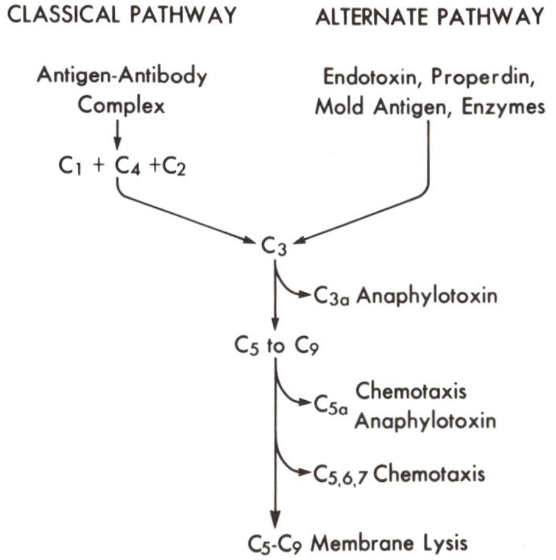

Figure 8.2. Activation of the complement cascade by the classic and alternate pathways.

system within the body. Primary consideration will be given here to how these immunological reactions involve the respiratory system. With the acceptance of an immunological reaction as the central pathogenetic mechanism in the generation of allergic diseases, it is necessary to identify an offending allergen (antigen), establish a relationship between exposure to the antigen and development of a lesion, and identify the immunological mechanism in the illness. Based on the nature of the immunological reaction involved, Gell and Coombs classified allergic disease into four main types of reactions (Table 8.1).

Type I. Also known as immediate-type hypersensitivity, type I hypersensitivity is produced by a specific class of immunoglobulin, immunoglobulin E or IgE. IgE antibody is commonly produced by the organism against a specific inhaled allergen such as pollens, molds, or animal danders. The IgE antibody then binds to surface receptors on tissue mast cells and/or circulating basophils and sensitizes these cells. Reexposure to the allergen results in allergen reacting with the cell-bound IgE, which causes the release of histamine and other mediators of inflammation that produce characteristic end-organ responses resulting in such allergic illnesses as asthma, hay fever, anaphylaxis, atopic dermatitis, and angioedema-urticaria. Asthma is discussed in greater detail below.

Type II. Also known as cytotoxic or cytolytic hypersensitivity, type II hypersensitivity is mediated by specific IgG or IgM antibody. This form of hypersensitivity most often occurs when circulating IgG antibody to exogenous antigens (streptococcal antigen) or to "self" antigens (thyroid antigen) react with antigenic determinants on a cell membrane. Once this reaction has occurred, complement becomes fixed at the antigen-antibody site and rapidly induces damage in the cell membrane, which leads to cytolysis of the cell. Many tissues in the body may be affected when IgG antibody reacts with antigenic determinants in the cell membrane and induces cytolysis and an

Table 8.1. Immunological Respiratory Diseases

	Mechanism	*Examples*
Type I	IgE on cell reacts with allergen-releasing mediator	Asthma, hay fever.
Type II	IgG or IgM directed against basement membrane; complement activated	Goodpasture's syndrome.
Type III	Circulating antigen-antibody complexes deposited in lung; complement activated; inflammatory reaction	Hypersensitivity pneumonitis, collagen vascular diseases.
Type IV	Cell-mediated (T-lymphocyte) immunity; lymphokines; inflammatory reaction	Tuberculosis, granulomatous diseases.

inflammatory reaction. This is illustrated in such illnesses as Goodpasture's syndrome and poststreptococcal glomerulonephritis.

In Goodpasture's syndrome, there occurs the development of antiglomerular basement membrane antibody. This antibody damages not only the basement membranes of the kidney but also those of the alveoli. Patients with Goodpasture's syndrome develop severe hemoptysis and renal failure and usually die within a few months of onset of symptoms. Recently, removal of the antiglomerular basement membrane antibody by plasmapheresis has improved survival in these patients.

Type III. Also known as immune-complex hypersensitivity, type III hypersensitivity may be mediated by IgG and IgM antibody. In this form of hypersensitivity, antigen enters the person by inhalation, injection, or ingestion. Antibody production is directed against the antigen. With continued exposure to antigen, the formation of antigen-antibody complexes occurs and these complexes circulate freely in the bloodstream. The circulating immune complexes may be deposited along the basement membranes of several target organs with the lung and kidney most commonly affected. Once the immune complexes are localized in a tissue, complement is fixed at that site, which induces cytolysis of the target cell and promotes an intense localized inflammatory reaction. The clinical symptoms that develop depend on the site of major organ involvement. Type III hypersensitivity contributes significantly to the pathogenesis of hypersensitivity pneumonitis such as farmer's lung, pigeon-breeder's lung, and other related inhalational lung diseases. These diseases are discussed in detail later in this chapter. Other illnesses produced by this mechanism likely include collagen vascular diseases such as systemic lupus erythematosis, polyarteritis nodosa, and rheumatoid arthritis. These illnesses may have significant lung involvement, presumably due to deposition of immune complexes in the lung and the resulting inflammation and fibrosis.

Type IV. Type IV hypersensitivity is also known as delayed type hypersensitivity or cell-mediated hypersensitivity. This form of hypersensitivity reaction is mediated by specifically sensitized T-lymphocytes without the involvement of the complement system. Exposure to antigen results in activation of the T-lymphocyte, and subsequent reexposure to antigen results in the release of several mediators or lymphokines. The lymphokines possess a wide variety of biological activities, which includes the attraction, localization, and activation of macrophages and polymorphonuclear cells as well as a direct cytotoxic effect on target cells. During acute cytotoxic reactions, intense inflammatory reactions may occur, for example, acute rejection reactions in transplant patients. As with type III hypersensitivity reactions, prolonged exposure to antigen may result in a chronic inflammatory process persisting that may progress to extensive organ fibrosis. This mechanism is thought to contribute largely to such reactions as tuberculosis, sarcoidosis, and chronic transplantation reactions.

Although specific mechanisms have been proposed to explain the immunopathogenesis of several hypersensitivity diseases, it is currently recognized that more than one of the above mechanisms may be involved in the development of a disease process. It is now appreciated that both humoral (immune complex) and cell-mediated immunity contribute to the pathogenesis of hypersensitivity pneumonitis and that a similar combination of mechanisms may also be present in the lung involvement in the collagen diseases such as systemic lupus erythematosis and polyarteritis nodosa.

ASTHMA

Asthma has been recognized since antiquity and was originally described by Hippocrates. Asthma is derived from a Greek word meaning "to pant" and was used to describe a condition manifested by episodic shortness of breath. From that time, no universally accepted definition has emerged, although most physicians will describe this illness as a disease characterized by increased responsiveness of the trachea and bronchi to various stimuli and manifested by a widespread narrowing of the airways (bronchoconstriction or bronchospasm) that changes in severity either spontaneously or as result of therapy. This increased responsiveness of the airways may result in acute, severe airway narrowing following exposure to a wide variety of stimuli such as inhaled pollens, mold spores, dusts, animal danders, noxious chemicals, drugs, exercise, and possibly psychological factors. In some patients, the bronchoconstriction is a manifestation of allergy. In many patients, allergic mechanisms cannot be implicated. Asthma tends to be an episodic disease, the acute exacerbations being interspersed with periods of complete well-being with minor symptoms present. However, severe unremitting symptoms may develop and persist despite intensive therapy over days or weeks. This is status asthmaticus.

Prevalence

Asthma is a common illness in western industrialized countries and is found in .2 to 1.0% of the total population. The incidence of asthma appears to be higher in groups with higher socioeconomic status. Asthma may affect all ages, but it occurs predominantly in early life. In childhood, boys are affected much more commonly than girls. Women become more commonly affected from age 30 years to age 60 years when men tend to predominate once again. The prognosis of this illness is extremely variable; complete resolution of symptoms may occur in later childhood or early adulthood. It may be expected that 50 to 80% of asthmatics whose illness has its onset before 16 years of age will have complete resolution or, at worst, will only have mild episodes of bronchoconstriction in later years. When the asthma has its onset during the adult years, the symptoms tend to be more chronic and unremitting, and somewhat less than 30% of this late onset group can be expected to have an eventual amelioration or resolution of their symptoms.

Etiology

A satisfactory definition of asthma has not been universally accepted, largely because of the diverse etiological factors that lead to bronchoconstriction. It is accepted, however, that a common facet to all forms of asthma is the presence of a nonspecific hyperirritability of the tracheobronchial tree. Those patients in whom a definite inciting stimulus can be identified and correlated to a specific IgE antibody have *allergic or extrinsic asthma.* Those patients with no definite inciting stimulus or with as yet no definable specific IgE antibody production to an allergen, have *idiosyncratic or intrinsic asthma.*

Allergic asthma is often associated with a positive family history of allergic disease such as eczema, rhinitis, urticaria, or asthma. Frequently symptoms are seasonal in nature, being correlated with allergens in the environment such as tree, grass, and weed pollens, and various airborne molds. These patients will demonstrate positive skin test reactions to the offending allergen and will have elevated titers of specific IgE antibody to the allergen. Other environmental allergens which may produce nonseasonal symptoms are animal dander, house dust mites, and molds.

A large proportion of the asthma population will have no discernible precipitating stimulus, a negative family history for allergic diseases, an absence of skin reactivity to the common allergens, and no discernible elevations of IgE antibody to any allergens. This group is termed the idiosyncratic or intrinsic asthmatic. Perhaps best considered here are those asthmatics whose clinical symptoms are precipitated by the ingestion of aspirin or other nonsteroidal anti-inflammatory agents such as indomethacin. These patients are usually adults with a triad of moderately severe asthma, nasal polyps, and sinusitis and who have a marked sensitivity to aspirin or related compounds. IgE antibody to these compounds has not been demonstrated, and this group of patients are, therefore, classified among the idiosyncratic group. Some occupationally related asthma is included in this group, because of the inability to demonstrate IgE antibody and/or a well-defined allergen, for example, meat-wrapper's asthma and baker's asthma. Finally, there are asthmatics who develop bronchoconstriction 1 to 10 minutes following periods of vigorous exercise. The clinical symptoms worsen for 30 to 60 minutes before improving spontaneously. The basis for this exercise-induced asthma remains largely unknown at the present. The inhalation through the mouth of large volumes of cold air may play a role, since breathing warmed, humidified air (as in nose breathing) is associated with less exercise-induced bronchoconstriction.

Pathology

The pathological alterations that have been described in asthma have been derived from postmortem examinations of patients who died with severe exacerbations of their asthma. As such, these findings are biased toward alterations that might be expected in more severe intractable asthma than would be seen in milder cases of this illness. Nevertheless, the alterations that are documented allow for a better understanding of the physiological alterations, which are also common to all forms of this illness. These alterations include:

- Smooth muscle hypertrophy.
- Mucosal swelling and cellular infiltration.
- Mucous plugging of airways.

Smooth Muscle Hypertrophy

The three essential alterations listed above may be seen illustrated in Figure 8.3. Examination of the airways reveals an increase in the smooth muscle mass within the tracheobronchial tree. Increasing experimental evidence suggests that this muscle is functionally different from normal tracheobronchial smooth muscle. This indicates that sensitized tracheobronchial smooth muscle has a higher resting tone than normal smooth muscle, contracts to a greater degree, and maintains contraction longer than normal smooth muscle when challenged by a sensitizing antigen.

Mucosal Alterations

A prominent finding is the degree of inflammation and swelling that involves the mucosa and submucosa of the airways. A striking and constant feature of these alterations is the shedding of the ciliated columnar epithelium, which is thought to occur secondarily to the development of submucosal inflammation and the production of excessive secretion from hypertrophied mucous glands and goblet cells. The shedding of epithelial cells may leave large areas of bronchial surface completely denuded of epithelium. Inflammation in the submucosa may be quite striking with marked infiltration by eosinophils,

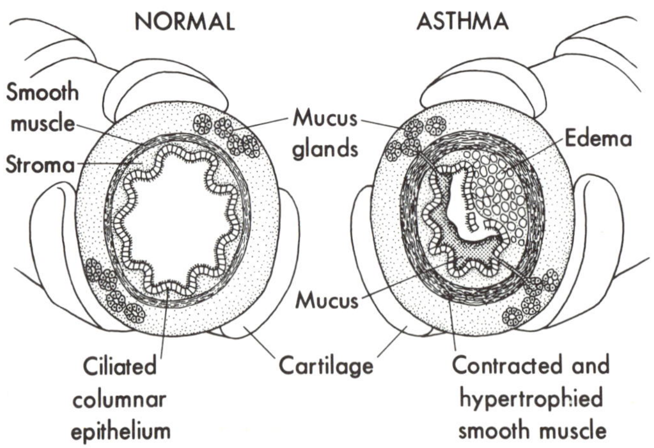

Figure 8.3. Smooth muscle hypertrophy and constriction, production of thick tenacious sputum and mucosal edema, producing airway obstruction in asthma.

lymphocytes, histiocytes, and plasma cells. Dilatation of capillaries and mucus gland enlargement may be prominent. All the above alterations are seen above a markedly thickened basement membrane, which is thickened to a greater degree in this illness than in any other form of obstructive lung disease.

Bronchial Secretions

Within the lumen of the tracheobronchial tree can be demonstrated the viscous bronchial secretions that contribute to the excessive sputum production in these patients. These secretions possess an increased content of protein and neuraminic acid, which increases viscosity. Another feature is the compact clusters of detached columnar cells, known as *creola* bodies. In addition may be seen crystalline structures, the *Charcot-Leyden* crystals, which are thought to be derived from degenerated eosinophil inclusion bodies. All these structures and substances are incorporated into the tenacious mucus plugs, which when compact enough to assume the shape of the tracheobronchial tree are referred to as *Curshman's* spirals.

The above features all contribute to the production of the airflow obstruction, which can be so readily documented during the life of the asthmatic patient. Another pathological feature noted at autopsy is the presence of atelectatic areas in the lung, principally involving secondary lung lobules. All the above features explain why the lungs fail to collapse from the chest wall as the pleural cavity is opened at autopsy. Despite widespread airway changes, it should be kept in mind that the alterations described in asthma are confined to the airways and no parenchymal changes are present.

Pathogenesis of Asthma

Immunological Release of Mediators

When the mechanism causing bronchoconstriction is immunological, the initial step involves the inhaled allergen bridging two specific IgE molecules on the surface of a mast cell either in the mucosa or in the submucosal layer of the airway. This interaction of antigen and antibody induces a series of biochemical reactions in the mast cell membrane, which causes the release of several mediators of inflammation from the mast cell (Figure 8.4).

Of major importance in this reaction sequence is the release of histamine, one of the preformed mediators stored in the basophilic granules within the mast cell. Histamine has many biological effects, including constriction of both large and small airways. The large airway bronchoconstriction is due to a direct effect of histamine on airway smooth muscle and reflex bronchoconstriction mediated by stimulation of irritant receptors in the airway mucosa acting via the vagus nerves (see below). In addition, histamine causes constriction of small peripheral airways. Other effects of histamine such as increasing capillary permeability likely contribute to the production of mucosal edema and further aggravate airway obstruction as the edematous mucosa further encroaches on the airway lumen.

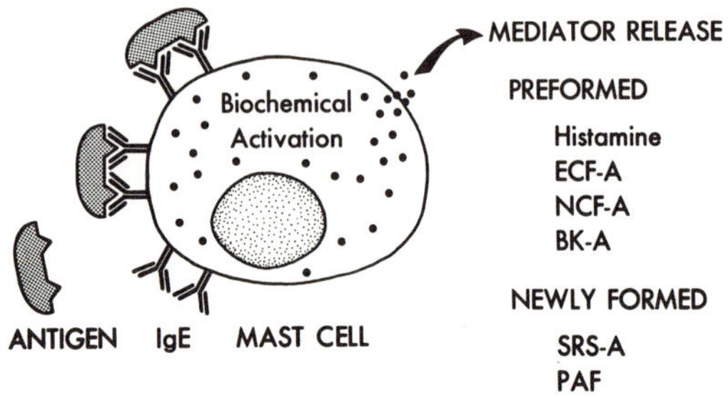

Figure 8.4. Release of preformed and newly synthesized mediators of inflammation from mast cells. Interaction between antigen and membrane-bound IgE results in biochemical activation and release of mediators from mast cells and circulating basophils.

A second major mediator released from mast cells is slow reacting substance of anaphylaxis (SRS-A), which is produced following activation of the mast cell by antigen-IgE interaction on the mast cell membrane. This substance can induce sustained smooth muscle contraction, and it has been hypothesized that SRS-A may act locally on airway smooth muscle to promote and sustain contraction of the airway smooth muscle. Several other mediators may be released as well, including an eosinophilic chemotactic factor (ECF-A), a platelet aggregating factor (PAF), a neutrophilic chemotactic factor (NCF-A), prostaglandins, bradykinin, and serotonin, but the role of these mediators in the pathogenesis of human asthma is not clearly established.

The above immunological mechanisms are well documented and may explain the mechanism of onset of the bronchoconstriction in allergen-induced asthma. As only 50% or less of asthmatics have a definable allergen to account for the onset of their symptoms, some other factor must be present to account for the onset of symptoms in the remaining patients. Several theories have been advanced to account for the onset of asthma in this latter group of patients and to account for the extreme hyperirritability of the airways to a wide variety of physical, chemical, and pharmacological stimuli. The hyperirritability is the most consistent feature of the asthmatic airway.

Hyperirritability of Cholinergic Irritant Receptor

The homeostatic control of airway tone and diameter is maintained under the balancing influence of the adrenergic and parasympathetic nervous systems. The parasympathetic nervous system tends to increase tone in the smooth muscle of the airway, promoting bronchoconstriction. The afferent limb of the reflex arc of the parasympathetic nervous system originates in "irritant" nerve receptors in the airway mucosa. Stimulation of these receptors will produce reflex bronchoconstriction, which acts through the vagus nerves. Airway smooth muscle cells are thought to have vagal receptors, which when stimulated produce cyclic GMP, which causes bronchoconstriction.

In antigen-antibody reactions within the airways, the local release of the chemical mediators of inflammation are thought to stimulate irritant receptors contributing to bronchoconstriction. In addition, inflammatory reactions may be produced within the bronchial mucosa by a variety of irritative stimuli. Disruption of the epithelial tight junctions occurs and allows exposure of the irritant receptors to the bronchial lumen. Hyperirritability, which may be documented following acute viral illness, is thought to occur as the exposed irritant receptors become stimulated by either chemical or physical stimuli. This may also explain the precipitation of asthma symptoms in asthmatics by viral infections and the prolonged period of bronchial hyperirritability in asthmatics following infections of the respiratory tract.

Partial Beta-Adrenergic Blockade

Not all the increased airway reactivity in asthmatics can be explained by an increased sensitivity of the parasympathetic nervous system since acute attacks of asthma cannot be completely reversed by the anticholinergic agent, atropine. The beta-adrenergic nervous system contributes to the maintenance of resting airway tone by producing a bronchodilator effect. It has been long considered that should this bronchodilator effect be reduced, a cholinergic bronchoconstriction could result. This may be seen clinically in some asthmatic patients who receive beta-adrenergic blocking agents such as propranolol for control of angina or hypertension. These blocking agents inhibit the adrenergic system and can cause severe bronchoconstriction to occur in asthmatics. The beta-adrenergic receptor, adenylate cyclase, is found in the cell membrane of numerous cells within the body, including airway smooth muscle and mast cells. Activation of this enzyme promotes the generation of cyclic AMP, which is known to relax airway smooth muscle and to inhibit the generation and release of the chemical mediators of inflammation from mast cells. A blockade or dysfunction of the adrenergic receptor could allow for mediator generation to occur in greater than normal amounts, and this could contribute to the generation of bronchoconstriction. This dysfunction of the adrenergic receptor has been embodied in the "partial beta-blockade" theory of asthma.

Pathophysiological Alterations in Asthma

Since airway obstruction is reversible in asthma, tests of airway function may be entirely within normal limits during symptom-free periods. During symptomatic intervals, the airflow obstruction may be documented by a wide variety of physiological measurements, which were outlined in Chapter 2 and will be reviewed below in relation to asthma.

Airflow Obstruction

The resistance to airflow within the lung (RL) is comprised of a component reflecting the frictional resistance between airflow and the wall of a conducting airway termed the resistance of the airways (Raw) plus a component reflecting the viscosity of the lung parenchyma, the resistance of the tissues to airflow (RTISS). As little parenchymal involvement of the lung is seen in uncomplicated asthma, the elastic properties of the lung are not altered greatly from normal and, therefore, do not contribute significantly to alterations in airflow parameters in the asthmatic patient. Measurements of airway resistance, Raw, can be readily obtained with the use of a body plethysmograph. Such measurements are obtained at low flow rates at or near end-expiration (i.e., at or near functional residual capacity, FRC). As FRC is the normal static or resting position of the lung, Raw at FRC gives an approximation of the resting tone or diameter of the airways. Resistance varies inversely as the 4th power of the radius of the airway, so that any decrease in the airway radius produces a profound increase in resistance to airflow in the affected airway. In addition, Raw is profoundly altered by changes in the radius of the large conducting airways and is relatively unaffected by changes in the radius of small peripheral airways, unless such changes are massive in extent. During the course of an acute asthmatic attack, the Raw can be expected to be increased in all patients with changes as much as 600% above the expected normal values for any patient. The use of the body plethysmograph to obtain this measurement however precludes its use except under special circumstances and has resulted in the use of simpler, although more indirect, assessment of airway function in the asthmatic patient.

One such approach is to assess the patient's ventilatory capacity during a forced maximal expiration. From this maneuver can be obtained the forced vital capacity (FVC), the forced expiratory volume in 1 second ($FEV_{1.0}$), the maximal expiratory flow rate (MEFR), the maximal midexpiratory flow rate (MMEF), and the $FEV_{1.0}$/FVC ratio. During an acute attack of asthma, the spirogram will characteristically show a prolonged forced expiratory time, a reduced FVC, and a marked reduction in the various flow parameters listed above. These features may be seen in Figure 8.5, which contrasts the spiro-

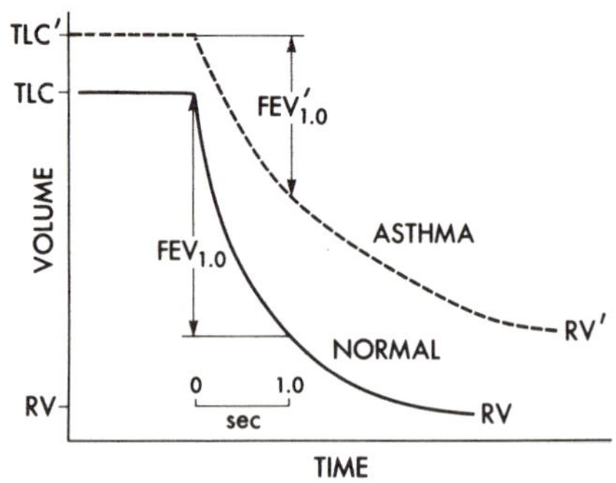

Figure 8.5. Change in forced expiratory volume in one second ($FEV_{1.0}$) in acute asthma. Solid line indicates normal tracing and the dashed line the reduction in $FEV_{1.0}$ and the prolongation of the forced vital capacity (FVC) in the asthmatic patient.

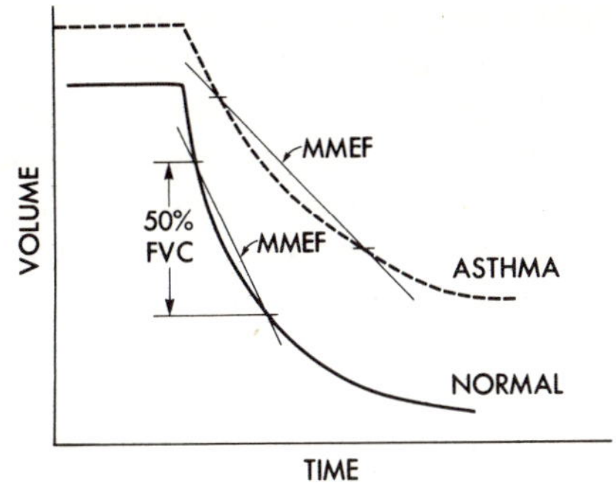

Figure 8.6. Maximum midexpiratory flow rate (MMEF) change in acute asthma. Solid line indicates the normal study with the dashed line representing the type of result seen in the asthmatic patient.

gram of a normal person with that of an asthmatic during an acute attack. The spirogram obtained from the asthmatic differs in several important aspects from the normal spirogram. The asthmatic initiates the maneuver from a higher lung volume (TLC) and ends the maneuver at a higher volume (RV) than the normal person (see below). The indices of expiratory flow, $FEV_{1.0}$, illustrated in Figure 8.5, and MMEF, illustrated in Figure 8.6, are reduced, and the time required to complete the FVC is prolonged.

Some of the measurements for assessing the degree of airway obstruction during the development of an acute asthmatic attack are more sensitive than others. The MMEF shows the most severe fall, followed by MEFR, $FEV_{1.0}$, and the FVC (Figure 8.7). As airway obstruction is reversed, either spontaneously or with treatment, the spirometric variables revert toward normal with the

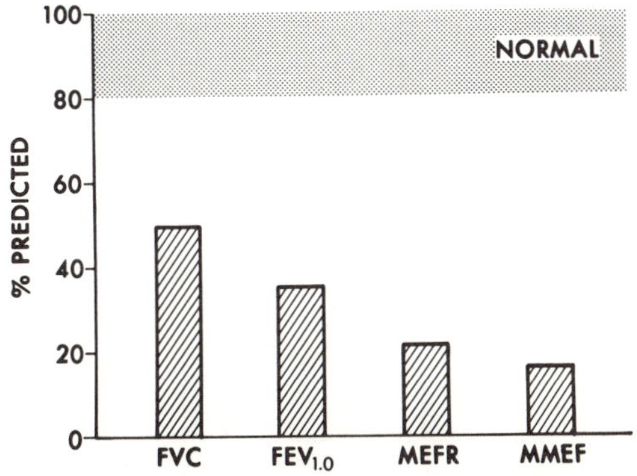

Figure 8.7. Alteration of spirometric variables during the acute attack of asthma in a patient. Spirometric variables are presented as a percentage of normal, with the bottom of the stippled area representing 80% of the predicted normal values.

most striking and earliest improvement noted for $FEV_{1.0}$, followed by MEFR and Raw. These tests parallel most closely alterations occurring within the larger conducting airways. The MMEF is relatively more sensitive to the effects of small airway narrowing. As this latter airflow parameter remains reduced for longer periods of time than the above spirometric parameters, it would appear that reversibility of airway involvement occurs first in the major airways, followed after some length of time by reversibility in the smaller peripheral airways. Indeed, although the $FEV_{1.0}$ may revert toward normal within hours of initiating treatment of an acute attack, the MMEF may show a persistence of flow limitation for up to 2 weeks after the onset of the acute episode.

Lung Volumes

The normal lung volumes and their determinants were discussed in Chapters 2 and 3. A wide spectrum of lung volume changes may be documented during an acute attack of asthma. It is common to see increases in residual volume (RV) and functional residual capacity (FRC). Total lung capacity (TLC) is more variable and may show a striking increase or little or no change in volume (Figure 8.8). At the present time it is not possible to predict the degree of increases in lung volumes in patients with acute exacerbations.

Several different mechanisms have been proposed to explain the increases in FRC and RV. As has been pointed out in Chapter 3, the FRC is determined by the balance of forces between the lung and the chest wall. At FRC, the normal tendency of the chest wall to retract outward is balanced by the normal tendency of the lung to retract inward. If the lung were to lose elastic recoil, the retractive forces causing the lung to collapse inward would be diminished. This would allow for a net increase in the retractive forces exerted outward. During the acute attack of asthma, elastic recoil of the lung has been documented to be reduced. This would be expected to result in an increase in

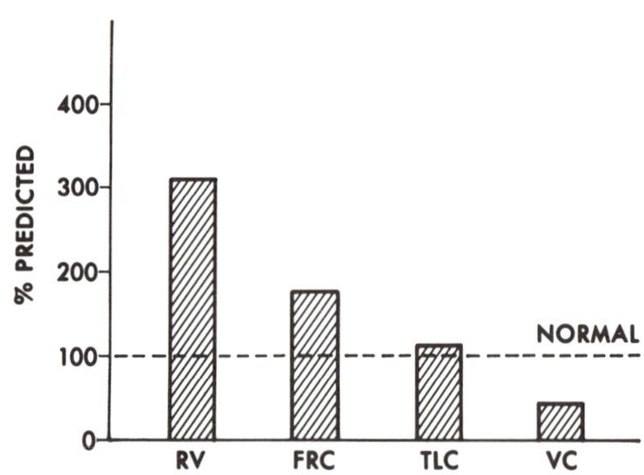

Figure 8.8. Alterations in subdivisions of lung volume during an acute attack of asthma in a patient. Volumes are expressed as a percentage of normal, with the dashed line indicating the predicted normal values for lung volumes.

alveolar size and FRC, since the balance of retractive forces between chest wall and lung increase outward to a more inspiratory position.

In addition to the above mechanism, it has been observed that pleural pressure during the acute attack remains more negative than would be expected during expiration. This indicates that inspiratory muscles such as the intercostal muscles and accessory muscles of respiration remain active even during the expiratory phase of respiration, which would tend to keep the lung inflated. This would increase FRC.

The increase in RV may be due in part to the loss in elastic recoil noted during the acute attack. In addition, however, premature closure of airways occurs secondary to mucosal swelling, mucous plug formation, and bronchiolar smooth muscle constriction. This premature closure results in an increased volume of air to be retained or trapped with each tidal breath, since airways close before complete emptying of alveoli occurs. An attempt to overcome such mechanical obstruction could occur as the asthmatic breathes at a higher lung volume, increasing FRC, which increases the retractive forces on airways and tends to keep them patent.

Abnormalities in Gas Exchange

The most commonly encountered blood gas alterations are hypoxemia with hypocapnea and a resulting respiratory alkalosis. The degree of hypoxemia will, in general, parallel the severity of the airway obstruction. The more severe the degree of obstruction, as assessed by the reduction in $FEV_{1.0}$, the more profound will be the degree of hypoxemia (Figure 8.9). The mechanism underlying the development of the hypoxemia is generally accepted as being due to ventilation-perfusion mismatching within the lung. The obstruction to airflow is nonuniformly distributed throughout the lung. Perfusion of the lungs may be altered and nonuniformly distributed throughout the lung due

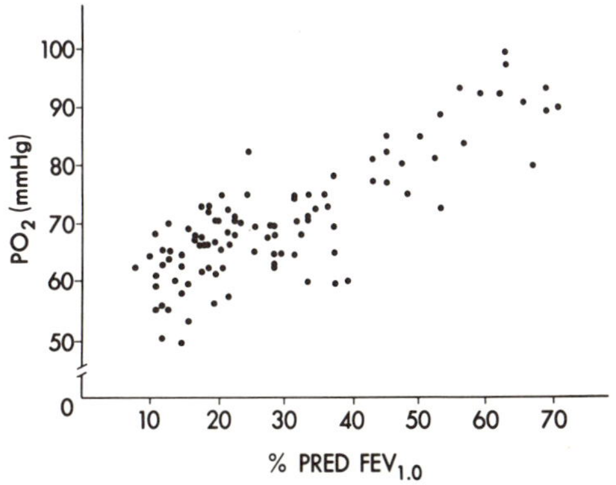

Figure 8.9. Relationship between $FEV_{1.0}$ and Pa_{O_2} during an acute attack of asthma. (Reprinted with permission, McFadden ER, Lyons H, Arterial blood gas tensions in asthma. *N Engl J Med* 278:1027, 1968).

to the presence of local hypoxic vasoconstriction or due to high intra-alveolar pressures. The resulting mismatching of ventilation and perfusion produces areas within the lung with low $\dot{V}/\dot{Q}$ ratios, and blood leaving such areas is poorly saturated with O_2, and this results in arterial hypoxemia.

During the early phase of an uncomplicated episode of asthma, patients will also present with hypocapnia caused by alveolar hyperventilation. This hypocapnia will be seen even in the face of severe airways obstruction. Alveolar hypoventilation with resulting hypercapnia only occurs when the $FEV_{1.0}$ falls below 20% of predicted for that person (see Figure 8.10).

The hyperventilation of these patients is mainly related to the activation of lung reflexes, which cause a rapid shallow breathing pattern (Chapter 6). The presence of normal alveolar ventilation indicated by normal Pa_{CO_2} is ominous. This indicates that the airflow obstruction is so severe that minute ventilation is insufficient to remove the produced CO_2 or that fatigue of the respiratory muscles is occurring. This may progress to the point of CO_2 retention, which indicates the patient is in grave danger.

PHARMACOLOGY OF ASTHMA

Receptors

Airway smooth muscle cells and mast cells have receptors on their surface. These interact with agonists, receptor stimulating hormones or chemicals, the "first messenger." In the case of airway smooth muscle, the interaction of agonist and receptor is the first in a series of events that results in either

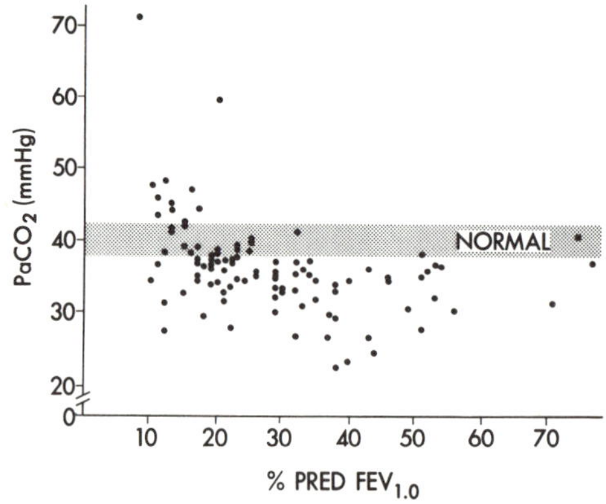

Figure 8.10. Relationship between $FEV_{1.0}$ and Pa_{CO_2} during an acute attack of asthma. (Reprinted with permission, McFadden ER, Lyons H, Arterial blood gas tensions in asthma. *N Engl J Med* 278:1027, 1968).

relaxation or contraction of smooth muscle. In the case of mast cells, agonist-receptor interaction may block the release of mediators.

After the first agonist-receptor interaction, a "second messenger" is believed to play a role. It is probably by changing the concentration of the "second messenger" in the cells that pharmacological agents have their effects on airway muscle tone. Cyclic nucleotides, cyclic AMP, and cyclic GMP are thought to be important "second messengers."

Airway smooth muscle cells have adrenergic receptors, cholinergic receptors, and receptors for histamine, serotonin, and other mediators.

Adrenergic Receptors

Airway smooth muscle cells have two types of adrenergic receptors, β_2 and α. β_2-Receptors are also found in other tissues. Stimulation of β_2-receptors on mast cells inhibits the release of mediators. Stimulation of these receptors on vascular smooth muscle causes vascular dilatation. β_2-Receptors are also found in skeletal muscle and in nervous tissue.

The β_2-receptor is the site of the enzyme *adenylate cyclase,* which when activated by agonist stimulation catalyzes the conversion of ATP to cyclic AMP. Intracellular accumulation of cyclic AMP causes airway smooth muscle relaxation by as yet unclear mechanisms. Some drugs, such as propranolol, can block the β_2-receptor and so can induce a reduction in cyclic AMP and thus cause bronchoconstriction.

Cyclic AMP is broken down by an enzyme, phosphodiesterase. Inhibition of this enzyme can thus increase intracellular cyclic AMP and cause smooth muscle relaxation (Figure 8.11).

α-Receptors are not as plentiful as β_2-receptors. α-Receptor stimulation causes only mild airway muscle contraction.

We will review the therapeutic agents changing intracellular cyclic AMP below.

Cholinergic Receptors

As mentioned above, efferent vagal fibers to airway smooth muscles play an important role in causing bronchoconstriction. The receptor is believed to be associated with the enzyme *guanylate cyclase,* which catalyzes a reaction that produces cyclic GMP. Intracellular accumulation of cyclic GMP produces an increase in smooth muscle tone. Anticholinergic drugs such as atropine and ipratropium can block the cholinergic receptors.

Glucocorticoids and Receptors

It has long been known that glucocorticoids are useful in the treatment of asthma. These agents do not appear to cause direct relaxation of airway smooth muscle; thus their effect is indirect. Their mechanism of action is not clear. There is some evidence that glucocorticoids increase the activity or the number of β-receptors and inhibit the cholinergic receptor. The first effect is

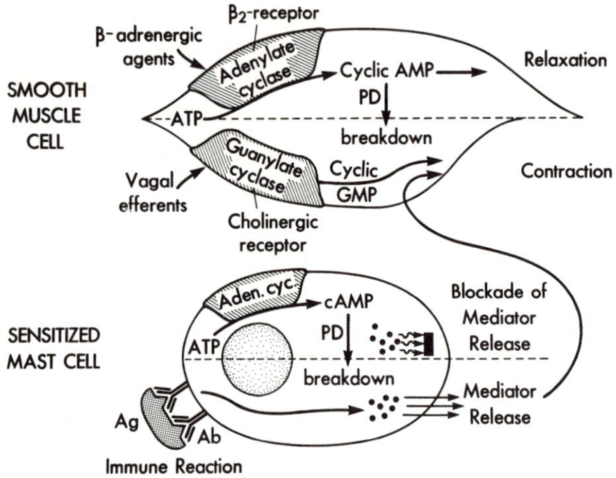

Figure 8.11. The role of receptors and cyclic nucleotides in relaxation and contraction of airway smooth muscle. β_2-Receptor stimulation in muscles and mast cells tends to relax smooth muscle. Cholinergic stimulation causes contraction. PD is the enzyme phosphodiesterase.

permissive making the muscle cells more responsive to β_2-agonists. The second could reduce cholinergic-mediated bronchoconstriction.

Therapeutic Agents

The important drugs most used in therapy of asthma are those that stimulate β_2-adrenergic receptors, those that inhibit phosphodiesterase, and glucocorticoids.

β_2-Receptor Agonists

Most agents that stimulate the β_2-receptor resemble the natural catecholamine epinephrine (adrenalin). Epinephrine, besides stimulating β_2-receptors, also stimulates β_1-receptors and α-receptors and so has widespread effects. This hormone is metabolized by an enzyme catechol-O-methyltransferase (COMT), which is found throughout the body. In addition, an enzyme, sulfatase, found in the gut inactivates this hormone.

Thus, as expected, epinephrine cannot be taken in pill form (inactivated by sulfatase), is short acting (inactivated by COMT), and has many side-effects (not a "pure" β_2-agonist). These problems with epinephrine have lead to "pharmaceutical manipulation" of the basic catecholamine structure in order to achieve the following aims: to make agents that are more specific (pure β_2-agonists), longer acting (not inactivated by COMT), and available in an oral form (not inactivated by sulfatase).

The side-effects of these drugs reflect the degree to which these drugs deviate from the ideal—that is, how much α-stimulation and β_1-stimulation also occur. On one extreme is epinephrine, which stimulates all adrenergic receptors (α, β_1, and β_2), and at the other extreme is salbutamol, which is at present the closest we have to a pure β_2-agonist.

When an agent has α-stimulant properties, it can cause slowing of the heart and an increase in blood pressure. When an agent has β_1-stimulant properties, it can increase the heart rate, make the heart irritable, and cause arrhythmias. β_2-Receptors are also found in the skeletal muscle and the central nervous system and so tremulousness and CNS excitation can occur. In addition, these agents are vascular dilators and can reduce pulmonary vasoconstriction. This can cause hypoxemia by increasing perfusion of low $\dot{V}/\dot{Q}$ lung units (see Chapter 9).

These drugs can be injected, inhaled, or swallowed depending on chemical structure. In general, when used as an aerosol a much smaller dose is used and bronchodilation is achieved with fewer side-effects than when used orally or by injection. Because of the deposition of some of the agent right on smooth muscle, aerosol inhalation causes rapid relaxation, often within 30 seconds.

Literally dozens of β-receptor agonists are available throughout the world. We will briefly mention some of the ones more widely used. Salbutamol and fenoterol are awaiting introduction in the U.S.A.

Epinephrine (*adrenaline*), as mentioned above, is a short acting agent that stimulates all adrenergic receptors.

Isoproterenol (*isoprenaline*) has marked β_1 and β_2 effects and no α effects. Its duration of action is very short, about a half hour. Because these two agents are so powerful and have so many side-effects, they are being supplanted in most outpatient treatment by "purer" β_2-agonists.

Isoetharine has a longer duration of action (3 to 4 hours) than the above agents. Although a "purer" β_2-agent, isoetharine does have some β_1-stimulant properties.

Metaproteronol is not degraded by COMT or sulfatase and so can be used orally and has a long duration of action (about 5 hours). This agent has both β_1-stimulant and β_2-stimulant properties.

Terbutaline is a powerful β_2-agonist, which may have side-effects related to the fact that it is also a powerful vasodilator and may thus reduce blood pressure. Side-effects are reduced when an aerosol form is used.

Salbutamol is at present the most potent and "purest" β_2-agonist, which is widely used clinically and has the fewest side-effects. It has almost no effect on the cardiovascular system. This agent is not deactivated by COMT or sulfatase and so can be used orally and has a long duration of action. It can be administered by aerosol, tablet, or injection.

Fenoterol is an agent that has properties very similar to salbutamol and may have a longer duration of action.

Phosphodiesterase Inhibitors

Cyclic AMP is broken down by an enzyme, phosphodiesterase; thus inhibition of this enzyme would increase cyclic AMP and lead to smooth muscle relaxation. The methylxanthines are agents that are clinically useful phosphodiesterase inhibitors. Theophylline is the most powerful smooth muscle relaxant of this family of drugs.

Although the effect on cyclic AMP is believed to be the way in which theophylline relieves bronchoconstriction, this may not be the whole answer. It is becoming clear that theophylline has other effects such as affecting calcium distribution, cyclic GMP, and prostaglandins.

Theophylline is available in a pure form or as loose complexes and salts. Aminophylline, the most widely used methylxanthine, is a mixture of 85% anhydrous theophylline and 15% ethylenediamine. Oxtriphylline is the choline salt of theophylline. Theophylline preparations can be used in tablet form; aminophylline can be injected intravenously.

The methylxanthines (which also include caffeine and theobromide) have many other effects besides bronchodilatation. They stimulate the central nervous system (including the respiratory center). They stimulate the heart. They reduce pulmonary arterial vasoconstriction. They are diuretic agents. These effects can be very desirable in treating respiratory failure. On the other hand, these agents can be highly toxic. This is because toxicity occurs at serum levels slightly above therapeutic levels. Toxic side-effects include nausea, vomiting, rapid heart rate, arrhythmias, reduction in cardiac output, and seizures. This last complication is caused by the CNS-stimulating effect.

Because these agents can be so toxic, blood levels are used to ensure that the correct dose is being used. The normal therapeutic range is 10 to 20 μg/ml of serum.

One of the reasons why toxicity is a problem is that the metabolism of methylxanthines is so variable. The normal serum half-life of theophylline is about 8 hours (range 3 to 9.5 hours) in adults. In children it is much shorter averaging 3.6 hours.

Theophylline is metabolized mainly by liver microsomal enzymes; thus when liver dysfunction is present the half-life is markedly prolonged and toxicity may occur. This occurs in primary liver disease and also when liver congestion due to right heart failure is present. The serum half-life of theophylline is reduced in cigarette smokers, perhaps because some chemical from cigarette smoke induces liver microsomal enzymes that enhances theophylline metabolism.

Glucocorticoids

Corticosteroids are classified into two general categories. Mineralocorticoids have their major effect on the kidney. Glucocorticoids have effects on many metabolic and inflammatory processes. Natural corticosteroids usually have both mineralocorticoid and glucocorticoid effects. Synthetic agents have been produced that have virtually pure glucocorticoid effects. Glucocorticoids are important drugs in the treatment of asthma, particularly when the β_2 or phosphodiesterase inhibitor bronchodilator cannot control the patient's disease.

Glucocorticoids are useful in asthma even when the bronchoconstriction is not caused by allergy. The mechanisms by which glucocorticoids ameliorate asthma are not well known, but two important classes of effects are probably involved: first, is the effect of these agents on the β_2-receptor, and second, are the effects of these agents on the inflammatory response.

Glucocorticoids potentiate the effect of β_2-agonists at the β_2-receptor site and, in addition, may inhibit both the α-receptor and the cholinergic receptor. These agents may also inhibit phosphodiesterase. All these effects can result in bronchodilation.

Glucocorticoids have a myriad of anti-inflammatory effects. Which effect(s) precisely is (are) the most important is not clear. Glucocorticoids stabilize lysosomal membranes, inhibit vasodilation at the site of inflammation, and reduce the numbers of eosinophils, mast cells, and lymphocytes. These agents also inhibit the formation, storage, and release of mediators including histamine, and in addition they may reduce the production of prostaglandin $F_2\ \alpha$. All these effects are potentially beneficial in asthma.

These drugs have many unwanted effects and when very large doses are used Cushing's syndrome is present. The patient develops truncal obesity, a "moon" face, and several skin problems including acne, striae, and easy bruising. In addition, patients develop muscular weakness, a metabolic alkalosis, high blood pressure, and osteoporosis. The effect on lymphocytes makes patients susceptible to infection (Chapter 15). In some patients the cure may be worse than the patient's asthma!

Since the complications of systemic steroid therapy are so severe, topical glucocorticoids that are inhaled directly into the lungs are now used. They are poorly absorbed, and so they have primarily a local effect in the lungs. Their use has resulted in many patients requiring much smaller doses of systemic glucocorticoids or none at all. The most widely used topical glucocorticoids are beclomethasone and triamcinolone.

The most widely used oral preparations are prednisolone and prednisone. The latter is converted into the former in the liver. The most widely used intravenous preparations are methylprednisolone and hydrocortisone.

The monograph by I. Ziment, listed in the references, is an excellent source for details concerning the use of all therapeutic agents in asthma.

Other Agents

Since the cholinergic nervous system can cause bronchoconstriction, by increasing cyclic GMP, anticholinergic agents can be used as bronchodilators. Inhaled anticholinergic agents are particularly useful in treating the bronchoconstriction that sometimes occurs in chronic bronchitis. This type of bronchoconstriction is in part initiated by irritant receptors and is mediated by vagal nerves. Atropine itself can be used by inhalation. Ipratropium has a longer duration of action than atropine and is widely used in Europe.

Finally, an agent has been developed that stabilizes mast cells, protecting them from the immune reactions that normally release mediators. The major use of cromolyn sodium is as a prophylactic agent when taken before allergen exposure or exercise. Why this agent should be effective in exercise-induced asthma is not known.

HYPERSENSITIVITY PNEUMONITIS

The inhalation of a wide variety of organic dusts may result in a distinctive group of interstitial lung diseases. These diseases may present in several forms. In the acute form, the person develops chills, fever, malaise, dyspnea, and cough within 2 to 8 hours following inhalational exposure to the offending antigen. Symptoms then resolve within 24 hours. In the chronic form of the illness, symptoms develop insidiously with fatigue, progressive dyspnea, and nonproductive cough. Both forms of this illness result in restrictive lung disease, since the pathological process involves the interstitium of the lung, alveoli, and the terminal airways. The way in which restrictive disorders disturb lung function are described in detail in Chapter 3. Here we will focus on the immune aspects.

Etiology and Immunopathogenesis

The organic substances capable of eliciting an immune reaction in the lung that results in a hypersensitivity pneumonitis (also called extrinsic allergic alveolitis) are continually increasing in number as new forms of this illness are recognized. Table 8.2 illustrates some of the more common causes of this illness, and it should be evident that a majority of these illnesses occur as part of an occupational exposure. It has been estimated that 3 to 15% of people exposed to the antigens listed in Table 8.2 will develop clinical disease when exposed to the antigen for an appropriate period of time. This period of sensitization of the person involves the inhalation of the antigen into the lung and the processing of the antigen by local immune tissue as outlined in the beginning of this chapter. This sensitization procedure initially involves the humoral immune system, since people produce precipitating antibody of the IgG and IgM classes against the antigen. Following sensitization, repeated exposure to the antigen results in the production of circulating antigen-antibody (immune) complexes. With the fixation of these immune complexes to mast cells and other submucosal cells, the complement cascade is activated and an inflammatory reaction is produced within the interstitium of the lung. In addition to activation of the classic complement pathway, some antigenic substances can activate the alternate pathway of complement activation, which

Table 8.2. Some Causes of Hypersensitivity Pneumonitis

Disease	*Etiological Agent*	*Source*
Farmer's lung	*Micropolyspora faeni* Thermophilic actinomycetes	Moldy hay
Bird-breeder's disease Poultry-worker's lung	Serum proteins of birds	Bird excreta
Bagassosis	*Thermoactinomycetes sacchari*	Sugar cane stalks
Humidifier lung	*Thermoactinomycetes vulgaris* *Thermoactinomycetes candidus*	Humidifiers Air conditioners
Mushroom-worker's lung	*Micropolyspora faeni* *Thermoactinomycetes vulgaris*	Mushroom compost
Maple-bark-stripper disease	*Cryptostroma corticale*	Maple tree bark
Cheese-washer's disease	*Penicillium caseii*	Moldy cheese
Sequiosis	*Aureobasidium rullulans*	Moldy Redwood sawdust

can act to amplify the inflammatory process. The resulting inflammatory response constitutes type III hypersensitivity or immune complex disease of the lung.

The majority of people with hypersensitivity pneumonitis have circulating antibody of the IgG class in their serum, which is specific for the offending antigen. This antibody will react with the specific antigen in agar to form a visible precipitin band and is called the *serum precipitin.* However, as many as 50% of asymptomatic people exposed to potentially sensitizing antigens also have precipitating antibody in their serum, which indicates that other host factors are necessary for the development of the clinical illness. It is perhaps most useful to consider the presence of the serum precipitin as indicating exposure to the antigen and as a contributor to the development of clinical illness in a susceptible person. Recently, it has been appreciated that cell-mediated immunity to organic dust antigens may also contribute to the pathogenesis of hypersensitivity pneumonitis. People with clinical disease can be demonstrated to have activated T-lymphocytes in their serum, which undergo blast transformation when exposed to antigen in vitro. The T-lymphocytes release several lymphokines such as migration inhibition factor (MIF) and macrophage activation factor (MAF), which potentiates immune reactions occurring within the lung. Exposed but asymptomatic people do not, as a rule, demonstrate any such cell-mediated immunity. Although it is not entirely clear at present how immune mechanisms operate to produce this illness, it appears that a combination of humoral immunity (type III reactions) and cell-mediated immunity (type IV reactions) occur in a susceptible person to produce hypersensitivity pneumonitis.

Pathology

The pathological changes in hypersensitivity pneumonitis are determined largely by the duration and intensity of exposure to the antigen and the immune reactivity of the patient. Lung biopsy specimens demonstrate small nodules throughout the lung parenchyma. These nodules consist of proliferating alveolar epithelial cells, prominent numbers of lymphocytes, plasma cells, and polymorphonuclear cells. There is also a prominent mononuclear cell infiltration with multinuclear giant cells. Inflammation involving the terminal bronchioles, bronchiolitis, may also occur. Immunoglobulin or complement deposits are not seen within the lesions, presumably because activated macrophages ingest immune complexes, complement and other cellular debris at the site of inflammation. Lung biopsy specimens obtained from people with the more insidious onset and chronic form of the illness tend to demonstrate a more marked granulomatous reaction within the lung parenchyma and a marked degree of fibrosis. Severe bronchiolitis obliterans may also be seen in the biopsy specimens.

Clinical Features

The development of symptoms in the patient with hypersensitivity pneumonitis depends on several factors: the characteristics, particle size, and antigenicity of the inhaled dust; the intensity, frequency, and duration of exposure; and the type and intensity of the immune response exhibited by the exposed patient. The manifestations of the illness tend to be the same for all the different forms of dust exposure and may present in an acute or chronic form of illness.

In the acute form, symptoms occur 4 to 6 hours following each exposure and consist of nonproductive cough, dyspnea, fever or chills, and malaise. The symptoms resolve spontaneously over a period of several hours and rarely persist for longer than 24 hours. Examination of the patient will reveal tachypnea and fine inspiratory bibasilar crackles. Laboratory examinations demonstrate a leukocytosis, arterial hypoxemia, and precipitating antibody against the offending antigen. The chest x-ray examination may be normal but often will show a nodular infiltrate involving predominantly the lower lobes. During the acute phase, pulmonary function tests will demonstrate a restrictive disorder—a decrease in forced vital capacity and forced expiratory volume in 1 second with an unchanged $FEV_{1.0}/FVC$ ratio. In addition, in keeping with the restrictive pattern of lung function involvement, the compliance of the lungs will be decreased and the diffusing capacity reduced.

The above pulmonary function abnormalities as well as many of the clinical features of the illness can be documented in the laboratory by subjecting the patient to a controlled inhalation challenge with the offending antigen. Such a

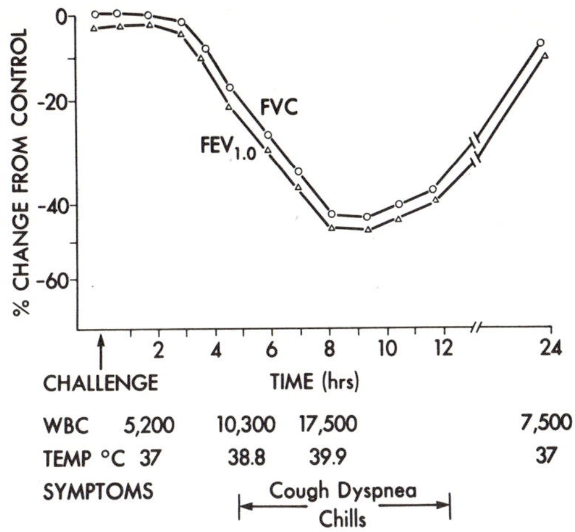

Figure 8.12. Graphic representation of the late onset reaction following inhalation challenge with antigen in a person with hypersensitivity pneumonitis. There occurs after 4 to 8 hours a fall in $FEV_{1.0}$, FVC, an increase in white cell count and body temperature, and an onset of symptoms that resolve by 24 hours.

procedure can be seen in Figure 8.12. At approximately 4 hours after the completion of the inhalation challenge, the $FEV_{1.0}$ and FVC begin to fall and reach a maximal fall at 8 hours. Simultaneously, the white cell count and body temperature increase to a maximum at 8 hours. At this point, the patient may develop chills and complain of general malaise. The $FEV_{1.0}$ and FVC, white cell count, and temperature return to normal by 24 hours and symptoms resolve.

In some forms of hypersensitivity pneumonitis such as pigeon-breeder's lung, a second form of response may be documented. Inhalation challenge with pigeon serum proteins in this illness may evoke an immediate-type response with an early fall in $FEV_{1.0}$ and FVC, which then revert to normal within 1 hour. These people will then develop the classic delayed response as already outlined (Figure 8.13). This immediate response as well as an immediate-type skin reaction in these patients is mediated by an IgE antibody specific for the antigen present, for example, pigeon serum protein.

In the chronic form of this illness, repeated exposure to antigen results in an insidious progression of cough, dyspnea, weakness, and weight loss. Serum precipitins will be present in only 50% of such patients, despite histories of adequate exposure to known antigenic dusts. In the chronic form of illness, fibrotic processes are the major pathological feature and this is reflected in the chest roentgenogram as linear fibrotic scarring with little evidence of nodule formation as is seen in the acute form of the illness. Pulmonary function testing reveals a primarily restrictive pattern because of the bronchiolitis; however, a reduction in flow rates may be seen. Hypoxemia is variable in this illness when measured at rest, but with exercise testing a fall in arterial oxygen saturation can be readily demonstrated in the majority of these patients.

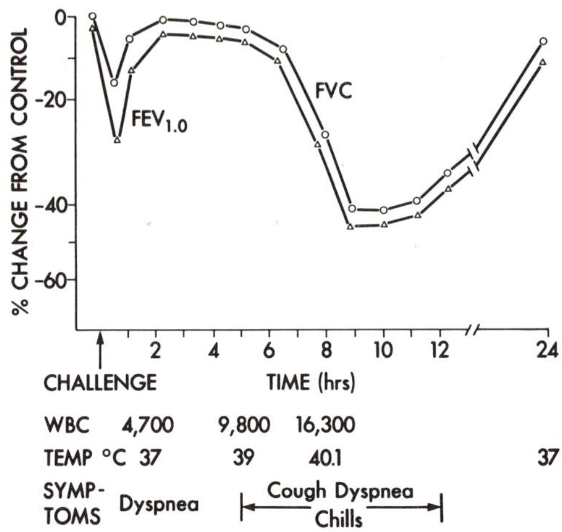

Figure 8.13. Graphic representation of a dual reaction demonstrating an early (at one hour) fall in $FEV_{1.0}$ with recovery to normal. This is followed by a late reaction at 4 to 8 hours with a fall in $FEV_{1.0}$, FVC, an increase in white cell count and body temperature, and an onset of symptoms. Complete resolution occurs by 24 hours.

Treatment

The most important aspect of treatment for patients with hypersensitivity pneumonitis is the identification of the offending antigen and the avoidance of the exposure and reinhalation of the antigen. Avoidance of exposure may entail total physical avoidance of sites known to contain the antigen, providing adequate ventilation systems and filter systems to remove airborne antigens, or the wearing of masks with adequate filters to remove particulate antigens.

The use of pharmacological agents in this illness is largely restricted to the use of glucocorticoids in those people with documented abnormalities in diffusing capacity. These agents will often reverse the abnormality in diffusing capacity as well as relieve the symptoms in the acute form of the illness. Results in the chronic form are not as striking presumably due to the presence of established fibrosis in the lung. Short trials of glucocorticoids may be used in these people with an attempt to improve the diffusing capacity, but they are discontinued once the diffusing capacity improves or is demonstrated not to be altered by this treatment.

BIBLIOGRAPHY

Boushey HA, Holtzman MJ, Sheller JR, et al: Bronchial Hyperreactivity. *Amer Rev Resp Disease* 121:389, 1980.

Fink JN: Hypersensitivity Pneumonitis, in Middleton E (ed): *Allergy: Principles and Practice.* St Louis, CV Mosby Company, 1979, p 855.

Plaut M, Lichtenstein LM: Cellular and Chemical Basis of the Allergic Inflammatory Response: Component Parts and Control Mechanisms, in Middleton E (ed): *Allergy: Principles and Practice.* St Louis, CV Mosby Company, 1979, p 115.

Roberts RC, Moore VL: Immunopathogenesis of Hypersensitivity Pneumonitis. *Amer Rev Resp Disease* 116:1075, 1977.

Weiss EB, Segal MS: *Bronchial Asthma: Principles and Practice,* Boston, Little Brown and Company, 1977.

Ziment I: *Respiratory Pharmacology and Therapeutics.* Philadelphia, WB Saunders, 1978.

9

Respiratory Failure 1: Oxygen

Meir H. Kryger

THE SEQUELAE OF HYPOXEMIA
Compensatory Responses to Hypoxemia
  Respiratory
  Cardiovascular
  Hematopoietic
Nervous System Dysfunction with Hypoxemia

The major function of the lung is to transfer oxygen from alveolar gas to blood and to transfer carbon dioxide from blood to alveolar gas. The purpose of gas exchange is to maintain arterial blood Po_2 and Pco_2 within certain limits. Many physiological mechanisms can disturb gas exchange and cause respiratory failure. Failure of the respiratory system is present when there occurs either failure to oxygenate the blood or failure to excrete carbon dioxide.

Why Cells Require Oxygen

For cells to be alive and function properly, they must have energy. Energy is required for generation of heat, mechanical work (as in muscle contraction), active transport against osmotic or ion gradients, nerve conduction, and synthesis of new molecules. Cells obtain energy from foodstuffs. The energy contained in covalent bonds of carbohydrates, lipids, and proteins can be liberated by combustion with oxygen (oxidative phosphorylation) and transformed into the high energy phosphate bonds of adenosine triphosphate (ATP). Although ATP can be produced by degradation of foodstuffs in reactions not requiring oxygen (anaerobic metabolism), the most efficient production of ATP occurs when oxygen does participate in the reactions (aerobic metabolism). In fact, when glucose is the substrate, 19 times more energy is produced by aerobic than anaerobic metabolism (Figure 9.1). The aerobic reactions occur in the mitochondria of cells. The Po_2 in mitochondria is quite low, and oxidative phosphorylation will continue when the mitochondrial Po_2 is as low as 1 to 2 mmHg. When mitochondrial Po_2 is reduced below

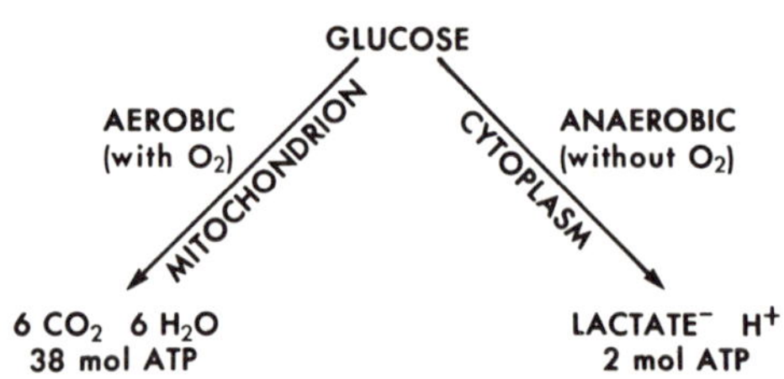

Figure 9.1. Aerobic metabolism generates 19 times as many high energy phosphate bonds as anaerobic metabolism when glucose is the substrate.

SENSITIVITY TO OXYGEN DEPRIVATION

NEURAL TISSUE CARDIAC MUSCLE KIDNEY SKELETAL MUSCLE	↓ DECREASING SENSITIVITY

Figure 9.2. Neural tissue dysfunctions rapidly when hypoxic; thus neurological symptoms are common with hypoxemia.

this level, anaerobic metabolism, which occurs in the cytoplasm, commences. Mitochondrial Po_2 is low because of continuous oxygen consumption. The Po_2 of blood is much higher than the Po_2 in the mitochondrion. Since the rate of diffusion of gases increases with an increased pressure gradient, the large blood-mitochondrion gradient for O_2 is advantageous, because oxygen must diffuse from the blood to mitochondria, a pathway that traverses interstitial space, cell membranes, and cytoplasm.

The survival of cells deprived of oxygen depends on the metabolic activity of the cells and the store of oxygen available to the cells. Cells with high metabolic rates, neural cells and contracting cardiac cells, cease to function rapidly after cessation of O_2 delivery (Figure 9.2). The brain is particularly vulnerable, because when anaerobic metabolism commences in neural cells, there is a rapid accumulation of H^+ and lactate ions due to the relative impermeability of the blood-brain barrier to charged particles. In contrast, when anaerobic metabolism occurs in other tissues, lactate$^-$ and H^+ can leave the cells.

Survival of hypoxic cells is prolonged when their metabolic rate is reduced. Hypothermia and anesthesia can lower the metabolic rate and thus lower the oxygen requirements of neural cells. A noncontracting heart, as in open heart surgery, requires one eighth the oxygen of a contracting heart. Resting skeletal muscle has a very low metabolic rate and may survive up to 6 hours of oxygen lack.

Oxygen lack in the tissues is called hypoxia. As discussed below, tissue hypoxia can be caused by a reduction in oxygen content of the blood, a reduction in the quantity of blood delivered to the tissues, impaired transfer of oxygen from blood to tissues, or impaired utilization of oxygen.

OXYGEN TRANSPORT

The main task of the lungs and cardiovascular system is to take oxygen from the air around us and to deliver it to metabolizing tissue, while excreting CO_2 (Figure 9.3). The process of transporting gas requires energy at each step. The first step is to initiate bulk flow of air into the lungs. This requires the respiratory muscles. Oxygen then *diffuses* from alveoli to blood, a process that depends on the kinetic energy of the O_2 molecules. Blood is then transported

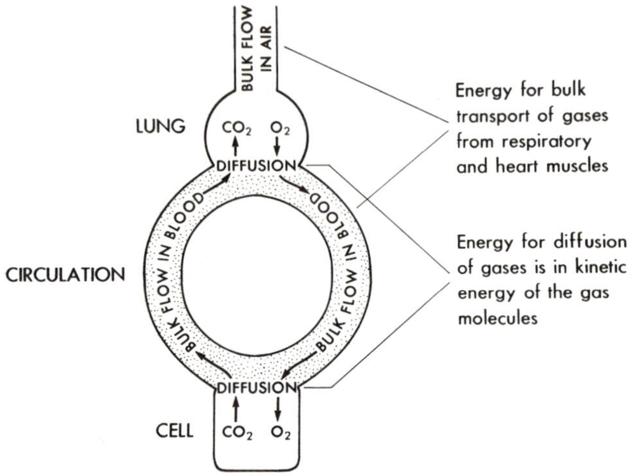

Figure 9.3. The transport of gases requires energy. The respiratory and cardiac muscles supply the energy for bulk transport, while the kinetic energy of molecules themselves supply the energy for diffusion.

by bulk flow to the tissues; this step requires cardiac muscle. Oxygen then diffuses to mitochondria. This final step also depends on the kinetic energy of the O_2 molecules. In summary, bulk transport of O_2 requires cardiac and respiratory muscle, while transport by diffusion depends on the kinetic energy of the molecules themselves. A measure of the kinetic energy of the molecules is the pressure of the gas.

A gas tends to fill completely any available space and is made up of molecules, which continually move about in all directions. Because of this continual motion, the molecules will collide with each other and the walls of the space. The collisions of the molecules on the walls cause the *pressure* exerted by the gas. In a sense, the pressure of a gas is an index of the tendency of its molecules to move. The molecules will tend to move from a region of high pressure to low pressure.

The *partial pressure* of each gas in a gas mixture is the pressure the gas would exert if it alone occupied the whole volume. The total pressure of a mixture of gases equals the total of the partial pressures of the individual gases. The total pressure of air at sea level is 760 mmHg and can be considered to contain nitrogen at a partial pressure (P_{N_2}) of about 600 mmHg and oxygen at a partial pressure (P_{O_2}) of about 160 mmHg.

In the gas phase, the partial pressure of a gas is proportional to the fractional concentration of the gas (e.g., $F_{I_{O_2}} = .21$ for air), which is then proportional to the volume of the gas. In other words, in the gas phase P_{O_2}, $F_{I_{O_2}}$, and volume of O_2 are *linearly related* to each other.

If a liquid such as blood were exposed to air, gases would diffuse into the liquid and from the liquid according to their own partial pressure gradients, until the partial pressure of each of the gases is the same in air and in the liquid (equilibrium). The quantity of gas *dissolved* in a liquid is proportional to the partial pressure of the gas in equilibrium with the solution.

Besides being dissolved in fluid, oxygen is transported by a specific carrier (hemoglobin). This carrier system may be saturated; once the carrier sites are filled no further oxygen can be carried by hemoglobin. Thus, the relationship between Po_2 and volume of O_2 in blood is *not linear.* Above a certain Po_2, increasing Po_2 has little effect on increasing the volume of O_2 in blood. As will be discussed in the next chapter, this is in sharp contrast to the situation of CO_2 transport; CO_2 does not "saturate" its transport system so that the volume of CO_2 in blood is linearly related to the Pco_2.

Oxygen is physically dissolved in plasma but is not very soluble in plasma (.003 ml O_2 being dissolved in 100 ml plasma/mmHg Po_2), and even at high Po_2 the quantity of oxygen dissolved is small. Hemoglobin, on the other hand, combines reversibly with a much greater quantity of oxygen. Each gram of hemoglobin is capable of combining with 1.34 ml oxygen.

The relationship between Po_2 and percent saturation of hemoglobin with O_2 (So_2) is sigmoid shaped (Figure 9.4). Above Po_2 60 mmHg, the curve is flat, and large changes in Po_2 result in small changes in So_2. Below Po_2 40 mmHg, the steep portion of the curve, small changes in Po_2 result in large changes in So_2. The oxyhemoglobin dissociation curve may be displaced to the right or to the left. One measure of the position of the curve is the Po_2 when the So_2 is 50%. This variable is called P_{50} and is usually about 27 mmHg.

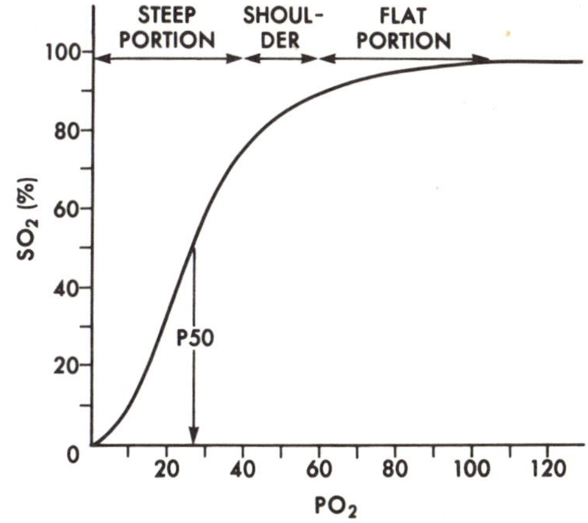

Figure 9.4. The oxygen-hemoglobin dissociation curve. When Po_2 exceeds 60 mmHg, the oxygen saturation increases little with changes in Po_2. Below Po_2 40 mmHg, a small fall in Po_2 results in a large fall in So_2. P_{50} is the Po_2 at which the So_2 is 50%. Po_2 is in mmHg.

Hemoglobin-Oxygen Affinity. Many factors can change the configuration of the hemoglobin molecule. This will change the ease with which oxygen can be bound and thus alter the affinity of hemoglobin for oxygen.

A *right shift* of the oxyhemoglobin dissociation curve (a higher P_{50}) indicates *reduced affinity* of hemoglobin for oxygen. This is because at a given Po_2 the hemoglobin is less saturated with oxygen. An increase in temperature, Pco_2, and H^+ concentration will all change the configuration of the hemoglobin molecule and reduce affinity for O_2.

2,3 Diphosphoglycerate, abbreviated 2,3 DPG, is produced in red blood cells in a side reaction of the main glycolytic pathway. 2,3 DPG production is increased when tissue hypoxia is present. Anemia and cyanotic heart disease are both associated with increased 2,3 DPG production. An increase in 2,3 DPG reduces hemoglobin-oxygen affinity, shifting the dissociation curve to the right (Figure 9.5). Acidosis (which itself reduces affinity) decreases 2,3 DPG concentration, which tends to offset the primary curve shifting effect of acidosis. 2,3 DPG is markedly reduced in stored blood bank blood. Changes in temperature and $[H^+]$ cause much larger shifts in oxyhemoglobin dissociation than changes in 2,3 DPG. Thus, 2,3 DPG may not play as important a role in oxygen transport as previously thought.

As will be discussed below, a right-shifted curve with reduced hemoglobin-oxygen affinity facilitates unloading of oxygen in the tissues.

Increased affinity of hemoglobin for oxygen occurs when the oxyhemoglobin dissociation curve is *left shifted*. This results in a *lower* P_{50}. Hypothermia, alkalemia, hypocapnia, and reduced levels of 2,3 DPG will all increase oxygen-hemoglobin affinity. Fetal hemoglobin also has increased affinity for oxygen. Carbon monoxide, besides displacing O_2 from hemoglobin (the affinity of

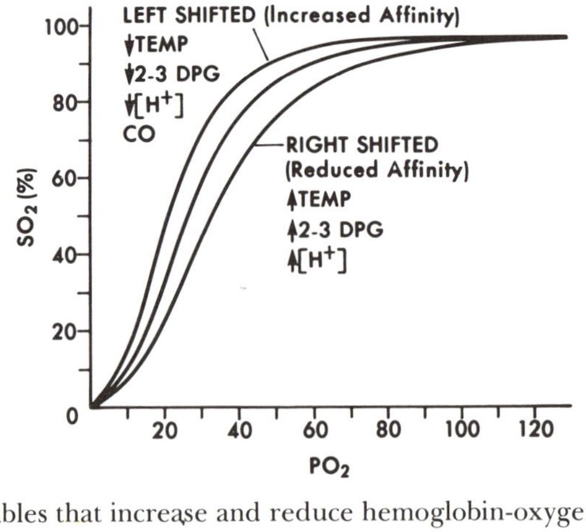

Figure 9.5. Variables that increase and reduce hemoglobin-oxygen affinity. Po_2 is in mmHg.

hemoglobin for carbon monoxide is 300 times greater than for oxygen) also markedly shifts the oxyhemoglobin dissociation curve to the left. A left-shifted curve facilitates loading of oxygen in the lungs but may interfere with O_2 unloading in the tissues.

Oxygen Delivery

The amount of oxygen delivered to the tissues depends on the quantity of blood delivered to the tissue (cardiac output) and the quantity of oxygen present in the blood (arterial oxygen content).

$$\text{Oxygen delivered} = \text{cardiac output} \times \text{arterial } O_2 \text{ content} \qquad \textbf{(1)}$$

One gram of hemoglobin when fully saturated with oxygen can combine with 1.34 ml O_2. Oxygen saturation is *actual* O_2 content divided by the maximal potential O_2 content, the oxygen-carrying capacity. Oxygen saturation is expressed as a percentage; when 100 ml blood contains 20 ml of oxygen and can only bind 20 ml, the oxygen saturation is 100%; if this 100 ml blood contains 15 ml oxygen, the oxygen saturation is 75%.

$$\text{Arterial oxygen content} = [(\text{hemoglobin concentration}) \times (1.34) \times (\text{arterial } O_2 \text{ saturation})] + (O_2 \text{ dissolved in plasma}) \qquad \textbf{(2)}$$

The O_2 dissolved in plasma ($.003 \times Po_2$) is small and in most instances can be ignored. Thus:

$$\text{Oxygen delivery} = (\text{cardiac output}) \times (\text{hemoglobin concentration}) \times (1.34) \times (\text{arterial } O_2 \text{ saturation}) \qquad \textbf{(3)}$$

Hypoxia can be caused by a reduction in one component (cardiac output, hemoglobin concentration, or So_2) of the O_2 delivery system. This last, very important equation also tells us that when one component of the oxygen delivery system is reduced, increase in the other components can restore oxygen delivery to normal. For example, if hemoglobin were reduced by half, doubling of the cardiac output restores oxygen delivery. On the other hand, if each of the components were reduced, the results could be catastrophic. For example, suppose there occurred a 20% reduction each in cardiac output, hemoglobin concentration, and So_2. Oxygen delivery would now be $.8 \times .8 \times .8 = .51$ or 51% of what it had been.

Under normal circumstances, not all the oxygen delivered to tissues is utilized. Usually only about 25% of delivered oxygen is used, so that blood returning to the right heart (mixed venous blood) will contain 25% less oxygen than blood going to the tissues (arterial blood). When oxygen delivery is reduced, the tissues can extract more oxygen from a given volume of blood and this will reduce the *mixed venous oxygen content* ($C\bar{v}_{O_2}$).

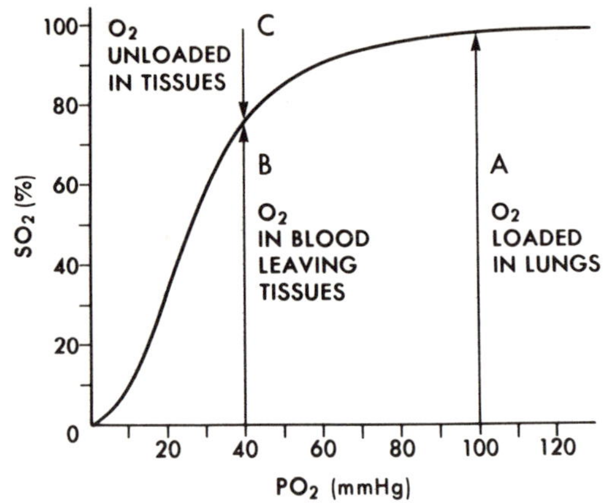

Figure 9.6. Oxygen loading of hemoglobin occurs at the high Po_2 of alveoli (A). Blood leaving tissues has a Po_2 of venous blood (B), thus the amount that has been unloaded in tissues equals C, which is A minus B.

Is It Better to Have Increased or Decreased Hemoblogin Affinity for Oxygen?

Oxygen loading of hemoglobin in the lung occurs when Po_2 is 90 to 100 mmHg and, therefore, occurs at the upper flat end of the oxyhemoglobin dissociation curve (Figure 9.6). At a Po_2 of 100 mmHg, there is little difference between the oxygen saturation (or the amount of O_2 loaded) of the blood with increased or decreased affinity.

Now consider the situation when loading must occur when the PA_{O_2} is low (Figure 9.7), as in the fetus, which must load oxygen onto its hemoglobin in the placenta, where the Po_2 is about 40 mmHg, and in a person at high altitude at 17,000 ft (5.2 km), where the alveolar Po_2 will be about 40 mmHg. In these situations, a left-shifted curve markedly increases Sa_{O_2} at Po_2 40 mmHg and, thus, increases oxygen loading. Indeed animals best suited to life in hypoxic environments (like the llama) have very left-shifted dissociation curves. Thus, increased oxygen-hemoglobin affinity is very advantageous when oxygen loading must occur when Po_2 is low.

Oxygen unloading occurs at the lower end of the oxyhemoglobin dissociation curve (Figure 9.8). The Po_2 of the tissues is usually about 40 mmHg. Blood leaving the tissues will have equilibrated with tissue Po_2 and will thus have a Po_2 of 40 mmHg. This is an important concept to remember; blood leaving the tissues will have a Po_2 of about 40 mmHg. If the blood leaving the tissues at Po_2 40 mmHg has increased affinity for oxygen, then the blood will have a higher So_2; therefore, less oxygen will have been unloaded. On the other hand, if affinity for oxygen is reduced, the blood leaving the tissues will have a lower So_2; therefore more oxygen will have been unloaded. Thus, reduced oxyhemoglobin affinity facilitates unloading of oxygen in the tissues. When

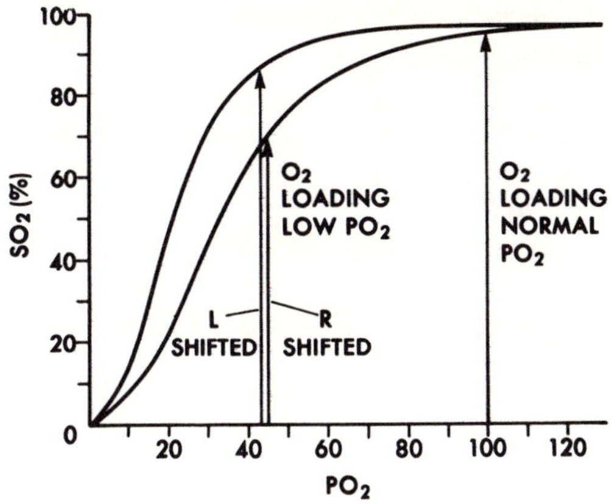

Figure 9.7. O_2 loading under normal circumstances occurs at a high alveolar Po_2, and it makes little difference if the oxyhemoglobin dissociation curve is right or left-shifted. If oxygen loading occurs when Po_2 is low (as in the fetus or at high altitude), a left-shifted curve (L) is advantageous.

there is increased hemoglobin-oxygen affinity, as in the llama or the fetus, tissue Po_2 is usually low, which helps to unload O_2.

Carbon monoxide both displaces oxygen from hemoglobin, reducing the available hemoglobin to combine with oxygen (a physiological "anemia"), and shifts the oxyhemoglobin dissociation curve to the left. This markedly impairs unloading of oxygen to the tissues even at low tissue Po_2. During exercise when tissue Po_2 may reach 20 mmHg, hemoglobin combined with carbon monoxide (carboxyhemoglobin) unloads little oxygen causing severe tissue hypoxia.

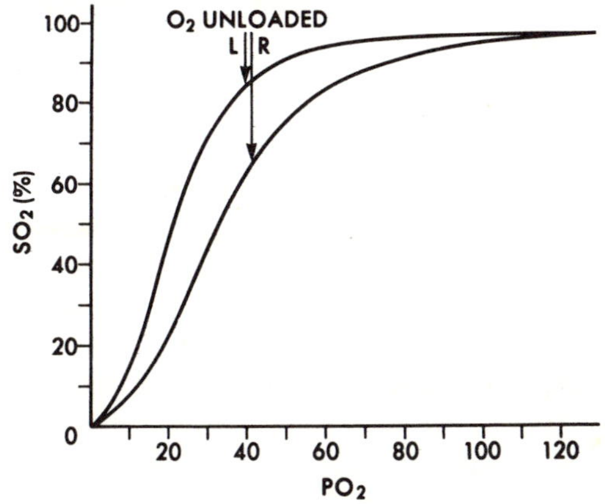

Figure 9.8. O_2 unloading is increased with a right-shifted (R) oxyhemoglobin dissociation curve (reduced O_2-hemoglobin affinity).

Table 9.1. Causes of Hypoxia

Reduced O_2 delivery
Low cardiac output (heart failure)
Low hemoglobin concentration (anemia)
Low arterial O_2 partial pressure (hypoxemia)
Reduced O_2 unloading in tissues
High oxygen-hemoglobin affinity
Impaired O_2 Utilization in mitochondrion
Enzyme poisons

Causes of Hypoxia

When tissue hypoxia is present, the cause must be established and an attempt must be made to improve the abnormal components of the oxygen transport system.

It is beyond the scope of this volume to review the causes of reduced cardiac output and reduced hemoglobin concentration as causes of hypoxia. If cardiac output is reduced, it can be increased by drugs that improve contractility or reduce the afterload of the heart. Transfusion of blood will correct reduced hemoglobin concentration. A reduction in arterial Po_2, a common cause of hypoxia, is discussed next.

CAUSES OF A REDUCTION IN Pa_{O_2}

Hypoxemia is a reduction in arterial oxygen content and can be caused by either a reduction in oxygen-carrying capacity (a reduction in hemoglobin concentration) or a reduction in the partial pressure of oxygen of arterial blood (Pa_{O_2}). A low Pa_{O_2} can be caused by hypoventilation, right to left shunt, mismatching of ventilation and perfusion, diffusion impairment, and breathing air with low Po_2.

Hypoventilation

At sea level barometric pressure is 760 mmHg. When air enters the upper airways, it is warmed and humidified. The partial pressure of the water vapor is 47 mmHg. Since the sum of partial pressures of all the gases (including water vapor) is 760 mmHg, the sum of the partial pressures of the gases not counting water vapor is 760 − 47 = 713 mmHg. Since oxygen is 20.93% of air, the Po_2 of warmed humidified air in the upper airway, the $P_{I_{O_2}}$ is .2093 × 713 = 149 mmHg. When this air reaches the alveoli oxygen is removed and CO_2 is added. If the amount of oxygen removed was exactly equal to the amount of CO_2 added to the alveoli then:

$$P_{A_{O_2}} = P_{I_{O_2}} - P_{A_{CO_2}}$$

where PA_{O_2} is the alveolar Po_2 and PI_{O_2} is 149 mmHg, the inspired oxygen partial pressure.

In fact less CO_2 is added than O_2 removed. The *respiratory exchange ratio* is the ratio of *CO_2 produced/O_2 consumed* and is used to predict more accurately *the ideal alveolar Po_2.*

$$\text{Ideal } PA_{O_2} = PI_{O_2} - \frac{PA_{CO_2}}{R} \quad (4)$$

Equation 4, a version of the alveolar gas equation, is described more fully in pp. 189 and 190 and in the appendix. The ideal alveolar PA_{O_2} of a patient is the Po_2 that would exist in the alveoli if his lung behaved as a perfect gas exchanger with a respiratory exchange ratio of R, which is determined by his metabolism. R is usually about .8 (range 0.7 to 1.0) and is determined by metabolism. At any given instant there occurs catabolism of carbohydrates, proteins, and lipids. A different respiratory exchange ratio (molecules CO_2 produced/molecules O_2 used) is present for each of these substrates (.7 for lipids, .85 for proteins, and 1.0 for carbohydrates), and the "whole body" respiratory exchange ratio depends on the contribution to overall metabolism of each.

The relationship of alveolar Pco_2 and alveolar ventilation is discussed more fully in the following chapter. As alveolar ventilation is increased, PA_{CO_2} decreases (Figure 9.9), and as expected from Equation 4, PA_{O_2} therefore increases. The alveolar Po_2 tends to plateau as ventilation increases. When the lungs are normal, arterial Po_2 will be only slightly less than ideal alveolar Po_2. When a reduction in alveolar ventilation, hypoventilation, is the only cause of

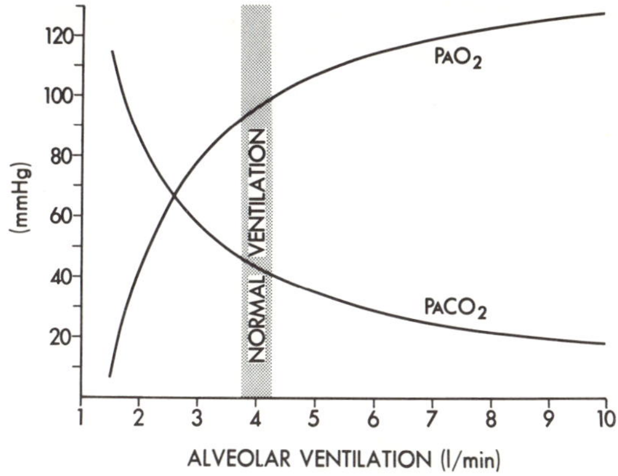

Figure 9.9. Increasing alveolar ventilation reduces PA_{CO_2}. PA_{O_2} is calculated from Pco_2 and R, the respiratory exchange ratio as described in the text. Notice that when ventilation is below normal, a small change in ventilation causes large changes in Po_2 and Pco_2. When ventilation is very high, much larger changes in ventilation are required to change Po_2 and Pco_2.

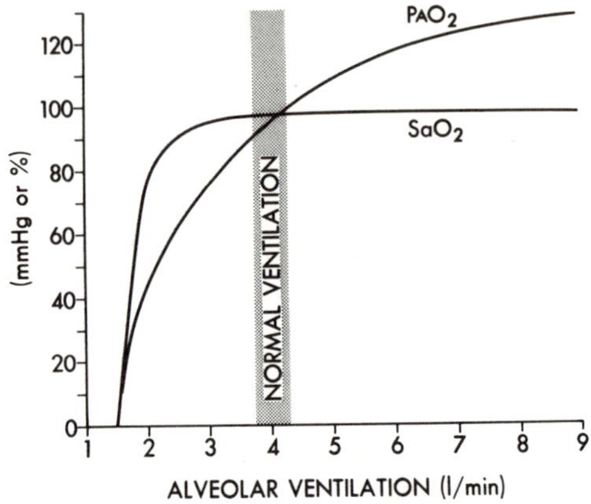

Figure 9.10. Because of the shape of the oxyhemoglobin dissociation curve, oxygen saturation is high when P_{O_2} exceeds 60 mmHg. Thus mild hypoventilation reduces P_{O_2} more rapidly than S_{O_2}. Severe hypoventilation causes both P_{O_2} and S_{O_2} to plummet.

hypoxemia, the difference between ideal alveolar P_{O_2} and arterial P_{O_2} will be small. Because of the shape of the oxyhemoglobin dissociation curve, Sa_{O_2} may be high when mild hypoventilation is present. When severe hypoventilation is present, Sa_{O_2} falls rapidly with small changes in ventilation (Figure 9.10).

Hypoventilation in the absence of lung disease occurs when the control of ventilation is abnormal or when weakness of the respiratory muscles is present. The causes of hypoventilation are reviewed in Chapters 6 and 9.

If hypoxemia is caused by hypoventilation, Equation 4 shows us two methods by which $P_{A_{O_2}}$ can be increased. First, inspired P_{O_2} may be increased; this can be done with oxygen therapy. Second, $P_{A_{O_2}}$ may be increased by reducing P_{CO_2} by increasing alveolar ventilation.

Shunt

A *shunt* is a communication between two parts of the circulation. Hypoxemia can occur when blood passes from the venous to the arterial circulation without taking part in gas exchange. The communication that causes shunt hypoxemia is usually from the right side of the circulation (great veins, right

Table 9.2. Features of Hypoxemia Caused by Hypoventilation

Pa_{CO_2} high
Normal (A − a) P_{O_2} difference
Improved by oxygen therapy
Improved by increasing alveolar ventilation

atrium, right ventricle, or pulmonary artery) to the left side of the circulation (pulmonary veins, left atrium, left ventricle, or aorta) and is called *a right to left shunt.*

When a communication exists between high and low pressure blood vessels, blood will flow from the high to the low pressure vessel. Thus, when a communication exists between the right and left ventricle, blood will flow from the high pressure circuit (left ventricle) into the low pressure circuit (right ventricle) and is called *a left to right shunt.* This shunt does not cause arterial hypoxemia, because all the blood that leaves the left ventricle (into the right ventricle and the aorta) has undergone gas exchange. In the presence of a left to right shunt, there may develop pulmonary arterial hypertension and increased pressure in the right ventricle. When right ventricular pressure exceeds left ventricular pressure, flow will be from right to left and thus cause hypoxemia. Thus, a left to right (nonhypoxemic) shunt may become a right to left (hypoxemic) shunt. This occurs in atrial septal defect, ventricular septal defect, and patent ductus arteriosus. In the tetralogy of Fallot, stenosis of the pulmonary outflow tract results in high pressures in the right ventricle from birth causing right to left flow from birth.

Abnormal vascular communications in the lung causing right to left shunt include congenital arteriovenous fistulae and acquired fistulae as may occur in chronic liver disease.

When lung tissue loses its gas-exchanging surface, as may occur with atelectasis or lobar pneumonia, but is still perfused, the perfusing blood does not participate in gas exchange and a shunt can be considered to be present.

Hypoxemia in right to left shunt is caused by mixing oxygenated and unoxygenated (or mixed venous) blood. An understanding of what happens when different blood samples are mixed is critical to the understanding of shunts.

Suppose we have a 100 ml sample of blood with a hemoglobin concentration of 15 gm/100 ml and with a Po_2 of 100 mmHg and a second sample identical to the first except the Po_2 is 40 mmHg. What would be the Po_2 if we mixed these two samples?

	Sample A	*Sample B*
volume (ml)	100	100
Hgb (gm)	15	15
Po_2 (mmHg)	100	40

The answer is not 70 mmHg. Let us examine the situation in more detail. Sample A's hemoglobin is 97.5% saturated with oxygen. Therefore, $15 \times 1.34 \times .975 = 19.6$ ml of oxygen are bound to the hemoglobin. In addition, $.003 \times 100 = .3$ ml of oxygen is physically dissolved. Therefore, sample A contains 19.9 ml O_2.

The hemoglobin of sample B is only 75% saturated with oxygen; therefore,

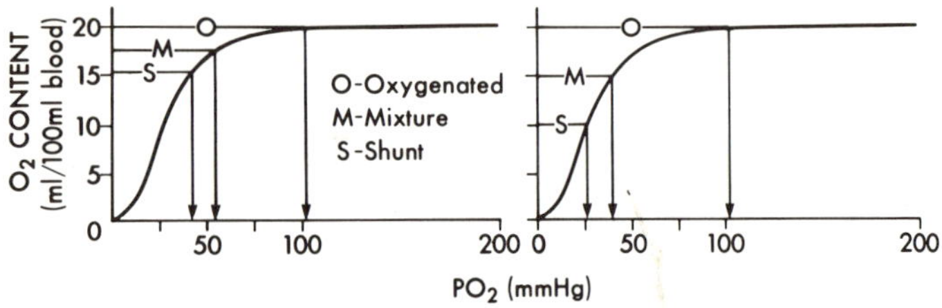

Figure 9.11. (*Left*) In a person breathing air, the effect of mixing 50% oxygenated blood and 50% shunted blood having a Po_2 of 40 mmHg. The oxygen contents determine the oxygen content of the mixture. In this example, the content of the mixture (M) is the mean of the contents of the oxygenated (O) and shunted (S) blood, thus content M is halfway between content O and S. (*Right*) This situation differs from the left figure in only one respect, venous O_2 content has been reduced from about 15 to about 10 ml/100 ml blood. Note that M, the content of the mixture, is still halfway between O and S, but because S is much lower, M is much lower. Mixed venous blood has its effect on the steep portion of the oxygen-hemoglobin dissociation curve.

$15 \times 1.34 \times .75 = 15.075$ ml O_2 are bound to hemoglobin. Only 0.12 ml O_2 are physically dissolved. Thus, sample B contains 15.195 ml O_2.

If we mix sample A and sample B, the mixture will contain $19.9 + 15.195 = 35.095$ ml O_2. The 30 gm of hemoglobin can bind 40.2 ml O_2. Therefore, the hemoglobin is $35.095/40.2 = 87.3\%$ saturated. From the oxyhemoglobin dissociation curve, we see that this is equivalent to a Po_2 of about 54 mmHg. *It is the oxygen content,* not the oxygen pressure, of samples A and B that *determines the state of oxygenation of the mixture* (Figure 9.11). This situation occurs because the relationship of oxygen pressure and oxygen saturation (and therefore oxygen content) is not linear. In the above example, sample A can represent the oxygenated blood and sample B the unoxygenated blood of a shunt.

Effect of Low Mixed Venous Po_2 on Shunt Hypoxemia

Low mixed venous Po_2 occurs when there is tissue hypoxia and occurs because the tissues extract more oxygen from a given volume of blood than usual. A reduction in cardiac output, anemia, or hypoxemia can cause tissue hypoxia and thus reduction in mixed venous Po_2.

In this situation, we are mixing oxygenated blood with blood having very low Po_2. Let us analyze the consequences of such a mixture:

	Sample A	*Sample B*
volume	100	100
Hgb	15	15
Po_2	100	20
Sa_{O_2}	97.5	40

In this situation, the oxygen saturation of the mixture (68.75%) is much lower than the mixed oxygen saturation in the last example in which sample B (the "mixed venous sample") had a Po_2 of 40 mmHg. This is because mixed venous blood has its effect on the steep portion of the oxyhemoglobin dissociation curve. Therefore in a shunt, *a low mixed venous O_2 content magnifies the effect of shunt on hypoxemia.* In other words, *tissue hypoxia, by causing low venous O_2 content, can cause arterial hypoxemia.* Even when a small shunt is present, a very low mixed venous O_2 content will cause hypoxemia. On the other hand, increasing mixed venous Po_2 markedly increases arterial Po_2 when shunt is present.

Effect of Breathing Oxygen on Shunt Hypoxemia

Breathing oxygen will raise the Po_2 of the blood participating in gas exchange, but will have no direct effect on the blood which does not participate in gas exchange (the shunted blood). This is equivalent to mixing a very high Po_2 sample with a sample with Po_2 40 mmHg (the normal mixed venous Po_2).

	Sample A	*Sample B*
volume	100	100
Hgb	15	15
Po_2	660	40
O_2 content	22.08	15.195

	Mixture
volume	200
O_2 content	37.275
O_2 capacity	40.2
Sa_{O_2}	92.7%

In this example, we note that increasing the Po_2 in sample A from 100 to 660 mmHg has had very little effect on the O_2 content of sample A, since the hemoglobin was already almost entirely saturated with oxygen when Po_2 was 100 mmHg (Figure 9.12).

Therefore, the only increase has been due to the O_2 that was physically dissolved. Thus the Po_2 of the mixture is found to be about 65 mmHg by referring back to the oxyhemoglobin dissociation curve for Sa_{O_2} = 92.7%. This situation is analogous to breathing O_2 in the presence of a shunt and shows that the *hypoxemia caused by a right to left shunt is relatively resistant to oxygen therapy.* Breathing O_2 has its effect on the flat portion of the oxyhemoglobin dissociation curve.

Figure 9.13 shows that with small shunts breathing O_2 may improve matters; when the shunt flow is 50% of the total blood flow, oxygen breathing has virtually no effect on Pa_{O_2}.

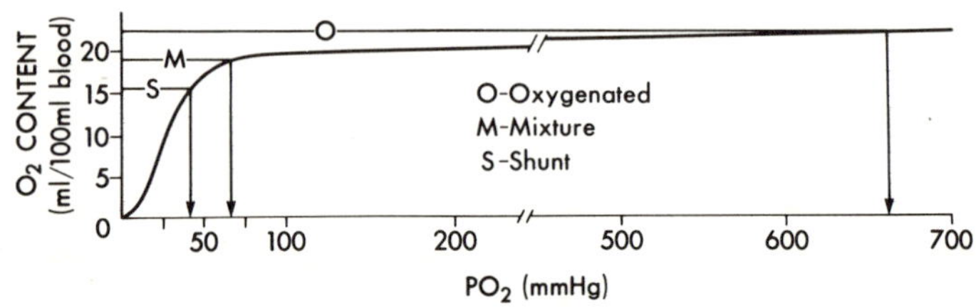

Figure 9.12. Effect of oxygen breathing on shunt. Increasing $P_{A_{O_2}}$ from 100 to about 660 mmHg has had very little effect on the oxygen content of (O) the oxygenated blood. Thus, content M and the P_{O_2} of the mixture is only increased slightly. This is because the effect of increasing $P_{A_{O_2}}$ is on the flat portion of the oxyhemoglobin dissociation curve.

Effect of Increasing Alveolar Ventilation on Shunt Hypoxemia

When the alveolar P_{O_2} is normal, the hemoglobin in the blood that takes part in gas exchange will be almost completely saturated with oxygen. Increasing ventilation above normal will result in an increase in alveolar P_{O_2} but will cause a very, very small increase in oxygen content of this blood. Increasing alveolar P_{O_2} will, of course, have no direct effect on the shunted blood. Thus, increasing ventilation will not improve the hypoxemia of shunt.

Calculation of Shunt

Calculation of shunt is basically the reverse of the process we have been using in the above examples. In the above examples, we knew the volume of

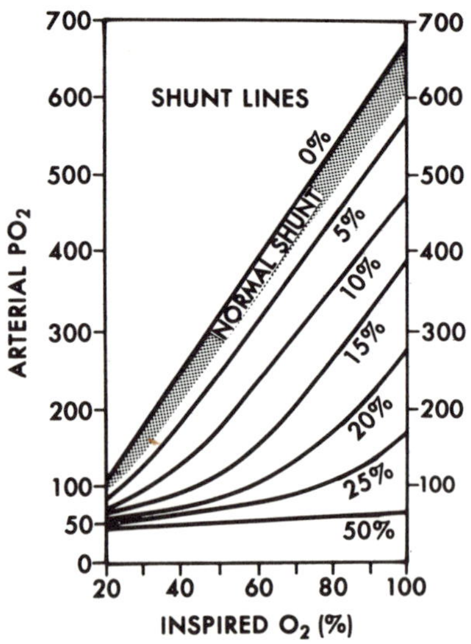

Figure 9.13. The effect of increasing inspired O_2 concentration on arterial P_{O_2} when different size shunts are present. Note that with large shunts, P_{O_2} does not increase much as inspired O_2 concentration is increased.

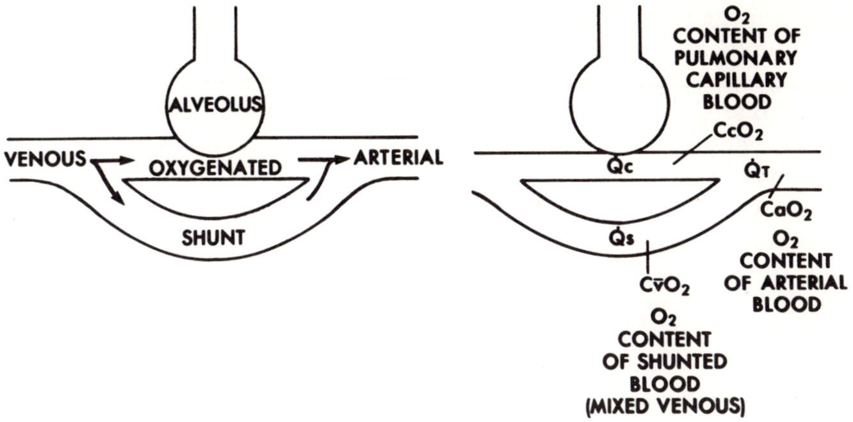

Figure 9.14. Variables used to calculate shunt. The shunt equation is $\dot{Q}s/\dot{Q}_T = Cc_{O_2} - Ca_{O_2}/Cc_{O_2} - C\bar{v}_{O_2}$ and is derived in the text.

the "shunted" blood and calculated arterial Po_2 and Sa_{O_2}. In calculating shunt, we measure arterial Po_2 and solve for the volume of the shunt (Figure 9.14).

The total cardiac output, $\dot{Q}t$, equals the sum of the shunt flow, $\dot{Q}s$, and the flow of blood taking part in gas exchange, $\dot{Q}c$. $\dot{Q}c$ is the abbreviation for pulmonary capillary flow.

$$\dot{Q}t = \dot{Q}s + \dot{Q}c$$

The product $\dot{Q}t \times Ca_{O_2}$ equals the total oxygen carried in the arterial blood and equals the sum of the total oxygen carried by the shunted blood ($\dot{Q} \times C\bar{v}_{O_2}$) and the total oxygen carried by the unshunted pulmonary capillary ($\dot{Q}c \times Cc_{O_2}$) blood.

$$\dot{Q}t \times Ca_{O_2} = \dot{Q}s \times C\bar{v}_{O_2} + \dot{Q}c \times Cc_{O_2}$$

since $\dot{Q}c = \dot{Q}t - \dot{Q}s$

$$\begin{aligned}(\dot{Q}t) \times (Ca_{O_2}) &= (\dot{Q}s) \times (C\bar{v}_{O_2}) + (\dot{Q}t - \dot{Q}s) \times (Cc_{O_2}) \\ &= (\dot{Q}s)\,(C\bar{v}_{O_2}) + (\dot{Q}t)\,(Cc_{O_2}) - (\dot{Q}s)\,(Cc_{O_2})\end{aligned}$$

rearranging

$$\dot{Q}s(Cc_{O_2}) - \dot{Q}s(C\bar{v}_{O_2}) = \dot{Q}t(Cc_{O_2}) - \dot{Q}t(Ca_{O_2})$$

or

$$\dot{Q}s(Cc_{O_2} - C\bar{v}_{O_2}) = \dot{Q}t(Cc_{O_2} - Ca_{O_2})$$

or

$$\frac{\dot{Q}s}{\dot{Q}t} = \frac{Cc_{O_2} - Ca_{O_2}}{Cc_{O_2} - C\bar{v}_{O_2}} \qquad (5)$$

Thus, the ratio of shunted blood to cardiac output ($\dot{Q}s/\dot{Q}t$) is calculated. In practice, shunt is measured in the following manner. While the patient breathes oxygen (for between 10 to 20 minutes), arterial and mixed venous blood samples are obtained. Hemoglobin concentration is measured, and then arterial oxygen content (Ca_{O_2}) and mixed venous oxygen content ($C\bar{v}_{O_2}$) are calculated. Cc_{O_2} is also calculated by assuming that the Po_2 of the pulmonary capillary blood equals ideal alveolar Po_2. Obtaining a mixed venous sample involves placing a catheter in the right ventricle or right pulmonary artery. In most people (who are not in heart failure or anemic), the arterial-venous O_2 content difference is about 5 ml/100 ml. Therefore, $\dot{Q}s/\dot{Q}t$ may be calculated by measuring Ca_{O_2}, by assuming that $C\bar{v}_{O_2}$ is 5 ml/100 ml less than Ca_{O_2} and using the shunt equation. In this situation, shunt may be estimated without resorting to right heart catheterization. A nomogram such as Figure 9.13 may also be used to obtain an estimate of shunt. Notice from this figure that normal people have a small shunt.

Therapy of Shunt Hypoxemia. As shown above, the hypoxemia of a large shunt will not be significantly improved by either breathing oxygen or increasing ventilation. When a smaller shunt is present, oxygen therapy may improve hypoxemia.

When shunt is present because of loss of gas-exchanging surface, as may occur with diffuse lung injury or pneumonia, positive end expiratory pressure has been used to treat hypoxemia. The rationale is that positive end expiratory pressure reverses microatelectasis or airway closure and may convert nongas-exchanging perfused units into gas-exchanging units.

Since the low mixed venous O_2 content caused by tissue hypoxia magnifies the effect of shunt, correction of tissue hypoxia may dramatically improve hypoxemia. Low cardiac output and anemia are reversible causes of tissue hypoxia.

Mismatching of Ventilation and Perfusion

Disease does not affect all airways and alveoli identically; some airways will be more obstructed than others; some alveoli will be more affected by disease than others. This means that some alveoli are hypoventilating relative to other alveoli. If perfusion of these hypoventilating alveoli is not reduced to exactly match the reduction in local ventilation, there will be hypoxemia. This is because blood leaving hypoventilated alveoli will have lower oxygen content

Table 9.3. Features of Hypoxemia Caused by Shunt

Increased (A − a) Po_2 difference
Improved by increasing $C\bar{v}_{O_2}$
Resistant to oxygen therapy if shunt is large
Not improved by increased ventilation

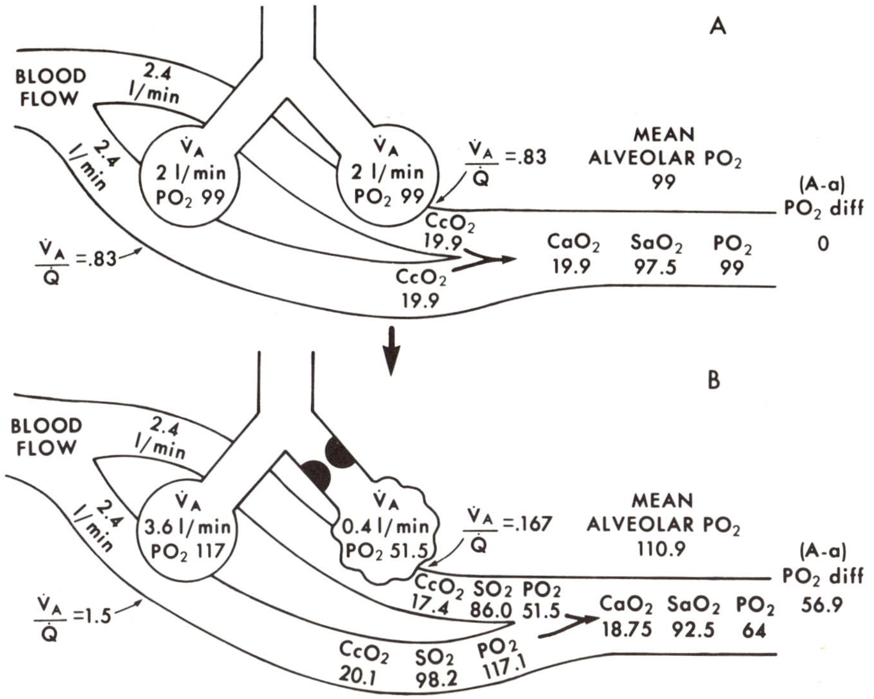

Figure 9.15. In A, there are two lung units each with a $\dot{V}/\dot{Q}$ ratio of .83, and arterial blood is normal. In B, there has been a reduction of ventilation of the right-hand unit, and an increase in ventilation of the left-hand unit. There has been no change in perfusion of the two units; thus the $\dot{V}/\dot{Q}$ ratio of the left unit is high (1.5) and in the right unit is low (.167). This has caused arterial hypoxemia. Although there has been no change in overall ventilation and overall perfusion, the mismatching of ventilation and perfusion has caused hypoxemia.

than relatively hyperventilated alveoli and will result in a *shunt-like* effect. The circulatory control of the lung is far from perfect; ventilation-perfusion mismatching is the most common cause of hypoxemia in lung disease. As discussed in Chapter 4, even in normal man there is some mismatching of ventilation and perfusion.

We have previously shown that alveolar Po_2 is related to inspired Po_2 and the quantity of CO_2 dumped into the alveolus and to the quantity of O_2 taken up by capillary blood. If a region of the lung is ventilating less than another region, reducing perfusion to that region will result in less oxygen uptake from these alveoli and less CO_2 output into these alveoli and can result in normal Po_2 of capillary blood leaving these alveoli.

Figure 9.15 shows a model in which 2 lung units, each with an alveolar ventilation of 2L/minute, are being perfused by a blood flow of 2.4 L/minute. Using Figures 9.16 and 9.17 we see that the end capillary oxygen content in each unit will be 19.9 ml/100 ml, and the mixed arterial oxygen content will be 19.9 ml/100 ml. This results in an Sa_{O_2} of about 97.5% and a P_{O_2} of 99 mmHg. Each unit contributes 50% of the alveolar ventilation, and the mean alveolar P_{O_2} is 99 mmHg, and the difference between mean alveolar P_{O_2} and arterial P_{O_2} is 0.

Now suppose that 1 lung unit becomes abnormal and that it now has a ventilation of only .4 L/minute and that the other lung unit increases its ventilation to maintain a total ventilation of 4 L/min. If perfusion to the two units remains unchanged, the hypoventilating hypoxic unit is being overperfused ($\dot{V}/\dot{Q} = .4/2.4 = .167$) and the hyperventilating hyperoxic unit is being underperfused ($\dot{V}/\dot{Q} = 3.6/2.4 = 1.5$). The blood leaving the low $\dot{V}/\dot{Q}$ unit will have a low O_2 content, while the blood leaving the high $\dot{V}/\dot{Q}$ unit will have increased its content by only a very small amount (Figure 9.16). The mixed arterial blood will have a content of 18.75 ml/200 ml, Sa_{O_2} 92.5%, and P_{O_2} of 64 mmHg. The left unit with a $P_{A_{O_2}}$ of 117.1 mmHg contributes 90% of the alveolar ventilation, while the right unit with a $P_{A_{O_2}}$ of 51.5 mmHg contributes 10% of the total alveolar ventilation. Thus, the mean alveolar P_{O_2} is 110.9 mmHg. There is now a difference between mean alveolar P_{O_2} (110.9 mmHg) and arterial blood P_{O_2} (64 mmHg) of 56.9 mmHg. Thus, there is now an increased alveolar-arterial P_{O_2} difference, called the (A − a) P_{O_2} difference. Thus, although total ventilation and total blood flow of the entire system is the same, mismatching of the two has occurred causing hypoxemia and increased the P_{O_2} difference between alveolar gas and arterial blood.

Mismatching of ventilation and perfusion causes hypoxemia because of the disproportionate effect of blood with low O_2 content from the low $\dot{V}/\dot{Q}$ units on the arterial blood. This is a *shunt-like effect*. Another lesson from this example is that high $\dot{V}/\dot{Q}$ regions cannot compensate for the reduction in content due to a low $\dot{V}/\dot{Q}$ region. This is because blood leaving a normal $\dot{V}/\dot{Q}$ region is already almost entirely saturated with O_2, and further increasing $\dot{V}/\dot{Q}$ only increases O_2 content by a trivial amount.

Since the blood leaving a low $\dot{V}/\dot{Q}$ unit is not well oxygenated, in terms of gas exchange, low $\dot{V}/\dot{Q}$ represents *wasted blood flow.* In fact, a $\dot{V}/\dot{Q}$ of zero represents a pure shunt.

Since the blood leaving a high $\dot{V}/\dot{Q}$ unit does not contain more oxygen than blood leaving a normal $\dot{V}/\dot{Q}$ unit, in terms of gas exchange, high $\dot{V}/\dot{Q}$ represents *wasted ventilation.*

Figure 9.16 shows the effect of changing the $\dot{V}/\dot{Q}$ ratio of a unit on the O_2 content of blood leaving that unit. As $\dot{V}/\dot{Q}$ decreases, the O_2 content of blood approaches the O_2 content of mixed venous blood. Thus, a unit with a very low $\dot{V}/\dot{Q}$ behaves as a shunt; hence the terms *shunt-like* and *venous admixture* are used to explain the effects of low $\dot{V}/\dot{Q}$ units on oxygenation of arterial blood. In addition, the figure shows that increasing $\dot{V}/\dot{Q}$ over the normal range has very little effect on O_2 content. As indicated below, the P_{O_2} of a high $\dot{V}/\dot{Q}$ unit is on the flat portion of the oxyhemoglobin dissociation curve.

As $\dot{V}/\dot{Q}$ is reduced to very low levels, the P_{CO_2} and P_{O_2} are the same as in the mixed venous blood (Figure 9.17). As $\dot{V}/\dot{Q}$ increases, P_{CO_2} decreases while P_{O_2}

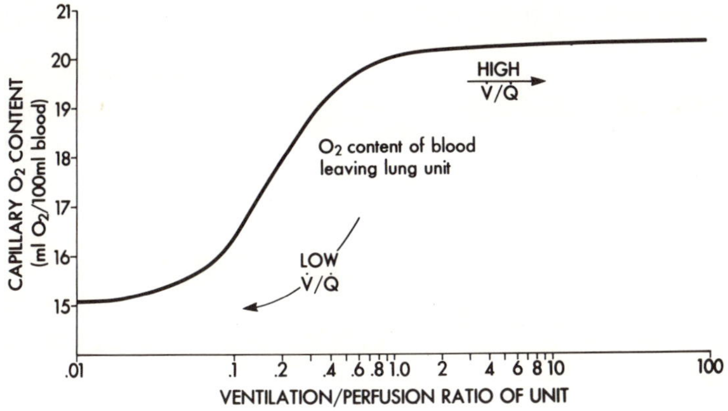

Figure 9.16. The O_2 content of blood leaving units with different $\dot{V}/\dot{Q}$ ratios. Increasing $\dot{V}/\dot{Q}$ over normal does not increase capillary O_2 content ("wasted ventilation"). When $\dot{V}/\dot{Q}$ is very low, the capillary blood has the same content as unoxygenated, mixed venous blood ("wasted perfusion"). A logarithmic x axis is being used. (Adapted, with permission, from West JB: Ventilation-Perfusion Relationships. *Am Rev Resp Dis* 116:919, 1977.)

increases. For very high $\dot{V}/\dot{Q}$ the Po_2 and Pco_2 are the same as inspired air; that is, the lung unit behaves like dead space or a nongas-exchanging unit. Thus, a region of very high $\dot{V}/\dot{Q}$ really represents a region of *wasted ventilation*.

Effect of Breathing Oxygen on $\dot{V}/\dot{Q}$ Hypoxemia

If there are high and low $\dot{V}/\dot{Q}$ units, we have seen that hypoxemia results. If in such a system the inspired gas were pure oxygen ($F_{I_{O_2}}$ = 1) instead of air ($F_{I_{O_2}}$

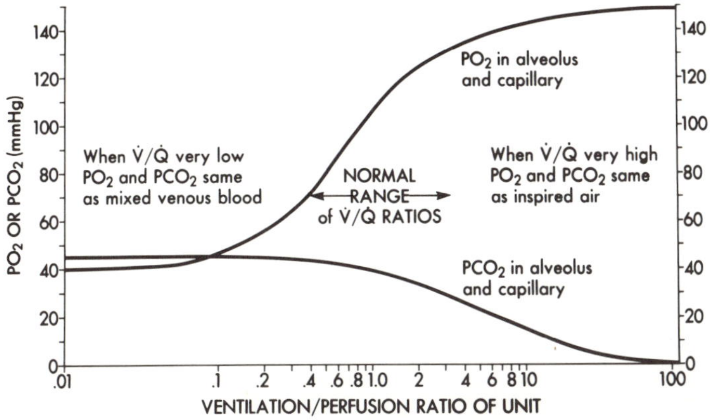

Figure 9.17. Effect of $\dot{V}/\dot{Q}$ ratio on Po_2 and Pco_2. When $\dot{V}/\dot{Q}$ is very high, Po_2 and Pco_2 are the same as inspired air; when the ratio is very low, they resemble mixed venous blood. (Adapted, with permission, from West JB: Ventilation-Perfusion Relationships. *Am Rev Resp Dis* 116:919, 1977.)

= .2093), eventually all the nitrogen would be washed out of all lung units and the low $\dot{V}/\dot{Q}$ unit would have a high P_{O_2}. Blood leaving this low $\dot{V}/\dot{Q}$ unit will, therefore, have a high P_{O_2} and high O_2 content. *Breathing 100% oxygen results in virtually identical arterial oxygen contents of blood leaving all lung units,* regardless of the $\dot{V}/\dot{Q}$ ratio. It has been mentioned that the hypoxemia of $\dot{V}/\dot{Q}$ mismatching is *shunt-like* because of the similarity of the effect of shunted blood and blood from low $\dot{V}/\dot{Q}$ regions on arterial oxygen content. An important difference between the two is that shunt-caused hypoxemia is resistant to oxygen breathing, while the hypoxemia of $\dot{V}/\dot{Q}$ mismatching is readily corrected by oxygen breathing. This fact is used clinically. Oxygen breathing will raise arterial P_{O_2} to about 600 mmHg in a patient with hypoxemia caused by $\dot{V}/\dot{Q}$ mismatching. If hypoxemia is caused by shunt, breathing oxygen does not raise the P_{O_2} to such levels, as is shown in Figure 9.13.

Although oxygen breathing improves hypoxemia caused by $\dot{V}/\dot{Q}$ mismatching, it can also actually worsen the matching of ventilation and perfusion by two mechanisms. First, as is discussed in Chapter 4, alveolar hypoxia causes pulmonary vasoconstriction that reduces perfusion of low $\dot{V}/\dot{Q}$ regions and redistributes blood flow to regions of higher $\dot{V}/\dot{Q}$. Thus, oxygen breathing (or any other vascular dilator) will relieve the vasoconstriction and thus increase perfusion of low $\dot{V}/\dot{Q}$ regions.

The second mechanism is related to the fact that the presence of nitrogen (which makes up about 80% of alveolar gas) helps keep alveoli from collapsing. The volume of nitrogen in alveoli is maintained because alveolar and blood P_{N_2} is similar, and so little diffusion of nitrogen occurs in either direction. When $\dot{V}/\dot{Q}$ ratios are very low (in the order of .001) the perfusion is so large relative to ventilation that more gas including N_2 is taken up by the blood than is put into the alveolar gas, and thus the alveolar volume will decrease until it collapses. Thus, a low $\dot{V}/\dot{Q}$ region of about .001 is unstable and may collapse and turn into a shunt. While oxygen breathing, the instability is worsened and regions with a $\dot{V}/\dot{Q}$ of .05 may collapse. This occurs because the alveoli become nitrogen-free during oxygen breathing, and the nitrogen "strut" supporting the alveoli is absent. In this situation, the only 2 gases in the alveoli are O_2 and CO_2. When perfusion grossly exceeds ventilation, the volume of gas taken up by the capillaries exceeds that added to the alveoli (CO_2 and inspired O_2), and without the nitrogen "strut," alveoli lose volume quickly and will collapse. Thus, oxygen breathing can turn a low $\dot{V}/\dot{Q}$ region into a shunt.

Effect of Mixed Venous Blood on $\dot{V}/\dot{Q}$ Hypoxemia

It has been shown that as $\dot{V}/\dot{Q}$ decreases, that the blood gases of the capillary blood leaving these regions approaches the blood gases of mixed venous blood. Thus, one potentially useful method to offset the deleterious effects of low $\dot{V}/\dot{Q}$ regions is to increase mixed venous O_2 content. Figure 9.18 shows the effect of increasing mixed venous O_2 content on end capillary O_2 content. As expected, for the low $\dot{V}/\dot{Q}$ regions, an increase in mixed venous O_2 content

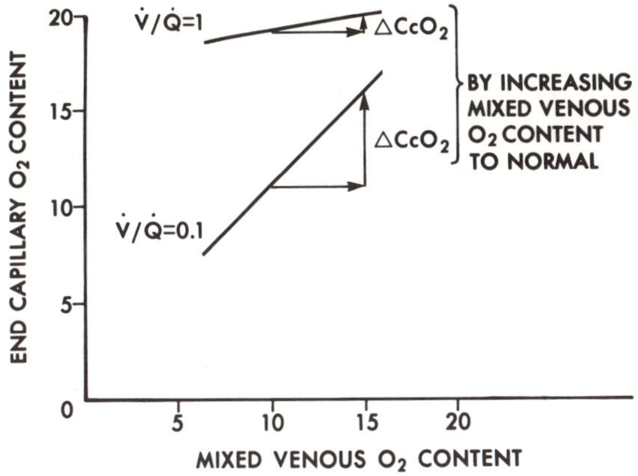

Figure 9.18. The effect of increasing mixed venous O_2 content with different $\dot{V}/\dot{Q}$ ratios. Note that when the ratio is low, increasing mixed venous O_2 content dramatically raises capillary O_2 content. This is similar to the situation with a true shunt. (Adapted, with permission, from West JB: Ventilation-Perfusion Relationships. *Am Rev Resp Dis* 116:919, 1977.)

results in a similar rise in end capillary O_2 content. Increasing mixed venous O_2 content thus can dramatically increase mixed arterial Po_2 by increasing the Po_2 of the low $\dot{V}/\dot{Q}$ regions. Low mixed venous O_2 content occurs when tissue hypoxia caused by anemia or low cardiac output is present. Correction of these two conditions will result in an increase in mixed venous O_2 content and will thus improve arterial Po_2.

Causes of Ventilation-Perfusion Mismatching

In normals some mismatching of ventilation and perfusion is present, accounting for a small difference (2 to 5 mmHg) between ideal alveolar and arterial Po_2. This occurs because of the different effects of gravity on ventilation and perfusion, and because even normal people have a small shunt.

Ventilation at the top of the lung is less than ventilation at the bottom of the lung. This is because pleural pressure at the top of the lung is more negative than at the bottom. Pressure is not uniform in the pleural space; going from top to bottom, it increases by about .25 cmH_2O for every centimeter distance down the lung. Because the lung is about 30 cm long, the pleural pressure is 7.5 cmH_2O (.25 × 30) more negative at the very top of the pleural space compared to the bottom. Because the upper zones always "see" a distending pressure 7.5 cmH_2O greater than the bottom, the upper lung zones are more distended and are on a flatter portion of the pressure-volume curve than the lower lung zones. Because of this, the volume of the upper lung zones change less with the same pressure change than the lower zones during breathing (Figure 9.19).

Blood flow, or perfusion, is also much less at the top than at the bottom of

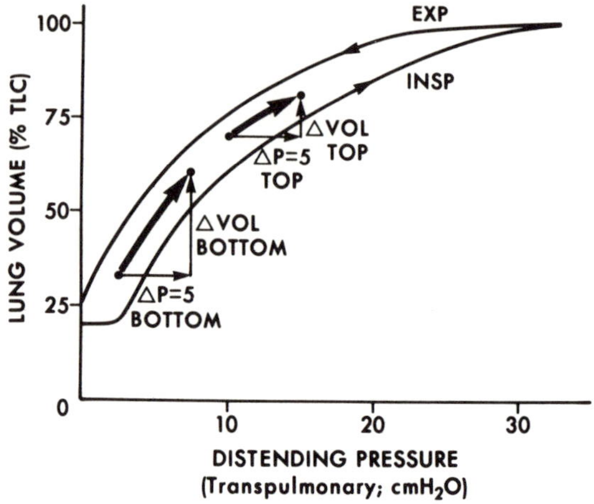

Figure 9.19. Ventilation at the top of the lung is less than on the bottom. During breathing, a given pressure difference (e.g., 5 cmH_2O) causes a greater volume change in the lower lung regions. This is caused by the fact that upper lung zones are more distended and on a flatter portion of the pressure-volume curve.

the lung. The reasons for this are also discussed in Chapter 4. Briefly, the pulmonary arterial pressure is less in the top than the bottom of the lung; hence flow is less at the top than the bottom of the lung. Blood flow increases more rapidly than ventilation going from top to bottom of the lung, and so even in normals there occurs some mismatching of ventilation and perfusion.

$\dot{V}/\dot{Q}$, the ventilation-perfusion ratio, in any region is ventilation divided by blood flow. In the top of the lung, ventilation exceeds perfusion and thus $\dot{V}/\dot{Q} > 1$. In the bottom of the lung, perfusion exceeds ventilation and thus $\dot{V}/\dot{Q} < 1$. $\dot{V}/\dot{Q}$ ranges from about 3 in the top of the lung to about 0.6 in the bottom of the normal lung (Figure 9.20).

$\dot{V}/\dot{Q}$ mismatching is the most common cause of hypoxemia in lung disease. Lung disease will result in ventilation-perfusion mismatching by one of 3 patterns: widening the normal distribution of $\dot{V}/\dot{Q}$ ratios, increased ventilation in high $\dot{V}/\dot{Q}$ regions, or increased blood flow in low $\dot{V}/\dot{Q}$ regions.

Widening of the distribution of $\dot{V}/\dot{Q}$ ratios occurs with most lung diseases and also even in normal elderly people. Instead of the normal range in $\dot{V}/\dot{Q}$ ratios (0.6 to 3), the range may be from 0.01 to more than 10 in the elderly.

Increased ventilation in high $\dot{V}/\dot{Q}$ regions implies increased wasted ventilation. In some patients half the total ventilation may go to regions of $\dot{V}/\dot{Q} > 10$. This results in a marked waste of ventilation. This pattern occurs in chronic airflow obstruction (the "pink puffer"), interstitial fibrosis, pulmonary embolism, and the respiratory distress syndrome.

Increased perfusion in low $\dot{V}/\dot{Q}$ regions implies wasted blood flow. This pattern occurs in chronic obstructive lung disease (the "blue bloater"), bronchial asthma, and pulmonary edema. The latter group may also demonstrate a large true shunt.

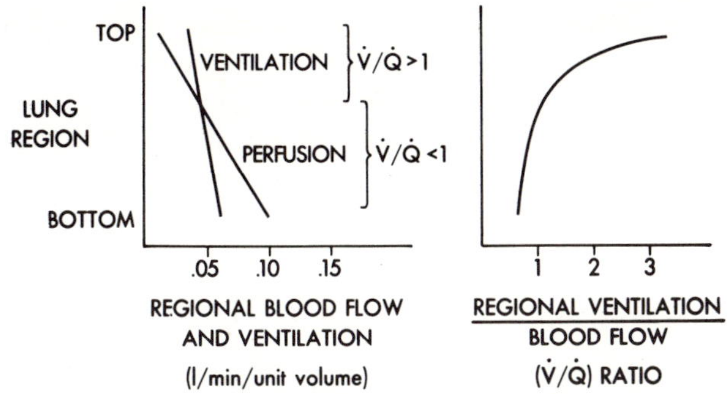

Figure 9.20. Ventilation and perfusion both increase going from the top to the bottom of the lung. Notice that the top of the lung is relatively overventilated ($\dot{V}/\dot{Q} > 1$), while the bottom of the lung is relatively overperfused ($\dot{V}/\dot{Q} < 1$).

As is often the case, a patient with any of the above disorders may demonstrate the combination of the three patterns.

Clinical Tests Indicating the Severity of $\dot{V}/\dot{Q}$ Mismatching

Tests that examine directly the distribution of ventilation-perfusion ratios are complex and are done in few institutions. To diagnose pulmonary embolism, the gross distribution of perfusion and the gross distribution of ventilation are examined by using radioactive trace substances. This test, the lung scan, is positive for the presence of embolism when a characteristic defect in perfusion is present. Absence of perfusion in a region known to be ventilating is highly suggestive of pulmonary embolism. The lung scan is useful when the patient does not have diffuse lung disease; when disease is present, regions of hypoperfusion or ventilation without perfusion might be due to the patient's underlying lung disease and not embolism.

As shown above, low $\dot{V}/\dot{Q}$ regions cause arterial hypoxemia, due to "wasted perfusion." On the other hand, high $\dot{V}/\dot{Q}$ regions do not cause hypoxemia but waste ventilation from the point of view of gas exchange, since the increase in ventilation is not accompanied by increased O_2 content of arterial blood.

Thus, we require tests that indicate the severity of wasted perfusion (low $\dot{V}/\dot{Q}$) and tests that indicate the severity of wasted ventilation (high $\dot{V}/\dot{Q}$).

Tests of Low $\dot{V}/\dot{Q}$ (Wasted Perfusion). The simplest indicator of low $\dot{V}/\dot{Q}$ is the ideal alveolar-arterial Po_2 difference, also abbreviated $(A - a)\ Po_2$ difference. The greater the contribution from low $\dot{V}/\dot{Q}$ regions, the greater the difference will be between alveolar and arterial Po_2. Ideal alveolar Po_2 is calculated from the alveolar gas equation and is the Po_2 that would be present in the alveoli if there were no ventilation-perfusion mismatching.

The alveolar gas equation is:

$$PA_{O_2} = PI_{O_2} - Pa_{CO_2}\left[FI_{O_2} + \frac{1 - FI_{O_2}}{R}\right] \tag{6}$$

$P_{A_{O_2}}$ is the ideal alveolar P_{O_2}; $P_{I_{O_2}}$ is the inspired P_{O_2}; Pa_{CO_2} is the arterial P_{CO_2} (which is substituted for alveolar P_{CO_2}); $F_{I_{O_2}}$ is the fraction of oxygen of air (.21 for air), and R is the respiratory exchange ratio (usually about .8). The extreme right hand part of the equation corrects for the difference in inspired and expired volume; inspired volume exceeds expired volume slightly because more O_2 is consumed than CO_2 produced. Notice what happens to this equation when $F_{I_{O_2}} = 1$:

$$P_{A_{O_2}} = P_{I_{O_2}} - Pa_{CO_2}\left[1 + \frac{1-1}{R}\right]$$

$$P_{A_{O_2}} = P_{I_{O_2}} - Pa_{CO_2} \qquad \text{(while breathing oxygen)} \qquad \textbf{(7)}$$

Thus when $F_{I_{O_2}}$ is 1 (breathing pure oxygen), the only gases in the alveolar gas are CO_2 and O_2, and whatever is not CO_2 must be oxygen.

The alveolar gas equation when breathing air can be simplified further:

$$P_{A_{O_2}} = P_{I_{O_2}} - \frac{Pa_{CO_2}}{R} + \left[\frac{Pa_{CO_2} \times F_{I_{O_2}}(1-R)}{R}\right] \qquad \textbf{(8)}$$

simplified equation correction factor

When R = .8 and $F_{I_{O_2}} = .21$, the correction factor is $.05 \times Pa_{CO_2}$. In other words when Pa_{CO_2} is about 40 mmHg, the correction factor is only about 2 mmHg. For most clinical purposes we may therefore ignore this correction factor and use the equation:

$$P_{A_{O_2}} = P_{I_{O_2}} - \frac{Pa_{CO_2}}{R} \qquad \textbf{(9)}$$

The (A − a) P_{O_2} difference would then be the alveolar P_{O_2} as calculated above minus the measured arterial P_{O_2}. In normal people the (A − a) P_{O_2} difference is less than 20 mmHg.

The other test that may indicate the contribution of low $\dot{V}/\dot{Q}$ regions is simply to treat the blood coming from low $\dot{V}/\dot{Q}$ regions as though it behaved like a true shunt and to use the shunt equation. We have previously seen that in fact with very low $\dot{V}/\dot{Q}$ regions the end capillary blood is similar to mixed venous blood. The *physiological shunt* equation is simply the shunt equation:

$$\frac{\dot{Q}ps}{\dot{Q}t} = \frac{Cc_{O_2} - Ca_{O_2}}{Cc_{O_2} - C\bar{v}_{O_2}} \qquad \textbf{(10)}$$

Cc_{O_2} is the O_2 content of end capillary blood equilibrated with ideal alveolar P_{O_2}. The physiological shunt $\dot{Q}ps/\dot{Q}t$ tells us that the effect of the low $\dot{V}/\dot{Q}$ regions on arterial blood is *as if* a shunt (or venous admixture) $\dot{Q}ps/\dot{Q}t$ were present.

Tests of High $\dot{V}/\dot{Q}$ (Wasted Ventilation). High $\dot{V}/\dot{Q}$ alveoli have lower P_{CO_2} than alveoli with a normal $\dot{V}/\dot{Q}$. Therefore, the greater the number of high $\dot{V}/\dot{Q}$

alveoli, the lower will be the mixed expired P_{CO_2}. High $\dot{V}/\dot{Q}$ regions behave like nonventilating dead space and thus contribute to the physiological dead space. One test of wasted ventilation is the *physiological dead space tidal volume ratio* which is calculated using the equation:

$$\frac{V_D}{V_T} = \frac{Pa_{CO_2} - P_{E_{CO_2}}}{Pa_{CO_2}} \quad (11)$$

V_D is physiological dead space, V_T is tidal volume, Pa_{CO_2} is arterial (equivalent to alveolar P_{CO_2}) and $P_{E_{CO_2}}$ is mixed expired P_{CO_2}. Note that as $P_{E_{CO_2}}$ becomes smaller (as happens with more contribution from high $\dot{V}/\dot{Q}$ regions), V_D/V_T becomes larger. For a more complete discussion of dead space see the following chapter.

Therapy of Hypoxemia Caused by $\dot{V}/\dot{Q}$ Mismatching

Hypoxemia caused by $\dot{V}/\dot{Q}$ mismatching can be treated by increasing alveolar P_{O_2}, increasing $C\bar{v}_{O_2}$, and by actually improving the matching of ventilation and perfusion.

As shown above, with oxygen breathing, even alveoli with very low $\dot{V}/\dot{Q}$ will eventually have a very high $P_{A_{O_2}}$; therefore, blood in the capillaries perfusing these alveoli will be saturated with oxygen.

Since blood leaving very low $\dot{V}/\dot{Q}$ regions resembles mixed venous blood, and since it is this low O_2 content blood that disproportionately causes hypoxemia, increasing $C\bar{v}_{O_2}$ will dramatically increase Pa_{O_2}. Thus if $C\bar{v}_{O_2}$ is low because of heart failure or anemia, correction of these will improve $C\bar{v}_{O_2}$ and therefore Pa_{O_2}.

In some disorders, there are low $\dot{V}/\dot{Q}$ regions with a significant portion of the blood flow perfusing these regions. This situation occurs in the adult respiratory distress syndrome. When such patients are treated by mechanical ventilation and positive end expiratory pressure (PEEP), there occurs a reduction in blood flow to low $\dot{V}/\dot{Q}$ regions.

Occasionally, a therapeutic maneuver can worsen ventilation perfusion matching. In bronchial asthma, hypoxemia occurs because a significant portion of blood flow occurs in units having low $\dot{V}/\dot{Q}$. When such patients are treated by bronchodilator, there may be worsening of hypoxemia. This occurs because bronchodilators may also dilate pulmonary blood vessels and thus increase perfusion to low $\dot{V}/\dot{Q}$ units.

Table 9.4. Features of Hypoxemia Caused by $\dot{V}/\dot{Q}$ Mismatching

Increased (A − a) P_{O_2} difference
Pa_{O_2} markedly increased by oxygen breathing
Pa_{O_2} markedly increased by increasing $C\bar{v}_{O_2}$

Impaired Diffusion

It seems evident that if there are impediments to the direct transfer of oxygen from alveolar gas to capillary blood, hypoxemia will result. In fact, this mechanism, impaired diffusion, is not an important cause of hypoxemia in most patients.

Transfer Between Inspired Air and Alveoli

Fresh air on its way to alveolar sacs must pass through the trachea, bronchi, terminal bronchioles, respiratory bronchi, and alveolar ducts. If mechanisms facilitating gas mixing did not occur, no air of a normal inspired tidal breath of 400 ml would reach alveolar sacs. Obviously, inspired air does reach alveolar gas and mixes with the gas that remains in the alveoli at the end of the last expiration. Several mechanisms facilitate this process. First, inspired air does not travel with a square wave front. In the small conducting airways, axial laminar flow occurs; the gas in the center of the stream travels faster than gas next to the airway wall; thus it travels further and can penetrate the alveoli. Second, the contracting heart actually shakes the lung, and this agitating action has an important effect on gas mixing. The third mechanism that helps gas mixing is diffusion.

Diffusion is the tendency of a gas to spread uniformly throughout the space available to it. This occurs because of the kinetic energy of the gas molecules. Gas will move from a region of higher kinetic energy to a region of lower kinetic energy. One measure of this moving tendency is the partial pressure of the gas. The Po_2 of the inspired air is greater than the Po_2 of alveolar air causing the movement of oxygen into alveoli. Similarly, CO_2 diffuses into the conducting airways. These mechanisms are so efficient that there are patients in whom the tidal volume is similar to the volume of the conducting airways (anatomical dead space) and in whom fresh air is clearly reaching alveoli!

Transfer Between Alveoli and Blood

Oxygen must traverse alveolar type 1 cells, basement membrane, the interstitial space of the lung, capillary endothelial cells, plasma, and the red blood cell membrane before combining with hemoglobin. Carbon dioxide makes the same trip in the opposite direction. In order for these gases to move between alveoli and red cells, they must diffuse through these structures, collectively called the *alveolar-capillary membrane.* The main constituent traversed is actually water, so that we are dealing with diffusion through liquid. The gases are dissolved in the water of these structures, and the dissolved gases diffuse from a region of high to low partial pressure.

The rate of gas diffusion is inversely proportional to the square root of its density. The density of a gas is proportional to its molecular weight. Thus, a light gas will diffuse more readily than a heavy one. Oxygen, which is lighter than carbon dioxide (molecular weight 32 vs 44), diffuses more easily than carbon dioxide in the alveolar gas. The diffusion through the alveolar-capillary membrane is diffusion through liquid, which depends on the surface area of the membrane and the solubility of the gases. *Carbon dioxide is much more soluble than oxygen,* with the end result that it diffuses 20 times more rapidly than oxygen through the alveolar-capillary membrane.

The last part of the journey that oxygen makes within the red blood cells is its binding with hemoglobin. This reaction appears normally to be the rate-limiting step in the transfer of oxygen from alveoli to blood.

In breaking down the transfer of oxygen into its component parts, we must account for two separate steps: the transfer of oxygen through the alveolar-capillary membrane and its binding with hemoglobin. The term diffusing capacity (abbreviated DL for *lung diffusing capacity*) has been used to describe both parts of this process. Since part of the process is not really diffusion, the term *transfer factor* has been suggested. Transfer factor may be thought of as the inverse of resistance to transfer of oxygen; in other words, the greater the transfer factor, the less the resistance for oxygen transfer. Thus 1/transfer factor is equivalent to resistance.

Using the electrical analogy of summing resistances in parallel, we may use the following equation:

$$\frac{1}{\text{Total transfer factor for } O_2} = \frac{1}{\text{transfer factor for } O_2 \text{ for crossing the alveolar-capillary membrane (membrane diffusing capacity)}} + \frac{1}{\text{transfer factor for } O_2 \text{ hemoglobin binding}}$$

The membrane diffusing capacity, abbreviated DM, is a function of the surface area available for diffusion, that is the surface area of the alveolar-capillary membrane. In addition DM, is a function of the Po_2 gradient between pulmonary capillary blood and alveolar gas. The transfer factor for O_2-hemoglobin binding is a function of how much blood comes in contact with alveolar gas (the pulmonary capillary volume, abbreviated Vc) and the rate of combining of O_2 and hemoglobin (abbreviated θ). Thus:

$$\frac{1}{\text{Total transfer factor for } O_2} = \frac{1}{\text{transfer factor for } O_2 \text{ for crossing the alveolar-capillary membrane (DM)}} + \frac{1}{\text{pulmonary capillary blood volume (Vc)} \times O_2\text{-hemoglobin reaction rate } (\theta)}$$

Using the diffusing capacity notation the equation is:

$$\frac{1}{\text{DL}} = \frac{1}{\text{DM}} + \frac{1}{\text{Vc} \cdot \theta} \qquad \textbf{(12)}$$

where DL is the total diffusing capacity and DM the membrane diffusing capacity.

Causes of Reduced Total Transfer Factor for Oxygen

Examination of Equation 12 reveals that transfer for oxygen can change if membrane diffusing capacity (DM) is reduced, pulmonary capillary blood volume (Vc) changes, or the O_2-hemoglobin reaction rate (θ) changes.

Reduction in membrane diffusing capacity can occur with loss of alveolar-capillary *surface area*. Diseases in which there is destruction of alveolar walls (emphysema) or surgical removal of lung tissue will, therefore, reduce O_2 transfer factor. Reduction in membrane-diffusing capacity can also occur with thickening of the alveolar-capillary membrane. Fluid and cells may accumulate in alveoli thickening the membrane. Fluid (interstitial edema), cells (inflammatory diseases such as viral pneumonia, carcinomatosis, and autoimmune disorders), and collagen in the interstitial space (sarcoid, diffuse interstitial pneumonitis) can also thicken the alveolar-capillary membrane.

Increase in pulmonary capillary blood volume can increase transfer factor for oxygen. In practice, this occurs when there is an increase in pulmonary venous pressure, which causes engorgement of the pulmonary capillaries. Heart diseases such as mitral valve stenosis commonly cause an increase in pulmonary venous pressure.

Changes in the O_2-hemoglobin reaction rate are caused by an increase in hemoglobin concentration (polycythemia), which increases O_2 transfer, and a decrease in hemoglobin concentration (anemia), which reduces O_2 transfer. An increase in the number of hemoblogin molecules passing through the pulmonary capillaries in a given unit of time will also result in an increase in O_2 transfer.

Table 9.5. Causes of Changes in Transfer Factor for Oxygen

$$\frac{1}{D_L} = \frac{1}{D_M} + \frac{1}{V_C \cdot \theta}$$

Decrease in DL	Decrease in DM
	Emphysema, surgical resection
	Fluid, cells in alveoli
	Fluid, cells, collagen in interstitium.
	Decrease in θ
	Anemia
Increase in DL	Increase in Vc
	Pulmonary venous hypertension
	Exercise
	Increase in θ
	Polycythemia
	Exercise

The movement of molecules from alveoli to blood depends on there being a difference in alveolar and capillary blood partial pressures. If the partial pressure of a gas is the same in capillary and alveolus, no gradient for diffusion is present.

Blood spends about .75 seconds in one trip through pulmonary capillaries. After about .25 seconds, the Po_2 of capillary blood is the same as the Po_2 of alveolar gas; therefore, beyond .25 seconds there does not exist a diffusion gradient for oxygen. Thus, the amount of oxygen taken up really depends on the number of hemoglobin molecules perfusing the alveoli. In a sense then, in normal people, oxygen uptake is limited by perfusion, not diffusion.

When lung disease is present there may be several reasons why diffusion should be impaired. The surface area of the alveolar-capillary membrane may be markedly reduced as in emphysema; the alveolar-capillary membrane may be markedly thickened as occurs with collagen overproduction in the interstitial space of the lung in diffuse interstitial fibrosis. Indeed, if we examine the time course of change of Po_2 when diffusion is abnormal, we see that Po_2 rises more slowly than when diffusion is normal, but the Po_2 of the capillary blood is still equal to that of alveolar gas when the blood leaves the pulmonary capillary. Thus, even in severe disease, diffusion does not limit the Po_2 of the blood leaving pulmonary capillaries (Figure 9.21).

There are two conditions that will potentially result in the red blood cells not being fully oxygenated when they leave the pulmonary capillaries. First, if the amount of time spent in the pulmonary capillary is reduced, there may not be enough time for complete oxygenation to occur. During exercise, red cells may spend as little as .25 seconds in the capillaries. As Figure 9.21 shows, this

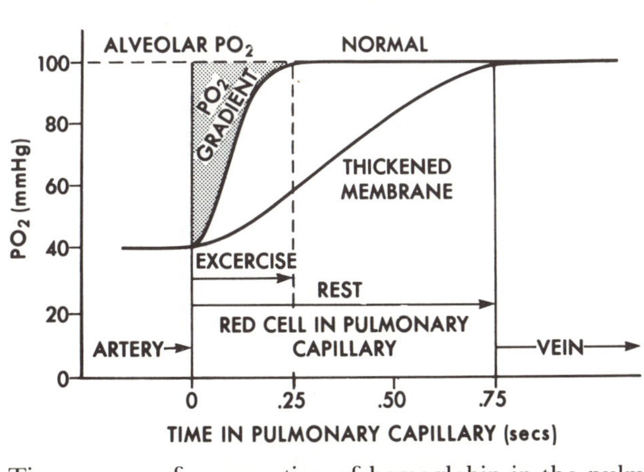

Figure 9.21. Time course of oxygenation of hemoglobin in the pulmonary circulation, in the presence of a normal alveolar-capillary membrane and with a thickened membrane. Notice that at rest Po_2 is normal in both situations. When transit time is reduced, as in exercise, there is insufficient time available to fully oxygenate hemoglobin when the membrane is thickened.

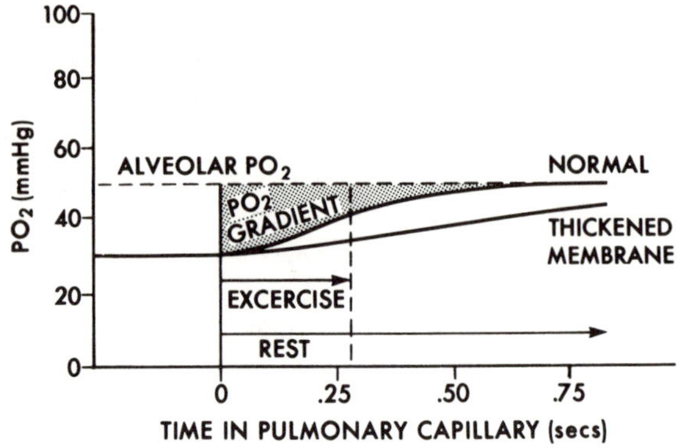

Figure 9.22. Time course of oxygenation of hemoglobin in the pulmonary capillary. When alveolar Po_2 is reduced, as in high altitude, the Po_2 gradient is reduced and there is insufficient time available to fully oxygenate hemoglobin, even at rest, when the alveolar-capillary membrane is thickened. Notice that a normal person may become hypoxemic during exercise when alveolar Po_2 is low.

results in no change in capillary Po_2 of normal people but a marked drop in capillary Po_2 of patients with impaired diffusion.

Second, if the gradient for diffusion is reduced, i.e., if *the difference* between the Po_2 of alveolar gas and the Po_2 of blood that has just entered the capillaries is reduced, hemoglobin may leave the capillaries not fully oxygenated (Figure 9.22). The *reductio ad absurdum* of this situation would occur if the alveolar Po_2 were the same as mixed venous Po_2. Oxygen would not diffuse at all into capillary blood. Thus, the lower the alveolar Po_2, the lower is the gradient for diffusion. At a high altitude of about 13,000 feet (4 km), alveolar Po_2 may be 50 mmHg lower than at sea level, but the mixed venous Po_2 is reduced by only about 10 mmHg. Thus, the gradient between alveolar and capillary Po_2 is about 40 mmHg less than at sea level.

Figure 9.22 shows that when alveolar Po_2 is reduced in a normal person, blood leaving pulmonary capillaries has had sufficient time to equilibrate with alveolar gas. But if that person should have a reduction in the amount of time blood spends in the capillaries, severe hypoxemia would occur. A patient, on the other hand, would be severely hypoxemic both at rest and during exercise if alveolar Po_2 were reduced. Thus, diffusion causes hypoxemia in patients when alveolar Po_2 is reduced or when pulmonary transit time is reduced. Oxygen breathing, by markedly increasing alveolar Po_2, increases the gradient between alveolar and capillary Po_2 and will substantially increase the end capillary Po_2.

Patients with interstitial lung diseases are hypoxemic at rest. *None of the mechanisms mentioned above adequately explain the hypoxemia.* Since in these disorders the alveolar Po_2 is normal or even high, how can end pulmonary capillary blood be hypoxemic? It is likely that mismatching of ventilation and perfusion explains virtually all of the hypoxemia at rest. If an alveolus is overperfused, it may be that the length of time that an individual red cell spends in the capillary is reduced. Thus, although the time blood spends in capillaries averages .75 seconds, the range may be much broader, particularly in disease. If some alveoli are perfused with capillaries having short transit time, blood leaving these units will be hypoxemic. Thus, in the presence of diseases that should impair diffusion, $\dot{V}/\dot{Q}$ mismatching has been shown to be the major mechanism explaining hypoxemia. During exercise, a significant portion of the hypoxemia is explained by impaired diffusion itself.

The Effect of Diffusion on Nonrespiratory Gas Transfer

Although not directly related to the subject of hypoxemia, it is appropriate now to discuss briefly nonrespiratory gas transfer. Inert gases are not bound to hemoglobin; therefore, their movement across the alveolar-capillary membrane is simply a function of density, water solubility, and partial pressure difference. The inhalational *anesthetic gases* have a density greater than oxygen, but they are much more water soluble and, therefore, diffuse much more readily than oxygen through the alveolar-capillary membrane. These gases (nitrous oxide, halothane, ether, etc.) are so water soluble that the partial pressure of these gases in capillary blood rises to the same partial pressure as in the alveoli in less than .1 second. For the remainder of the time that blood remains in the capillary no partial pressure gradient for the gas is present, so that, in a sense, transport of these gases into the body is limited by pulmonary capillary blood flow.

It is critical to remember that the *direction* of movement of gas molecules is determined by the partial pressure gradient. If the gradient is such that the partial pressure of a gas is greater in capillary blood than in the alveoli, gas molecules will travel into the alveoli. Consider what happens with nitrous oxide anesthesia. During anesthesia, the alveolar P_{N_2O} equals end capillary P_{N_2O}. If the patient is no longer given nitrous oxide by inhalation, there is an abrupt drop in alveolar P_{N_2O}, and thus N_2O will pour out of capillary blood into the alveoli. This may dilute the oxygen remaining in the alveoli and cause severe alveolar hypoxia.

Tests of Diffusion Impairment

Because oxygen transfer from alveolus to capillary at rest is perfusion- and not diffusion-limited, measures of oxygenation are not specific for diffusion impairment. The exception is that a drop in arterial P_{O_2} *during exercise* characteristically occurs in patients with an abnormal alveolar-capillary membrane. This is useful in following the course of patients with interstitial lung disease. Indeed, in patients with early disease, the only abnormality present may be a drop in Pa_{O_2} with exercise.

Carbon monoxide is so well bound by hemoglobin that an enormous number of carbon monoxide molecules can be "soaked up" by hemoglobin keeping the pressure of CO in blood low. Thus when CO is inhaled, the P_{CO} of capillary

Table 9.6. Features of Hypoxemia Caused by Impaired Diffusion

At rest seldom the major cause of hypoxemia
In patients causes hypoxemia during exercise and if $P_{I_{O_2}}$ reduced
Hypoxemia improved by O_2 breathing

blood never rises to the P_{CO} of alveolar gas. Therefore, a P_{CO} gradient is present the whole time blood is in the pulmonary capillaries. Thus, CO uptake is limited by diffusion, which depends on the P_{CO} gradient being present. This property of CO is used in tests of diffusion.

Because carbon monoxide transfer is diffusion-limited, tests of carbon monoxide transfer have been used to document impaired diffusion. Several different methods are used to measure carbon monoxide diffusion, the $D_{L_{CO}}$. All the tests involve measurement of CO uptake as a function of the CO driving pressure (the alveolar-capillary P_{CO} difference), which is alveolar P_{CO}, because capillary P_{CO} is so low. The test is interpreted as if diffusion is the only variable affecting CO transfer; mechanisms causing changes in CO transfer are similar to those causing reduced O_2 transfer (see Table 9.5). However, it must be kept in mind that reduced transfer of O_2 or CO is most often caused by ventilation-perfusion mismatching. This should not detract from the usefulness of this test in following the progress or response to treatment of patients with lung disease. $D_{L_{CO}}$ is a sensitive test, but it should be interpreted not simply as an index of impaired diffusion but as an index of impaired transfer that may be caused by impaired diffusion and ventilation-perfusion mismatching.

Treatment of Hypoxemia Caused by Impaired Diffusion

Since diffusion depends on the magnitude of the difference between alveolar and capillary P_{O_2}, diffusion may be increased by increasing this difference. Alveolar P_{O_2} can be markedly increased by simply breathing oxygen.

Reduced Inspired Oxygen Pressure ($P_{I_{O_2}}$)

We have previously discussed how ideal alveolar P_{O_2} is determined by inspired P_{O_2}, alveolar P_{CO_2}, and the respiratory exchange ratio using the simplified alveolar air equation:

$$P_{A_{O_2}} = P_{I_{O_2}} - \frac{P_{a_{CO_2}}}{R}$$

Reduction in inspired P_{O_2} will reduce alveolar P_{O_2}. Oxygen makes up 21% of air. Reduction in barometric pressure causes a reduction in oxygen partial pressure, since the P_{O_2} of ambient air is .21 × barometric pressure (PB). Since

Table 9.7. Features of Hypoxemia Caused by Reduced $P_{I_{O_2}}$

Caused by reduced $P_{A_{O_2}}$
Causes severe hypoxemia when diffusion is impaired
Responds to oxygen breathing

air is always humidified as it enters the respiratory system, the water vapor pressure must be subtracted from the barometric pressure before calculating the oxygen partial pressure of inspired (humidified) air. Thus:

$$P_{I_{O_2}} = .21 \times (PB - 47)$$

Barometric pressure is reduced at high altitude, and $P_{I_{O_2}}$ will be reduced. Patients with lung disease may develop severe hypoxemia when $P_{I_{O_2}}$ is reduced, because the reduction in $P_{A_{O_2}}$ will magnify hypoxemia caused by other mechanisms. In particular, diffusion of oxygen depends on the magnitude of the alveolar-pulmonary capillary P_{O_2} gradient, and the diffusion of O_2 may be seriously impaired when $P_{A_{O_2}}$ is reduced. Thus, patients with impaired diffusion and normal people exercising at high altitude may become seriously hypoxemic. See Chapter 16, which deals in more detail with the problems of high altitude.

OXYGEN STORES

If breathing suddenly stopped, the stores of oxygen in the body can be utilized. Unfortunately, the oxygen stores of the body are small, are rapidly depleted, and can be used as an emergency source of oxygen for only short periods.

Oxygen is stored in the lungs, hemoglobin, body water, and myoglobin. Very little oxygen is stored in body water because of the low solubility of oxygen in water. Myoglobin is a poor emergency store of oxygen, because the oxygen-myoglobin affinity is so high that oxygen is not unloaded from myoglobin until almost lethal hypoxemia is present. Thus, the only useful stores of oxygen are in the lungs and those bound to hemoglobin.

Normally the lungs contain about 400 ml of oxygen, and the hemoglobin binds about 850 ml oxygen. Thus, the total usable oxygen stores are about 1250 ml. Since oxygen consumption is about 200 to 300 ml per minute, it is clear that oxygen stores would be depleted in about 5 minutes of apnea. If preexisting alveolar hypoxia or hypoxemia were present, oxygen stores would be much lower. If alveolar P_{O_2} were 50 mmHg instead of the normal 100 mmHg, the lung would now store about 200 ml of oxygen and hemoglobin about 750 ml of oxygen. Thus, a hypoxic patient has much lower oxygen stores than a normal person and would deplete oxygen stores much more rapidly during apnea. An easy way to increase oxygen stores is to fill up the lungs with oxygen by breathing pure oxygen. This maneuver will increase oxygen stored in the lungs to 2000 to 3000 ml.

Because oxygen stores are usually so small, changes in ventilation or $P_{I_{O_2}}$ will result in rapid changes in alveolar P_{O_2} with half the change in $P_{A_{O_2}}$ occurring within the first minute. In contrast, because of the huge body stores of CO_2, P_{CO_2} changes much more slowly when ventilation is changed. Thus, early during apnea or hypoventilation, P_{O_2} falls much more rapidly than P_{CO_2} rises.

THE SEQUELAE OF HYPOXEMIA

Hypoxemia will result in compensatory responses by the organ systems concerned with oxygen transport (respiratory, cardiovascular, and hematopoietic systems) and dysfunction of tissues most sensitive to oxygen lack (nervous tissue). These responses to hypoxemia (polycythemia and pulmonary vasoconstriction) may themselves cause severe problems and may become *maladaptive.*

Compensatory Responses to Hypoxemia

Respiratory

Arterial hypoxemia stimulates the carotid body, which sends impulses to the respiratory pacemaker in the medulla. This causes an increase in ventilation (Chapter 6). The increase in ventilation will lower P_{CO_2} and thus increase alveolar P_{O_2}, since ideal alveolar $P_{O_2} = P_{I_{O_2}} - (Pa_{CO_2})/R$. It now appears that hypoxemia itself may blunt this response and that this blunting is related to the severity and the duration of hypoxemia. When hypoxemia is especially severe (P_{O_2} less than 30 mmHg), there may occur within minutes direct depression of the neural cells in the respiratory pacemaker, which depresses ventilation. Less severe hypoxemia also causes blunting of the ventilatory response; it may take years to decades of mild hypoxemia for this to occur (see Chapter 6).

Cardiovascular

Since it takes several days for newly produced red blood cells to begin to appear after exposure to hypoxia, this response cannot compensate for an acute reduction in oxygen delivery. This leaves the cardiovascular system to play a critical role in improving oxygen delivery when acute hypoxemia is present. The cardiovascular system responds to hypoxemia in two ways. First, there is an increase in cardiac output due to an increase in stroke volume and heart rate. This response, however, may diminish after several days of hypoxemia. Second, there occurs a redistribution of blood flow, so that the flow to the heart and brain is increased out of proportion to the increase in

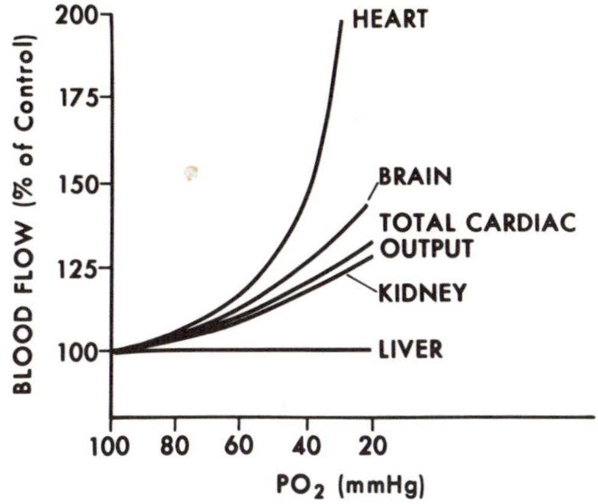

Figure 9.23. Blood flow to various organs with hypoxemia. Notice that the organs most sensitive to oxygen lack (the brain and heart) show the greatest increase in flow, and the changes are out of proportion to the changes in cardiac output.

cardiac output (Figure 9.23). This is advantageous, since the beating heart and the brain have high metabolic rates and are particularly vulnerable to oxygen lack. In spite of the increase in cerebral blood flow, hypoxemia still regularly causes brain dysfunction (see below).

Pulmonary arteriolar constriction occurs when airway hypoxia is present. If there are regions in the lung that are more hypoxic than others, this mechanism will redirect blood to the better ventilated regions, improve ventilation-perfusion matching, and thus increase arterial Po_2. However, when all lung regions are hypoxic, as often occurs with diffuse lung diseases, this response will lead to generalized pulmonary vasoconstriction, which causes *pulmonary hypertension* (Figure 9.24). Hypercapnia also causes pulmonary vasoconstriction and has a synergistic effect on hypoxic vasoconstriction. Pulmonary hypertension represents an increased afterload to the right ventricle. Thus, to maintain cardiac output there must be an increase in the work of the right ventricle. Ultimately there may occur right ventricular failure resulting in venous hypertension and edema formation in the dependent portions of the body. Heart failure caused by lung disease is called *cor pulmonale.*

Hematopoietic

A reduction in tissue Po_2 results in the elaboration of a factor, erythropoietin, which increases red blood cell production (Figure 9.25). About 90 to 95% of erythropoietin production is dependent on the kidney; the remainder is dependent on the liver. These organs do not actually produce erythropoietin but may elaborate an enzyme that changes an inactive circulating precursor of erythropoietin into active erythropoietin. Another hypothesis gaining favor is that under normal circumstances the kidney produces an inhibitor that inacti-

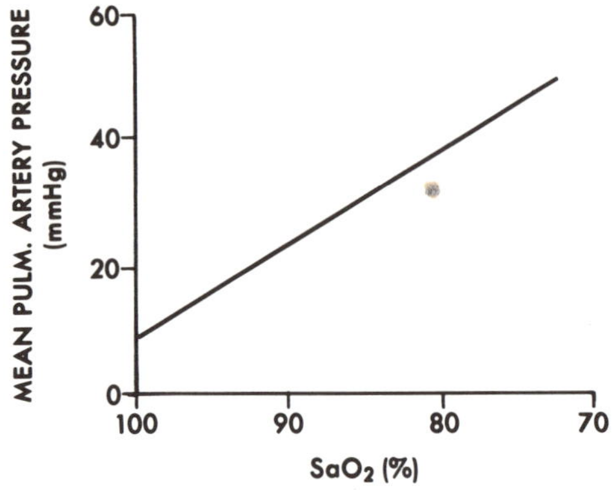

Figure 9.24. Mean pulmonary artery pressure in hypoxemic patients with chronic airflow obstruction. (Adapted from Enson Y, Giuntini C, Lewis ML, et al: *J Clin Invest* 43:1146, 1964.)

vates erythropoietin and that with an hypoxic stimulus there occurs inactivation of the inhibitor.

An increase in red blood cell production results in an increased hemoglobin concentration and, therefore, an increased oxygen-carrying capacity. An increased red cell mass is called *polycythemia*, or more correctly, *erythrocytosis.* Initially the increased oxygen-carrying capacity is beneficial, since oxygen delivery may be maintained with a lower Sa_{O_2}. The problem is that when polycythemia is severe, the blood becomes viscous and literally attains the consistency of molasses, which increases the work load of the right ventricle and causes a marked reduction in cerebral blood flow.

Nervous System Dysfunction with Hypoxemia

The nervous system is very sensitive to oxygen lack (see Chapter 16). Only 10 to 15 seconds after cessation of cerebral blood flow (as occurs with cardiac asystole) unconsciousness occurs. Hypoxemia when mild causes reversible abnormalities in neural function. Hypoxemia when severe and prolonged causes death of neural cells. Because these cells do not regenerate, anoxic brain damage is permanent.

Hypoxemia causes an increase in cerebral blood flow that is out of proportion to the increased cardiac output. In spite of this, deficits in neurological function can be detected even with mild hypoxemia. Most of the data available was obtained in persons made acutely hypoxemic (see Figure 16.2).

The rods of the retina are highly sensitive to hypoxemia. A detectable reduction in night vision (which is mediated only by the rods) occurs when Po_2 is reduced to 65 to 75 mmHg (Sa_{O_2} 91 to 94%). This degree of hypoxemia is encountered at altitudes of 5,000 to 6,000 feet (1.5 to 2 km). With more severe hypoxemia (Po_2 about 50 mmHg, Sa_{O_2} about 85%), there occurs constriction of the visual fields, enlargement of the blind spot, and decreased color discrimination involving primarily loss of red sensitivity.

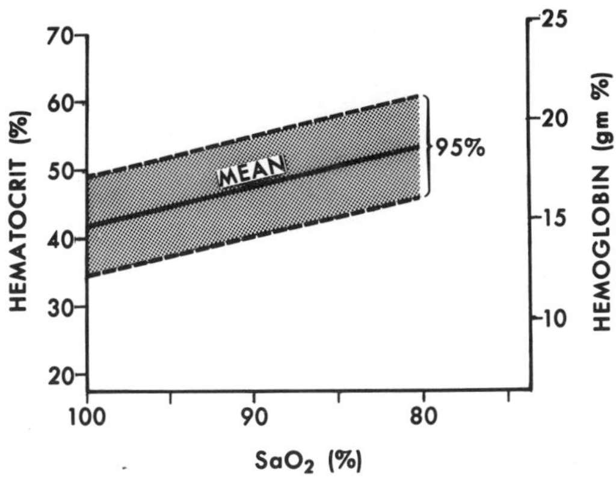

Figure 9.25. Red cell response to hypoxemia. This data was obtained from normal persons living at different altitudes. (Figure redrawn from Weil J, Jamieson G, Brown DW, et al: *J Clin Invest* 47:1627, 1968.)

With still more severe hypoxemia (Po_2 35 to 50 mmHg), serious but reversible deterioration in cerebral cortical function (orientation, arithmetic tasks, memory, psychomotor tasks) occurs and restlessness and confusion are common. When Po_2 falls below 30 mmHg, loss of consciousness occurs. When PO_2 falls below 20 mmHg for just a few minutes, *irreversible* damage of neural cells occurs.

BIBLIOGRAPHY

Comroe JH, Forster RE, Dubois AB, et al: *The Lung*, ed 2. Chicago, Year Book Medical Publishers, 1962, p 77.

Finch CA, Lenfant C: Oxygen transport in man. *New Engl J Med* 286:407, 1972.

Nunn JF: Distribution of pulmonary blood flow, in Nunn JF: *Applied Respiratory Physiology*. London, Butterworth, 1977, p 274.

Nunn JF: Diffusion, in Nunn JF: *Applied Respiratory Physiology*. London, Butterworth, 1977, p 310.

Nunn JF: Oxygen, in Nunn JF: *Applied Respiratory Physiology*. London, Butterworth, 1977, p 375.

Robin ED: Of men and mitochondria: Coping with hypoxic dysoxia. *Am Rev Resp Dis* 122:517, 1980.

West JB: *Ventilation/Blood Flow and Gas Exchange*, ed 3. Oxford, Blackwell Scientific Publications, 1977.

West JB: Ventilation-perfusion relationships. *Am Rev Resp Dis* 116:919, 1977.

10

Respiratory Failure 2: Carbon Dioxide

Meir H. Kryger

Gas exchange occurs not only at the lung-pulmonary capillary interface but also at the tissue-systemic capillary interface. Gas exchange in the tissues involves transfer of O_2 from red cells to metabolizing cells and transfer of CO_2 from the metabolizing cells to red cells. Carbon dioxide is by far the major waste product of metabolism. CO_2 is then carried in venous blood to the lungs.

CARBON DIOXIDE TRANSPORT

Aerobic metabolism occurs in mitochondria. Membranes are freely permeable to CO_2 which traverses by diffusion, the mitochondrial membrane, the cellular cytoplasm, the cell membrane, and interstitial space before entering blood. Diffusion depends on the presence of a partial pressure gradient for CO_2 for each of these steps.

When CO_2 diffuses into the blood, most enters red blood cells, while the remainder stays in the plasma (Figure 10.1). In the plasma CO_2 may take part

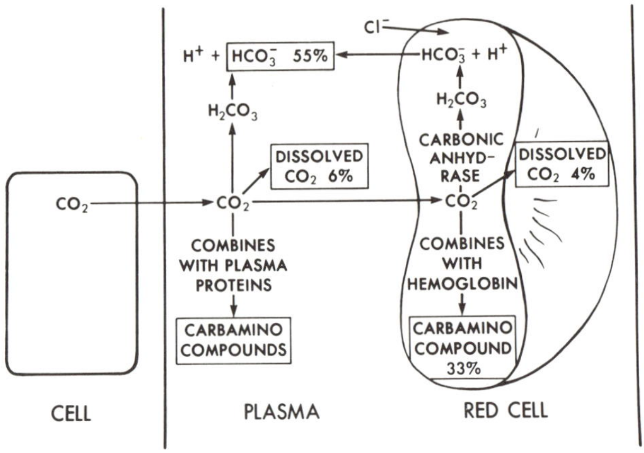

Figure 10.1. CO_2 produced by metabolism is transported in the blood in several forms. 55% of the produced CO_2 that is excreted is carried as the HCO_3^- ion; 33% is combined with hemoglobin, and the remainder is dissolved or combined with plasma proteins. (Data obtained from Table 26 in Nunn JF: Carbon Dioxide, in Nunn JF: *Applied Respiratory Physiology*. London, Butterworth, 1977, p. 334.)

in one of three reactions. First, CO_2 may dissolve in the plasma. The volume of CO_2 taken up by blood in solution is small (100 ml of plasma will dissolve about .067 ml of CO_2 for each 1 mmHg P_{CO_2}). Since arterial P_{CO_2} is about 40 mmHg and venous P_{CO_2} is 46 mmHg, the amount of CO_2 taken up by 100 ml plasma is only $(46 - 40) \times .067 = .4$ ml. Second, the CO_2 may be hydrated by the reaction $CO_2 + H_2O \rightleftharpoons H_2CO_3 \rightleftharpoons H^+ + HCO_3^-$. This is a slow reaction, since plasma lacks the enzyme carbonic anhydrase, which can increase the reaction rate 13,000 times. Finally, CO_2 can be bound by plasma proteins forming *carbamino compounds*. These three reactions occurring in plasma only account for a small fraction of the CO_2 taken up by the blood.

Most of the CO_2 diffusing into the blood enters red blood cells. A small quantity of the CO_2 dissolves. Red blood cells contain the enzyme carbonic anhydrase, which catalyzes the reaction:

$$CO_2 + H_2O \xrightleftharpoons[\text{anhydrase}]{\text{carbonic}} H_2CO_3 \rightleftharpoons H^+ + HCO_3^-$$

The H^+ formed is soaked up and buffered by hemoglobin. When this occurs the configuration of the molecule changes in such a way as to reduce the affinity of hemoglobin for oxygen, thus facilitating oxygen unloading. This is called the *Bohr effect*. The HCO_3^- formed by the above reaction leaves the red cell, because the red cell membrane is very permeable to negatively charged particles (HCO_3^- or Cl^-) but not very permeable to positively charged ions. As HCO_3^- diffuses out of the cell into the plasma, the interior of the cells has an excess of positive ions. Chloride ions (Cl^-) shift from the plasma into the red blood cells to re-establish electroneutrality.

Hemoglobin, besides being able to buffer H^+, can also combine directly with CO_2 forming carbamino groups:

$$\text{Hb}-\underset{|}{\overset{\text{H}}{\text{N}}}-\text{H} + CO_2 \rightleftharpoons \text{Hb}-\overset{\text{H}}{\underset{}{\text{N}}}-\underset{\|}{\text{C}}\text{OH} \rightleftharpoons \text{Hb}-\overset{\text{H}}{\text{N}}-\underset{\underset{\text{O}}{\|}}{\text{C}}-\text{O}^- + H^+$$

Thus, hemoglobin can combine with CO_2 and then buffer the hydrogen ions produced. The amount of CO_2 that can combine with hemoglobin and the amount of hydrogen ions that can be buffered are both affected by the state of oxygenation. Unoxygenated hemoglobin combines more readily with CO_2 to form carbamino compounds (the *Haldane effect*) and is a better buffer (can accept more H^+ ions) than oxygenated hemoglobin.

Thus, carbon dioxide affects hemoglobin-oxygen affinity and, therefore, the loading and unloading of O_2 (Bohr effect). Conversely, oxygen affects the loading and unloading of CO_2 (Haldane effect). These interactions are complementary in the tissues and the lung and facilitate gas exchange at both locations (Figure 10.2).

In the lungs, CO_2 leaves mixed venous blood (P_{CO_2} 46 mmHg) and enters alveolar gas (P_{CO_2} 40 mmHg) by diffusion. Since most of the CO_2 is carried as bicarbonate, the reverse of the processes described in Figure 10.1 occurs. Bicarbonate ions (HCO_3^-) shift back into the red cells where carbonic anhy-

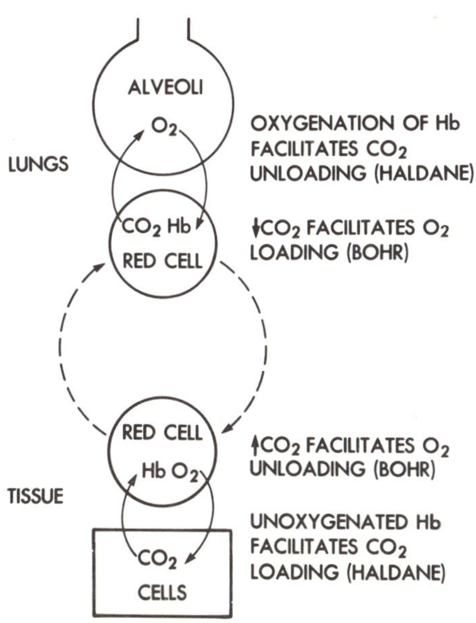

Figure 10.2. The Bohr and Haldane effects are complementary both in the lung and tissues in facilitating gas exchange.

drase catalyzes the reverse reaction to form CO_2. Oxygenation of hemoglobin reduces the amount of CO_2 that can be kept as carbamino groups. The CO_2 that "appears" by these mechanisms rapidly diffuses into alveolar gas.

Since CO_2 is carried by a system of different "carriers," CO_2 cannot saturate its transport system as oxygen saturates the O_2 combining sites on the hemoglobin molecule. The CO_2 carrying system is so efficient that even a severe reduction in hemoglobin will not result in reduced CO_2 transport. This is because red blood cells have an excess of carbonic anhydrase (even in anemia), and so, when anemia is present more CO_2 is carried as HCO_3^- in the plasma. When carbonic anhydrase effect is reduced (as with acetazolamide), CO_2 still is hydrated in the plasma but more slowly. The problem is that when blood reaches the pulmonary capillaries there may be insufficient time for the conversion of HCO_3^- to CO_2 to occur, and so there may be reduced transfer of CO_2 from blood to alveoli.

As we have seen (Figure 9.10), increasing ventilation above normal increases $P_{A_{O_2}}$ but does not increase S_{O_2} or arterial O_2 content. This is because O_2 saturates its carrier system; this is shown by the flat portion of the oxyhemoglobin dissociation curve. This contrasts with the effect of increasing ventilation, which reduces both $P_{A_{CO_2}}$ and the CO_2 content of blood. CO_2 cannot saturate its carriers; there is no flat portion of the CO_2 dissociation curve. P_{CO_2} and CO_2 content are linearly related in the entire physiological range (Figure 10.3). The importance of these differences is that a well-ventilated region will be able to compensate for the reduced CO_2 transfer but not the reduced O_2 transfer of a poorly ventilated region.

Carbon Dioxide Stores

In contrast to the small oxygen stores in the body, carbon dioxide stores are much, much larger, exceeding 100 liters. CO_2 is dissolved in body water and is also stored as HCO_3^- in plasma, cells, and interstitial fluid. In addition, CO_2 is stored in bone as CO_3^{--}. Because of the very large stores, and because some of

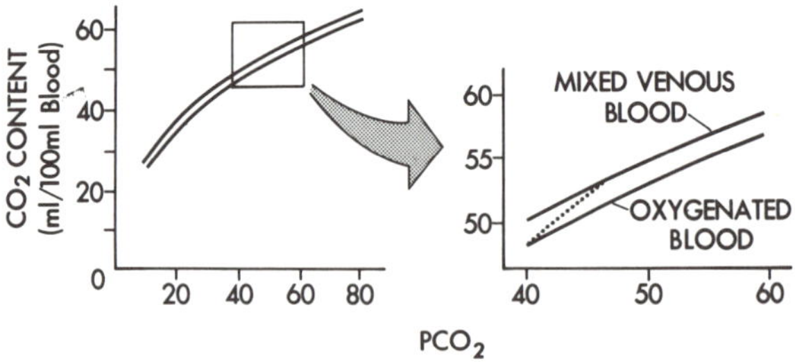

Figure 10.3. The relationship of P_{CO_2} in mmHg to CO_2 content of blood. The right-hand figure represents data in the physiological range and shows that the relationship is linear. The dotted line connects the venous and arterial lines and represents the change in CO_2 content of blood on undergoing gas exchange in the lung.

the stores (bone) have slow turnover of CO_2, a change in ventilation results in a much slower change in P_{CO_2} than P_{O_2}.

CAUSES OF HYPERCAPNIA

Hypercapnia, an elevation of arterial P_{CO_2} is caused by hypoventilation and mismatching of ventilation and perfusion. CO_2 is a very soluble gas, which diffuses so rapidly across the alveolar-capillary membrane that its diffusion is not limited by diseases in which the alveolar-capillary membrane is grossly abnormal.

Hypoventilation

Hypoventilation is present when alveolar ventilation is inadequate to meet the metabolic requirements of the body. By metabolic requirements is meant oxygen uptake and carbon dioxide elimination. Hypoventilation will result in elevation of alveolar P_{CO_2} and a reduction in alveolar P_{O_2} and, therefore, hypercapnia (elevated arterial blood P_{CO_2}) and hypoxemia. Hypoventilation as a cause of hypoxemia is described in the previous chapter.

Regardless of the level of ventilation, in the steady state CO_2 elimination must equal CO_2 production. If ventilation is reduced but CO_2 production is constant, this means that in order for CO_2 output to remain constant, more CO_2 must be eliminated for every liter of alveolar ventilation. Similarly, if CO_2 production is increased but ventilation remains constant, more CO_2 must be eliminated for every liter of alveolar ventilation. How can more CO_2 be eliminated for every liter of alveolar ventilation? This can be accomplished by increasing the concentration of CO_2 in alveolar gas. Since the concentration of a gas is linearly related to the partial pressure of the gas, this can be accomplished by increasing alveolar P_{CO_2}.

In the steady state, CO_2 output = alveolar ventilation × alveolar CO_2 concentration or;

$$\text{alveolar } CO_2 \text{ concentration} = \frac{CO_2 \text{ output}}{\text{alveolar ventilation}}$$

The relationship may be expressed in terms of alveolar P_{CO_2}:

$$P_{A_{CO_2}} \text{ (mmHg)} = \frac{CO_2 \text{ output}}{\text{alveolar ventilation}} \times .863 = \frac{\dot{V}_{CO_2}}{\dot{V}_A} \times .863$$

where .863 is the factor that compensates for the different units used to express the variables in this equation, $\dot{V}_{CO_2}$ is ml/min and $\dot{V}_A$ is l/min.

This important equation says that if ventilation does not rise proportionately as CO_2 output rises, P_{CO_2} will rise. Thus, P_{CO_2} is an index of the adequacy of ventilation in meeting the metabolic requirement of CO_2 elimination. Since arterial P_{CO_2} (Pa_{CO_2}) equals alveolar P_{CO_2}, Pa_{CO_2} is an index of alveolar ventila-

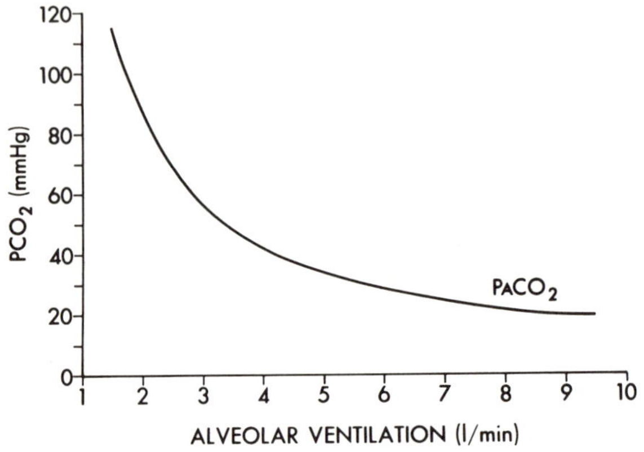

Figure 10.4. The relationship between alveolar ventilation and Pco_2 in mmHg when CO_2 production is 200 ml/minute. Note that the relationship is steep when ventilation is low and flat when ventilation is high.

tion. Pa_{CO_2} is elevated above the normal range (Pco_2 35 to 45 mmHg) when alveolar hypoventilation is present.

The relationship between alveolar ventilation and Pco_2 is shown in Figure 10.4. The relationship is not linear. An identical change in alveolar ventilation will have a dramatically different effect on Pco_2 depending on whether hypoventilation or hyperventilation were initially present. Thus, when hypercapnia is present, Pco_2 is very sensitive to small changes in ventilation. When hypocapnia is present, Pco_2 is not sensitive to small changes in ventilation. The importance of these facts is that a patient who has a high Pco_2 will have large changes in Pco_2 with small changes in ventilation. Thus, a small decrease in ventilation in a hypercapnic patient can have disastrous effects. On the other hand, a small increase in alveolar ventilation can dramatically lower the Pco_2.

Hypoventilation occurs when the control of ventilation is abnormal or when weakness of the respiratory muscles is present (Chapter 6).

Diseases of abnormal control of ventilation (Table 10.1) include disorders involving the chemoreceptors and the respiratory center (or pacemaker). Drugs are a common cause of a depressed chemical drive. Weakness of the respiratory muscles occurs when the efferent neural pathways from the medulla to the respiratory muscles are abnormal, when the neuromuscular function is abnormal, or when the muscles themselves are abnormal.

Diseases of the airways and of the thoracic cage may also cause hypoventilation. As will be discussed below, a $\dot{V}/\dot{Q}$ disturbance can cause the hypercapnia, which is then permitted to persist by depressed or absent hypercapnic drive.

Mismatching of Ventilation and Perfusion

Mismatching of ventilation and perfusion can cause hypercapnia. Capillary blood leaving a low $\dot{V}/\dot{Q}$ region will have a low Po_2 *and* a high Pco_2. The Pco_2

Table 10.1 Causes of Hypoventilation

Reduced drive to breathe
Disorders of medulla
Idiopathic hypoventilation, infections, drugs, bleeding, trauma, syringomyelia
Muscle weakness
Disorders of spinal cord
Transection
Anterior horn cell dysfunction
Disorders of nerves
Guillain-Barré
Disorders of neuromuscular junction or muscle
Myasthenia gravis
Myotonic dystrophy
Reduced drive and abnormal lungs or chest wall
Airways obstruction (blue bloater)
Obesity
Kyphoscoliosis

of very low $\dot{V}/\dot{Q}$ regions is similar to the mixed venous P_{CO_2}. Figure 10.5 shows what may occur to CO_2 homeostasis when there occurs $\dot{V}/\dot{Q}$ mismatching. In this example, CO_2 production is 200 ml per minute and the alveolar P_{CO_2} of the lung units is 40 mmHg.

Each blood vessel dumps 100 ml of CO_2 into each lung unit. Now suppose one unit becomes very obstructed but is still being perfused and that its $\dot{V}/\dot{Q}$ approaches zero. Virtually no CO_2 will be dumped into the unit, and the capillary blood leaving the unit will have a P_{CO_2} of 46 mmHg. The blood flow to the normal unit will dump 100 ml of CO_2 into that lung unit, and the capillary blood leaving the unit will have a P_{CO_2} of 40 mmHg. The immediate result of this is that arterial P_{CO_2} has gone up by 3 mmHg, but also that only 100 ml of the 200 ml of CO_2 that were produced were eliminated. In the steady state, CO_2 elimination must equal CO_2 production. In this situation, CO_2 elimination can be increased to normal by one of three mechanisms.

First, an increase of blood flow to the normal region will increase CO_2 elimination by that region, since every 100 ml/minute of blood flow will dump 4.1 ml (52 − 47.9) of CO_2 into the well-ventilated alveolus.

Second, if ventilation of the normal region were increased, the CO_2 content of the blood leaving the unit would be reduced. The greater the ventilation of that unit the lower will be the CO_2 content of blood leaving the unit. This can compensate for the high CO_2 content of blood leaving the low $\dot{V}/\dot{Q}$ region. Thus, a high $\dot{V}/\dot{Q}$ region can compensate for a low $\dot{V}/\dot{Q}$ region as far as CO_2 is concerned. This is in contrast with the situation for O_2. When ventilation is normal, S_{O_2} is almost 100%, an increase in ventilation will not materially increase the O_2 content of blood leaving that region. Thus, a high $\dot{V}/\dot{Q}$ region can compensate for the hypercapnia but not for the hypoxemia caused by low $\dot{V}/\dot{Q}$. What then will stimulate ventilation when $\dot{V}/\dot{Q}$ mismatching is present?

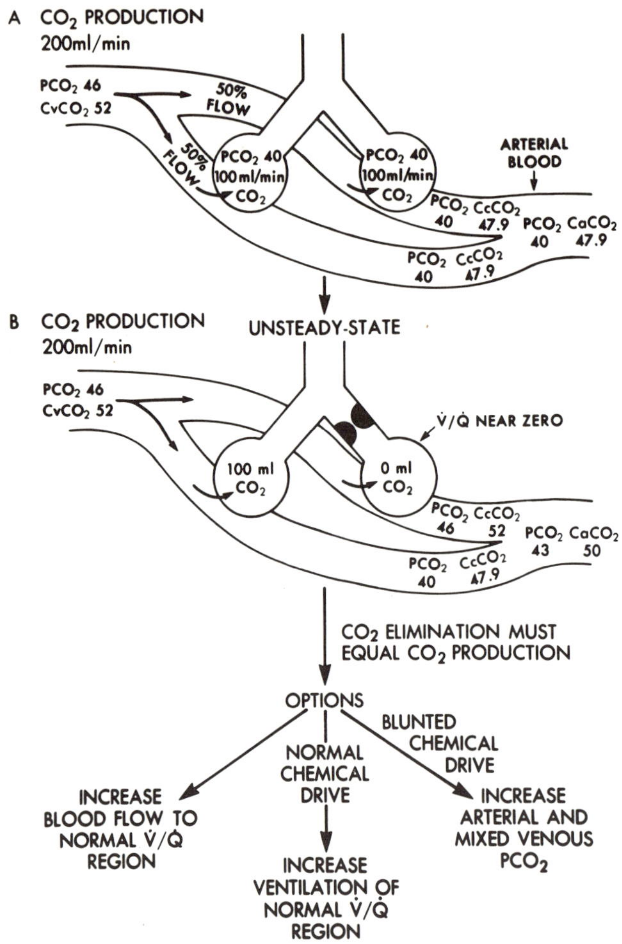

Figure 10.5. In the presence of $\dot{V}/\dot{Q}$ mismatching, in order for CO_2 elimination to equal CO_2 production, one of three things may occur: blood flow to normal $\dot{V}/\dot{Q}$ regions may increase, ventilation may increase, or an increase in P_{CO_2} of blood is allowed to occur. The last sequence is allowed to occur when the chemical drive to breathe is depressed.

The cause of the increased ventilation is the ventilatory control system. When disease of the interstitial space is present, ventilation is "driven" by vagally mediated reflexes (see Chapter 6). Hypercapnia is unusual in diseases of the interstitial space. When airway disease is present, the hypoxemia and hypercapnia stimulate chemoreceptors, which results in an increase in ventilation. The most common blood gas abnormality in lung disease is this pattern; normal Pa_{CO_2} and low Pa_{O_2}. In such patients, hypercapnia usually only occurs as a terminal event.

The third mechanism that will restore CO_2 elimination to normal is simply not changing ventilation or blood flow. Arterial and mixed venous P_{CO_2} will increase until CO_2 elimination equals CO_2 production, i.e., until 200 ml CO_2 are eliminated in the ventilating region. When this occurs, twice as much CO_2 is being eliminated in that region and $P_{A_{CO_2}}$ will rise from 40 to 80 mmHg. Thus, one way to allow CO_2 elimination to return to normal is to simply allow hypercapnia to occur. Clearly this course is dependent on an absent or depressed hypercapnic drive to breathe. This combination, $\dot{V}/\dot{Q}$ mismatching and blunted hypercapnic drive, is found in some patients with chronic airflow obstruction with the "blue-bloater" profile and in patients who have the obesity-hypoventilation syndrome. Persons with absent chemical drive such as those with idiopathic hypoventilation may develop fulminant respiratory failure with mild respiratory infections because of the inability to respond to the hypercapnia. In summary, lung diseases cause $\dot{V}/\dot{Q}$ mismatching, which causes hypercapnia. The presence or absence of chemical drives to breathe determines whether the hypercapnia is allowed to persist.

Dead Space

Not all inspired air reaches alveoli. Therefore not all inspired air participates in gas exchange. One reason is, of course, that no gas exchange occurs in the conducting airways. The volume of gas that does not mix with alveolar gas is called *anatomic dead space.* The volume of the conducting airways is roughly about 1 cc per pound weight of the subject.

Occasionally, a patient may have a very low tidal volume that is only slightly greater than the volume of the conducting airways; yet gas exchange in this circumstance may be adequate. The reasons for this apparent paradox are as follows: in small airways flow is laminar with the center of the stream traveling faster and "penetrating" further into the lung; the contracting heart actually shakes the lung facilitating gas mixing; gas diffusion down a concentration gradient is a rather rapid process. Recently it has been shown that entirely normal gas exchange may be obtained by simply applying a high frequency pressure wave to the lungs, that is, shaking the lung with no measurable tidal volume!

Artificial airways, tracheostomy tubes and endotracheal tubes, can markedly reduce the size of the anatomic dead space.

Because of maldistribution of ventilation and perfusion, even air reaching alveoli may not take part in gas exchange at all (if the alveoli are unperfused) or the ventilation may be "wasted" if the alveoli are underperfused (high $\dot{V}/\dot{Q}$ regions). The *physiological dead space* is the volume of gas that behaves as if it did not participate in gas exchange. Figure 10.6 shows that the gas of air that is "wasted" in the conducting airways or in alveoli contains little CO_2. The more wasted ventilation present, the lower will be the mixed expired P_{CO_2}. The proportion of the tidal volume that does not participate in gas exchange, the physiological dead space/tidal volume ratio (V_D/V_T), is calculated using the equation:

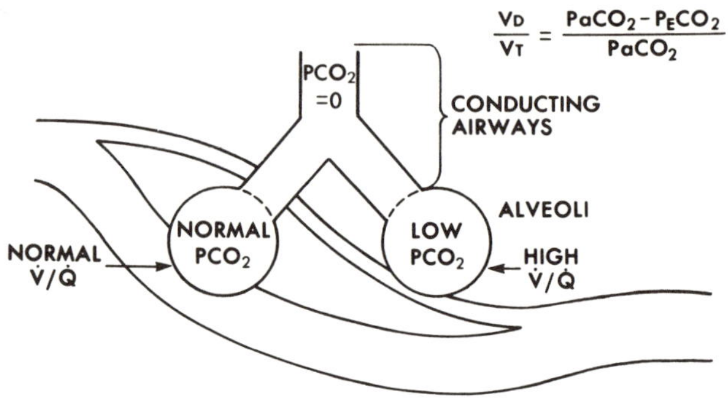

Figure 10.6. Anatomical deadspace and low $\dot{V}/\dot{Q}$ regions have very low P_{CO_2}. Thus the greater the wasted ventilation, the smaller will be the mixed expired P_{CO_2} ($P_{E_{CO_2}}$), and the higher will be the deadspace tidal volume ratio V_D/V_T.

$$\frac{V_D}{V_T} = \frac{Pa_{CO_2} - P_{E_{CO_2}}}{Pa_{CO_2}}$$

where $P_{E_{CO_2}}$ is the mixed expired P_{CO_2}. If we had perfect alveoli simply connected to the outside without conducting airways, $P_{E_{CO_2}}$ would be Pa_{CO_2} and therefore V_D/V_T would be 0.

SEQUELAE OF HYPERCAPNIA

Acidosis

The effect of CO_2 on acid-base regulation is also discussed in Chapter 12. CO_2 in the gas phase (alveolar gas) is in equilibrium with the CO_2 in aqueous solution. CO_2 dissolved in water is in equilibrium with carbonic acid, H_2CO_3:

$$CO_2 + H_2O \rightleftharpoons H_2CO_3$$

Carbonic acid dissociates by the equation:

$$H_2CO_3 \rightleftharpoons H^+ + HCO_3^-$$

The overall reaction can be written as:

$$\text{alveolar } CO_2 \rightleftharpoons CO_2 + H_2O \rightleftharpoons H_2CO_3 \rightleftharpoons H^+ + HCO_3^-$$

Thus, an elevation in P_{CO_2} drives the reactions to the right and causes an increase in $[H^+]$ or a reduction in pH.

Because CO_2 crosses cell membranes so easily, an elevation in P_{CO_2} causes an elevation in intracellular P_{CO_2} and hence in intracellular $[H^+]$. Since transfer of H^+ across membranes is much slower than CO_2, the H^+ ions are at least temporarily "trapped." Thus, CO_2 is an acid capable of raising the intracellular concentration of hydrogen ions. The intracellular acidosis interferes with many enzymatic reactions requiring a normal pH.

The effect of changes in P_{CO_2} on pH can be calculated from the Henderson-Hasselbalch equation:

$$pH = pK' + \log \frac{[HCO_3^-]}{[CO_2 + H_2CO_3]}$$

where CO_2 is the dissolved CO_2. The squared brackets ([ ]) indicate concentration. The quantity of dissolved CO_2 (in mmoles) is several hundred times greater than the H_2CO_3 concentration, so the latter term may be ignored. The quantity of CO_2 dissolved equals $\alpha \times P_{CO_2}$, where α is a specific solubility factor for CO_2 and equals .03 and $pK' = 6.1$. Thus, we may rewrite the above equation as:

$$pH = 6.1 + \log \frac{[HCO_3^-]}{[.03 \times P_{CO_2}]}$$

Thus, raising P_{CO_2} will lower the pH (Figure 10.7).

Buffering. Defense of pH occurs in several phases when respiratory acidosis occurs. The first line of defense, chemical buffering, is rapid. Buffering by the blood is instantaneous. Buffers are substances that minimize changes in pH when H^+ is added. Buffers consist of a weak acid and its conjugate base, a

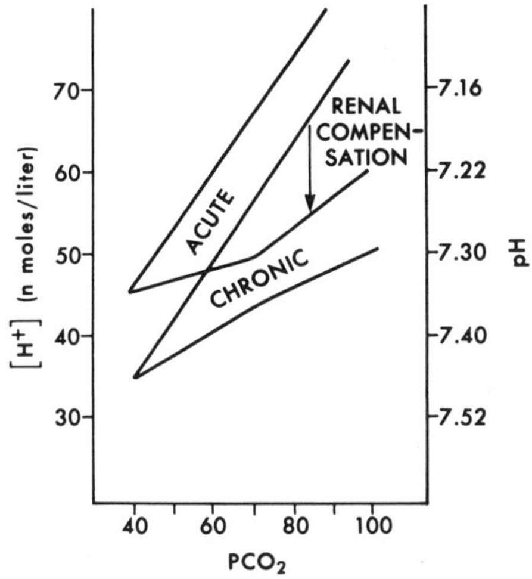

Figure 10.7. Effect of hypercapnia on $[H^+]$ and pH. Acute hypercapnia causes severe acidemia, because renal compensation, which is slow, has not had a chance to occur. (Adapted, with permission, from Weiss EB, Dulfano MJ: Quantitative Acid-base Dynamics in Chronic Pulmonary Disease. Defense of pH During Acute Respiratory Acidosis Superimposed upon Chronic Hypercapnia. *Ann Intern Med* 69:263, 1968).

buffer pair. The H^+ ion of a strong acid reacts with the conjugate base to form a weak acid:

H^+X^-	+	A^-	→	HA	+	X^-
Strong acid		Conjugate base		Weak acid		Anion

In this example, A^- and HA are the buffer pair (conjugate base and weak acid). The major buffer pairs in the blood are:

Plasma	*Red Blood Cells*
HCO_3^-/H_2CO_3	HCO_3^-/H_2CO_3
$HPO_4^=/H_2PO_4^-$	Hb^-/HHb
Pr^-/HPr	$HbO^-/HHbO$

Pr^- is plasma protein; Hb^- is unoxygenated hemoglobin; HbO^- is oxygenated hemoglobin. Functionally, the buffer pairs may be divided into two groups, the carbonic acid-bicarbonate buffer pair and the so-called nonbicarbonate buffer pairs that are made up of all the remaining buffer pairs. This group can be abbreviated the $HBuf/Buf^-$ pair. Not all the buffer pairs can buffer carbonic acid. As will be discussed in the next chapter, a buffer pair cannot buffer one of its own components. Thus, the HCO_3^-/H_2CO_3 buffer pair cannot buffer the H^+ produced by carbonic acid, because if the HCO_3^- buffered this H^+, this would merely produce more H_2CO_3.

Thus, buffering of carbonic acid is accomplished by the *nonbicarbonate buffers* (abbreviated Buf^-) by the reaction:

$$CO_2 + H_2O \rightarrow H_2CO_3 + Buf^- \rightarrow HBuf + HCO_3^-$$

In this reaction, the carbonic acid is buffered by the nonbicarbonate buffer, but notice, that for every molecule of Buf^- used, one molecule of HCO_3^- is generated. This elevation in $[HCO_3^-]$ reflects the buffering that has occurred with an acute elevation of P_{CO_2}. $[HCO_3^-]$ rises only about 1 mEq/L for every 10 mmHg rise in P_{CO_2}. Almost all the buffering of H_2CO_3 is done by hemoglobin, proteins, and phosphates. It has been shown that buffering by blood is much different than buffering by the whole body. At the same P_{CO_2}, the rise in $[HCO_3^-]$ is less when the whole body rather than blood is used as a buffer (Figure 10.8). In the body, the interstitial space fluid (which occupies a much larger space than the vascular space) contains no hemoglobin and very little protein. Its main buffer is HCO_3^- which, as we have said, does not buffer H_2CO_3. Thus the interstitial space does not experience a direct increase in $[HCO_3^-]$ from buffering H_2CO_3. The $[HCO_3^-]$ *of the blood* rises with H_2CO_3 buffering, and this HCO_3^- leaks into the interstitial space. This explains why the whole body has a lower than expected $[HCO_3^-]$ with hypercapnia.

Renal Compensation. The second defense against respiratory acidosis involves the kidney. The kidney can secrete H^+ directly, and for every mole of H^+ secreted, one mole of HCO_3^- is generated. In addition, the kidney can resorb

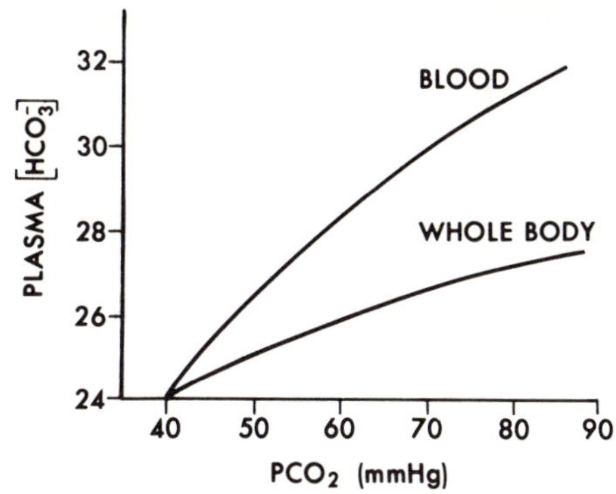

Figure 10.8. Buffering by the blood alone compared with buffering by the whole body. The difference can be explained by the fact that a significant part of the body is interstitial space, which contains mainly bicarbonate, which cannot buffer rises in P_{CO_2}.

virtually all the HCO_3^- in the glomerular fluid. These mechanisms are slow, requiring hours to days to become apparent. Maximal compensation may require a week. As a result of the increase in $[HCO_3^-]$, pH will return toward normal. When compensation is complete, $[HCO_3^-]$ usually will have risen by about 4 mEq/liter for every 10 mmHg increase in P_{CO_2} (see Figure 12.7).

Acute on Chronic Respiratory Acidosis

Patients with chronic respiratory acidosis often develop an acute exacerbation of their disease, usually caused by an infection or a narcotic-sedative drug that depresses the drive to breathe. Because the $[HCO_3^-]$ is already high, the pH will be higher at a given P_{CO_2} than with a pure acute respiratory acidosis alone. This is called *acute on chronic respiratory acidosis.*

Circulation

The effect of hypercapnia on the circulation is complex. In addition to a direct relaxing effect on vascular smooth muscle, hypercapnia causes an increase in the activity of the sympathetic nervous system. This causes vascular smooth muscle contraction and has an inotropic effect on the heart. Thus with hypercapnia, a hyperkinetic circulation, an increased cardiac output with bounding pulses, is common. When hypercapnia becomes very severe, the effect of acidosis predominates and a reduction in cardiac output and blood pressure may occur. Although hypercapnia usually causes an increase in cardiac output, cerebral blood flow rises far out of proportion to the increase in cardiac output (Figure 10.9). At first glance, this is advantageous in a hypoventilating patient who is also hypoxemic, since this will increase O_2 delivery to the brain. As we shall see below, this may also cause cerebral edema. Hypercapnia and the associated acidosis causes *pulmonary arterial con-*

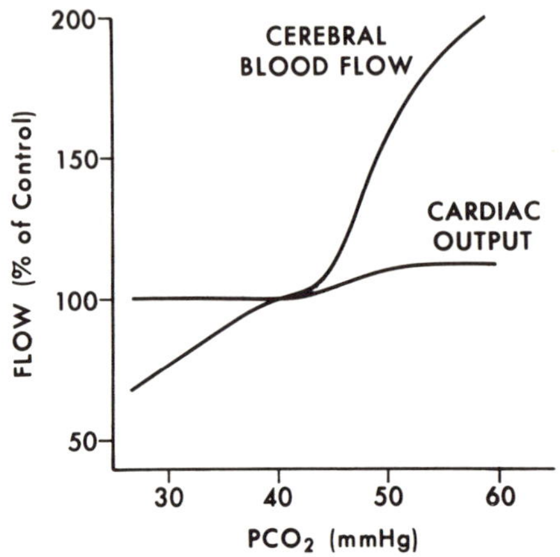

Figure 10.9. Hypercapnia causes an increase in cardiac output, but proportionally a much greater increase in cerebral blood flow. Note also that reduction in P_{CO_2} markedly reduces cerebral blood flow.

striction and thus plays an important role in the development of pulmonary hypertension and cor pulmonale.

Cerebral Cortex

An acute increase in P_{CO_2} can cause abnormalities in higher brain function ranging from confusion to coma. There are several reasons for this (Table 10.2). First, an increase in blood P_{CO_2} causes an increase in intracellular $[H^+]$ in all cells. CO_2 easily traverses the barrier between blood and brain extracellular fluid, the blood-brain barrier. The increase in cerebral cell P_{CO_2} causes the increase in $[H^+]$. Second, an increase in blood P_{CO_2} causes a greater increase in brain extracellular fluid $[H^+]$ than blood $[H^+]$. This occurs because extracellular fluid contains HCO_3^- but virtually no protein buffer. As has been mentioned the HCO_3^-/H_2CO_3 buffer pair cannot buffer carbonic acid. The correction of pH can be accomplished by an increase in extracellular fluid $[HCO_3^-]$ or by transfer of H^+ from the extracellular fluid. The blood-brain barrier is much less permeable to HCO_3^- and H^+ than to CO_2. Thus, correction

Table 10.2. The Brain in Hypercapnia

Major Manifestation	*Caused by*
Cerebral edema	Cerebral vasodilation
Intracellular acidosis	CO_2 diffusibility
Extracellular acidosis	CO_2 diffusibility and lack of protein buffer

of the extracellular fluid acidosis is delayed. The third reason why CO_2 may cause cerebral dysfunction is because it is such a powerful cerebral vasodilator, and the increase in cerebral blood flow may cause edema and increase brain extracellular fluid pressure. This is manifested as an increase in cerebrospinal fluid (CSF) pressure and even as swelling of the optic discs. Finally, CO_2 has anesthetic properties. The P_{CO_2} at which this occurs is not entirely clear, since some patients with *chronic* hypercapnia, whose P_{CO_2} is close to 100 mm Hg may have normal cerebral function. Probably most cases of "CO_2 narcosis" are caused by cerebral acidosis and not the anesthetic properties of CO_2.

BIBLIOGRAPHY

Bouhuys A: Respiratory dead space, in Fenn WO, Rahn H (eds): *Handbook of Physiology, Section 3, Respiration.* Washington, DC, American Physiological Society, 1964, p 699.

Nunn JF: Carbon Dioxide, in Nunn JF, *Applied Respiratory Physiology.* London, Butterworth, 1977, p 334.

West JB: Causes of carbon dioxide retention in lung disease. *N Engl J Med* 284:1232, 1971.

West JB: Ventilation-perfusion relationships. *Am Rev Resp Dis* 116:919, 1977.

11

Respiratory Failure 3: The Patient

Meir H. Kryger

In the previous two chapters, we reviewed the physiological features of hypoxemia and hypercapnia as though they were unrelated entities. In reality, a patient with respiratory failure may present with both abnormalities. Indeed, the patient with alveolar hypoventilation must have both hypoxemia and hypercapnia. Patients with respiratory failure usually present with one of two patterns: hypoxemia alone, or hypoxemia and hypercapnia. Hypoxemia always occurs in respiratory failure. It is the hypoxemia that causes *irreversible* brain damage and kills patients.

In trying to sort out patients with respiratory failure, it must be remembered that signs and symptoms may be caused by the disease itself or by the accompanying blood gas abnormalities.

SYMPTOMS, SIGNS, AND LABORATORY FEATURES OF HYPOXEMIA AND HYPERCAPNIA

Dyspnea, an uncomfortable awareness of difficulty in breathing, occurs in the presence of hypoxemia or hypercapnia. When hypoxemia or hypercapnia are present but dyspnea is absent, the inappropriate *lack* of dyspnea suggests that the chemical drives to breathe are depressed.

Personality change, confusion, somnolence (sleepiness), and coma all represent severe cerebral dysfunction and can be caused by either hypoxemia or hypercapnia.

Headache and papilledema (optic disc swelling) are caused by cerebral edema due to cerebral vasodilation of hypercapnia.

Tremors and asterixis resembling the "flap" of liver disease are most likely caused by cerebral acidosis.

Rapid heart rate, bounding pulses, and warm skin, indicating a hyperkinetic circulation, are caused by the direct effect of hypoxemia and hypercapnia on the circulation, compounded by the effect of catecholamines released when respiratory failure is present.

Cyanosis, a bluish tinge of the skin and mucous membranes, indicates hypoxemia. Hemoglobin has a color that ranges from blue to red. The color of any pigment is related to the wavelengths of light absorbed and reflected. The configuration of the hemoglobin molecule changes when it is oxygenated, and as a result of this, less light in the red part of the spectrum is absorbed. This causes oxygenated hemoglobin to be red. Cyanosis is a bluish hue that is present on the skin and mucus membranes, which usually occurs when the concentration of unoxygenated hemoglobin in these capillary beds is greater than about 5 gm%. If capillary blood is half venous and half arterial blood and hemoglobin concentration is 15 gm%, the mean capillary So_2 will be about 67% when cyanosis is present. When capillary So_2 is 67%, in every 100 ml of blood 10 gm hemoglobin will be oxygenated and 5 gm will be unoxygenated. A capillary So_2 of about 67% occurs when arterial So_2 is about 80%. Thus, when hemoglobin concentration is normal, cyanosis is not a sensitive index of hypoxemia.

Since capillary So_2 is determined by arterial and venous So_2, it is clear that a reduction in either venous or arterial So_2 can cause cyanosis. Low venous So_2 occurs when tissue hypoxia is present. A low arterial So_2 is the most common cause of cyanosis, because it reduces So_2 in both the arterial and venous capillary beds.

When anemia is present, capillary So_2 must be even lower for cyanosis to be apparent. If hemoglobin concentration is 10 gm%, capillary So_2 must be 50% for there to be 5 gm% of unoxygenated hemoglobin. With very severe anemia (hemoglobin about 5 gm%), cyanosis does not occur, because the capillary So_2 cannot drop low enough to cause cyanosis. Conversely, when hemoglobin concentration is elevated, less severe hypoxemia causes cyanosis.

Pulmonary hypertension occurs in the presence of alveolar hypoxia and hypercapnia. This represents an increased afterload to the right ventricle, which eventually causes an increase in right ventricular end diastolic pressure, right atrial pressure, and venous pressure. The increase in hepatic venous pressure, when acute, causes the liver to be enlarged and tender. The increase in venous pressure also causes edema formation in the dependent portions of the body. This sequence of events is called *cor pulmonale.* Acute pulmonary hypertension responds rapidly to treatment. Chronic pulmonary hypertension may be fixed, that is, unresponsive to treatment.

Arterial blood gases must be done to confirm the presence of respiratory failure. This is because some of the features described above may occur in disorders of other organ systems or may not be sensitive enough to indicate the severity of respiratory failure. Arterial blood gases must be done when respiratory failure is suspected.

Respiratory failure is always associated with hypoxemia but not always with hypercapnia. Three patterns of blood gas abnormality are commonly seen.

Low Pa_{O_2}, Normal or Low Pa_{CO_2}, Normal or High pH. This is the most common pattern observed in chronic obstructive lung disease (the pink puffer), interstitial lung disease, bronchial asthma, and the adult respiratory distress syndrome.

Low Pa_{O_2}, High Pa_{CO_2}, Normal or Slightly Reduced pH. These are the blood gases that occur with *chronic hypoventilation.* The normal pH indicates there has been sufficient time for the kidney to regenerate HCO_3^- to compensate for the high Pa_{CO_2}. This pattern occurs in chronic obstructive lung disease (the blue bloater), the obesity-hypoventilation syndrome, and other disorders associated with abnormal drive to breathe or weakness of the respiratory muscles.

Low Pa_{O_2}, High Pa_{CO_2}, and Low pH. This pattern, which occurs with acute hypoventilation, indicates there has been insufficient time for renal compensation to occur. This finding occurs with overdoses of drugs that reduce the drive to breathe or with paralysis of the respiratory muscles. Patients with chronic hypoventilation may have a sudden reduction in alveolar ventilation (usually caused by an infection or drug ingestion) that gives the pattern of acute on chronic hypoventilation: mainly a low Pa_{O_2}, a very high P_{CO_2}, a low pH, but an elevated [HCO_3^-]. The magnitude of the acid-base changes is discussed in the following chapter.

In any lung disease, even one that usually produces only hypoxemia (without hypercapnia) such as asthma, or interstitial disease, hypercapnia will occur when the disease becomes severe enough or is terminal. In bronchial asthma, even a slightly elevated P_{CO_2} indicates impending disastrous hypoventilation.

Polycythemia indicates that hypoxemia is chronic, since it takes weeks to months for hemoglobin production to respond completely to a low P_{O_2}.

SYMPTOMS, SIGNS, AND LABORATORY FEATURES OF DISEASES CAUSING RESPIRATORY FAILURE

The history is the secret weapon in the physician's arsenal and will usually indicate the cause of the respiratory failure and help decide therapy.

Chronic *cough and expectoration* in a cigarette smoker suggest chronic bronchitis, a form of chronic airflow obstruction. A recent change in quantity or color of sputum suggests an exacerbation of the disease and suggests that *acute or chronic hypoventilation* may be present.

Other features in the patient's history may indicate the cause of respiratory failure: a history of reversible paroxysmal dyspnea suggests bronchial asthma; severe dyspnea unresponsive to correction of blood gas abnormalities suggests that it is related to reflexes arising from the lungs, the usual finding in severe interstitial disease, and often in bronchial asthma; a history of suicide attempts suggests drug depression of the ventilatory control system; a past history of poliomyelitis may also indicate the presence of depressed ventilatory drive; weakness worsening with repeated activity (with associated weakness of the extraocular muscles) suggests myasthenia gravis. Evidence of airflow obstruction is found in patients with bronchial asthma and chronic obstructive lung disease. Crackles are found in alveolar edema or interstitial disease.

Laboratory tests also help indicate the cause of respiratory failure. The chest x-ray is a critical test, which surprisingly often has unexpected results; air in the pleural space (pneumothorax), a collapsed lobe, diffuse alveolar filling, and pleural effusion are some "unexpected" findings in patients in respiratory failure, which are actually quite common.

The measurement of vital capacity (VC) and forced expiratory volume in one second (FEV_1) are useful bedside tests in patients who are cooperative enough to do them. A normal FEV_1 and VC (i.e., normal lungs) in a patient who is hypoventilating is characteristic of patients with depressed drives to breathe. A low VC with a proportionately lower FEV_1 indicates airflow obstruction. A low VC with a proportionately high FEV_1 suggests restriction. Patients with muscular weakness have a low VC, but the most characteristic finding is a reduction in the amount of force their respiratory muscles can generate. When such patients are asked to suck as hard as they can, they usually generate less than -10 cmH_2O pressure; other patients can usually generate much more negative pressure.

An exciting development in laboratory evaluation of patients in respiratory failure concerns the diagnosis of respiratory muscle fatigue. This test is an electromyogram, which may tell us when the respiratory muscles are no longer capable of sustaining increased work.

PRINCIPLES OF TREATMENT

It is hypoxemia that kills patients. The first principle is that there must be correction of hypoxemia, and then specific therapy is instituted. The most important variables guiding therapeutic decisions are the patient's mental status and arterial blood gases. These must be continuously evaluated to monitor progress. Is the situation an emergency? Sometimes the patient must be treated before any evaluation. Features indicating an emergency situation are recent nervous system dysfunction (somnolence, stupor, coma), episodes of apnea, and an unstable cardiovascular system. Such a patient cannot breathe on his own. The patient must receive ventilatory support (see below). The aim of emergency therapy is to reverse life-threatening hypoxemia and acidosis.

When the situation is less emergent, hypoxemia may be treated by increasing the inspired P_{O_2}. This can be achieved with low-flow nasal cannulae delivering 1 to 5 L/minute of oxygen, or Venturi masks, which deliver oxygen at certain concentrations (24, 28, 35, and 40%). Using such delivery systems, the oxygen delivery can usually be controlled within limits. This is important because increasing Pa_{O_2} to high levels in patients with CAO may substantially worsen hypercapnia (see p. 113); the use of controlled O_2 lessens this problem.

In patients with diffuse lung injury, severe hypoxemia may not respond to oxygen administration, because of perfusion of unventilated regions. Continuous positive airway pressure (CPAP) may be used to treat this. In this system, the airway pressure is maintained continuously at greater than atmospheric pressure. This "opens up" closed nonventilating lung units.

Once the hypoxemia has been dealt with, specific therapy can be instituted. When airflow obstruction is present, bronchodilators are used. When an infection is present, antibiotics are used. If a pneumothorax or a pleural effusion is present, drainage of the pleural space may be necessary. If a narcotic has been taken, a narcotic antagonist can be used. In a few selected instances, respiratory stimulants may be used.

Once the acute episode is controlled, decisions about chronic therapy are made. Some patients may require long-term oxygen therapy; patients with respiratory muscle weakness may require long-term mechanical ventilation.

Mechanical Ventilation

It was shown in the chapter on hypoxemia that the most effective way to increase Pa_{O_2} is to increase inspired P_{O_2}; this is true even when mild alveolar hypoventilation is present. Thus, the vast majority of patients are treated with oxygen. Mechanical ventilation by itself (i.e., without PEEP) has little role in improving Pa_{O_2} unless hypoventilation is playing an important role. Mechanical ventilation is used mainly to increase alveolar ventilation or for the application of positive end expiratory pressure (PEEP).

Under normal circumstances, air moves into the lungs when alveolar pressure is less than atmospheric pressure. Contraction of the inspiratory muscles causes the reduction of alveolar pressure. When the pressure gradient between the lungs and atmosphere is too small, there will occur a reduction in inspiratory airflow. This is the situation that occurs when the inspiratory muscles are not contracting properly or when severe obstruction is present. With severe obstruction, there is a large pressure drop across the obstruction so that the pressure on the mouth side of the obstruction might not be very negative, even though the alveolar pressure itself may be very negative. A very stiff (nondistensible) lung needs much more pressure to increase its volume. When the respiratory muscles cannot generate the necessary pressure to maintain ventilation, in these circumstances there occurs, in essence, respiratory pump failure (Figure 11.1).

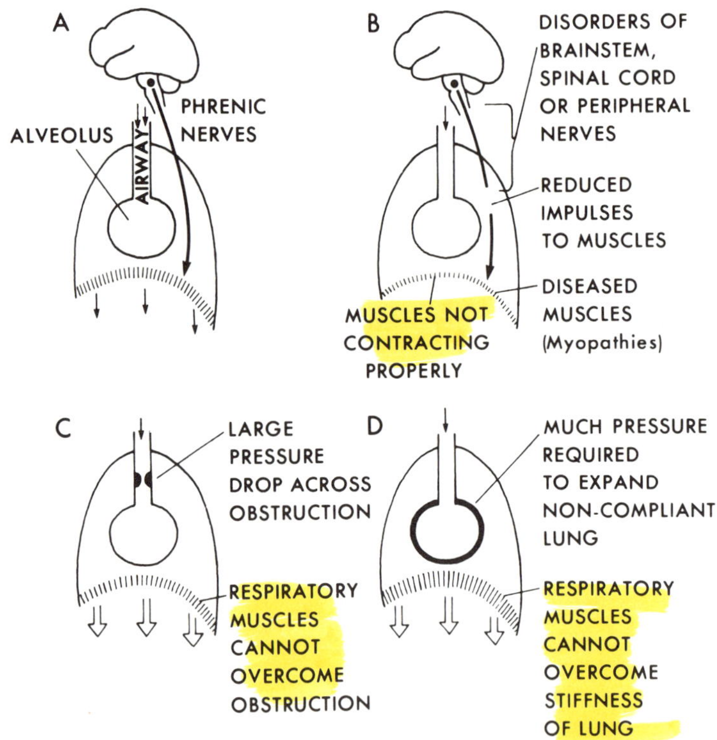

Figure 11.1. Major indications for mechanical ventilation. (*a*) The normal respiratory system. (*b*) The respiratory muscles are not contracting properly. This can be due to disorders of the muscles themselves, nerves, or the brainstem (*c*). With very severe airflow obstruction, the inspiratory muscles cannot generate sufficient pressure to generate adequate airflow. (*d*) When the lung is noncompliant (stiff) the respiratory muscles cannot overcome the lung stiffness.

Mechanical ventilation simply applies intermittent positive pressure at the upper airway, so that a pressure gradient necessary to maintain airflow into the lungs is present. The ventilator acts as a pump that can be adjusted to deliver a certain volume of air (volume-cycled ventilation) at a certain rate. Most machines in use today are volume-cycled; in other words the machine delivers a set volume. Previously, pressure-cycled machines were popular; these machines generate a set airway pressure. This latter system has disadvantages, because as the mechanical properties of the lung change, the pressure required to maintain ventilation also changes.

The patient is connected to the ventilator using an artificial upper airway. Usually, an endotracheal tube is inserted through the nose or mouth into the trachea. This tube has a balloon cuff, which prevents leaking during ventilation.

Mechanical ventilators have become very sophisticated; they have alarms, which indicate that the patient is not receiving the set tidal volume or that the pressure required to deliver the set tidal volume is excessive. In addition, inspiratory time and expiratory time can be adjusted. The latter setting is particularly useful in patients with airway obstruction who require a long expiratory phase. Another important feature of these machines is that they can be used simply to assist the patient. When the patient tries to initiate a breath, this triggers the machine to deliver the tidal volume. Thus, the patient and the machine are working in synchrony. The patient controls the machine and not vice versa. If the patient's respiratory control system is normal, P_{CO_2} will be kept close to normal. Another important feature of modern ventilators is that inspired P_{O_2} can be precisely controlled to maintain an adequate Pa_{O_2}. This is important in the prevention of oxygen toxicity (see below).

Positive end expiratory pressure (PEEP) may be used with a ventilator. Instead of the pressure at the mouth being atmospheric at the end of expiration, it is kept slightly positive. PEEP tends to open "closed lung units," which behave like a shunt, and thus improves $\dot{V}/\dot{Q}$ matching and improves Pa_{O_2}. PEEP may also allow the lung to operate at a higher lung volume and on a more compliant portion of its pressure-volume curve. The main advantage of PEEP is that it allows a lower $P_{I_{O_2}}$ to be used to maintain Pa_{O_2} at adequate levels. How much PEEP is used? The *minimal* amount of PEEP that does the job is the best amount of PEEP. The vast majority of patients seem to do well on 2.5 to 10 cmH_2O of PEEP.

COMPLICATIONS OF THERAPY OF RESPIRATORY FAILURE

The physician on treating the patient may cause new problems. It is beyond the scope of this volume to review in detail the unwanted effects of drugs used. Any drug that has sedative properties may cause depression in the drive to breathe and hypoventilation. These drugs must be avoided in the patient in respiratory failure who is not being mechanically ventilated. Toxic doses of bronchodilators may cause tachycardia and cardiac arrhythmias; in addition, the methylxanthine bronchodilators may cause nervous system excitability ranging from nervousness to seizures. We will briefly review complications of oxygen, the artificial airway, the ventilator, and PEEP.

Unwanted Effects of Oxygen

Increasing Pa_{O_2} to above normal levels may cause hypoventilation in patients with chronic airflow obstruction. Commonly, P_{CO_2} will rise when such patients are treated with *controlled* oxygen, but in the vast majority of patients, the rise in P_{CO_2} is not a problem and is a tolerable consequence of increasing Pa_{O_2}. When Pa_{O_2} rises excessively, severe hypoventilation and hypercapnia may ensue and cause "CO_2 narcosis," which is discussed elsewhere (p. 113).

Oxygen breathing can also worsen the matching of ventilation and perfusion by two mechanisms: relief of hypoxic vasoconstriction may increase perfusion of low $\dot{V}/\dot{Q}$ regions, and oxygen may induce alveolar instability by removing the nitrogen strut and cause alveolar collapse (p. 186).

Oxygen Toxicity

One of the points repeatedly stressed in this volume is the importance of oxygen in the maintenance of cellular function. It is ironic that too much oxygen can be toxic and that organisms have mechanisms to defend themselves against the toxic effects of excess oxygen.

Oxygen (O_2) is converted to a potent free radical, the superoxide anion (O_2^-), by the addition of an electron to oxygen. A large number of enzymes in various cells produce large amounts of O_2^-, although it may only exist for microseconds. This free radical is toxic to cells, because it inhibits certain enzymes, can damage cell membranes, and can kill cells.

Very high P_{O_2} (exceeding 1000 to 2000 mmHg), as is encountered in compression chambers and underwater divers, causes nervous system toxicity and seizures, which may begin minutes after exposure.

In the clinical setting, two aspects of oxygen toxicity are important. First, newborns with an arterial P_{O_2} exceeding about 150 mmHg may develop damage of capillaries in the retina. This may cause obliteration of these capillaries and a fibroblastic repair reaction. The resulting *retrolental fibroplasia* can cause irreversible blindness. Second, with the advent of oxygen delivery systems capable of delivering very high concentrations of oxygen, *pulmonary oxygen toxicity* has become a problem. It seems most likely that the superoxide anion first damages pulmonary capillary endothelial cells. This causes a pulmonary capillary leak with accumulation of fluid in the interstitial space. The epithelial (type I) cells are then damaged, and the epithelium is denuded. In an attempt to repair the damage, the type II cells (which also produce surfactant) proliferate and line the basement membrane. It is likely that these type II cells can then differentiate into type I cells. This process may result in disordered collagen deposition in the interstitial space, causing interstitial fibrosis.

While the above process is going on, severe hypoxemia occurs. Thus, a vicious cycle is started; oxygen that was initially treating hypoxemia is now causing hypoxemia.

How much oxygen is safe? Within one day (6 to 30 hours) of pure oxygen breathing, pulmonary oxygen toxicity may occur. It takes about 7 days to develop toxicity breathing 55% oxygen. People can probably tolerate 35% oxygen indefinitely.

Superoxide dismutase (SOD) is an enzyme that "detoxifies" the superoxide anion and thus is protective against the toxic effects of oxygen. There are actually several forms of SOD, and these enzymes are found in life forms ranging from bacteria to algae to man. The concentration of this enzyme increases when hyperoxia is present. Higher concentrations of SOD may increase the tolerance to high Po_2.

Artificial Airway

The major problems associated with the endotracheal tube occur because of two reasons, the location of the tube and the cuff of the tube. If a *nasotracheal* tube is used, the tube may obstruct the Eustachian tube and cause an ear infection. If an oral endotracheal tube is used, it loops over the tongue and the patient cannot eat. The most serious problem caused by the location of the tube occurs when it is pushed too far into the tracheobronchial tree. When this occurs, the distal orifice of the tube will be in the right bronchus and only the right lung will be ventilated.

Tracheal tubes have cuffs near the distal orifice. When these cuffs are inflated, all the air driven into the tube by the mechanical ventilator goes into the lungs. When the cuff is deflated, some of the air can leak out of the trachea. The problem with these cuffs is that when they are inflated with too great a pressure, they can compress blood vessels in the trachea and thus injure it. Months after such an injury and after the tube has been removed, scar formation may cause stenosis of the trachea.

Mechanical Ventilation

Ventilators work because they pump air into the upper airway. This increases the pressure encountered by the airways and lungs. When a very high pressure is generated, there may occur damage (barotrauma) to the respiratory system. The most common injury is the tearing of lung parenchyma causing an air leak into the pleural space, a pneumothorax. Less commonly, air will dissect into the lung interstitial space and centrally into the mediastinum, a pneumomediastinum. Air may then dissect into the fascial planes of the neck and thorax, subcutaneous emphysema.

PEEP

Positive end expiratory pressure increases mean intrathoracic pressure and reduces the pressure gradient between the right atrium and the great veins. This reduces the gradient for venous return and can cause a reduction in cardiac output (Chapter 4). PEEP also markedly increases the incidence of barotrauma.

BIBLIOGRAPHY

Deneke SM, Fanburg BL: Normobaric oxygen toxicity of the lung. *N Engl J Med* 303:76, 1980.

McCord JM, Fridovich I: The biology and pathology of oxygen radicals. *Ann Intern Med* 89:122, 1978.

Petty TL: *Intensive and Rehabilitative Respiratory Care. A Practical Approach to the Management of Acute and Chronic Respiratory Failure*, ed 2. Philadelphia, Lea and Febiger, 1974.

Roussos C, Grassino A, Macklem PT: Inspiratory muscle fatigue and acute respiratory failure. *Can Med Assoc J* 122:1375, 1980.

Sykes MK, McNicol MW, Campbell EJM: *Respiratory Failure*, ed 2. Philadelphia, Lippincott, 1976.

Zwillich CW, Pierson DJ, Creagh CE, et al: Complications of assisted ventilation. A prospective study of 354 consecutive episodes. *Am J Med* 57:161, 1974.

Zwillich CW, Kryger M, Weil J: Hypoventilation: Consequences and management, in Stollerman (ed): *Advances in Internal Medicine.* Chicago, Year Book Medical Publishers, vol 23, 1978.

12

The Lung in Acid-Base Regulation

Meir H. Kryger

Because the respiratory system controls P_{CO_2}, and because most of the acid produced in the body is CO_2, the respiratory system plays a pivotal role in the regulation of the acid-base status of the body. The respiratory system can both cause an acid-base disorder and compensate for an acid-base disorder caused by another organ. Although in this chapter we will emphasize the role played by the respiratory system, to understand acid-base physiology the function of both the respiratory and renal systems must be understood.

DEFENSE OF pH

Most enzymatic reactions require an optimal H^+ concentration (abbreviated $[H^+]$). The body has mechanisms that regulate $[H^+]$ within a very narrow range. Acid-base status may be expressed in terms of $[H^+]$ or pH. pH is $-\log[H^+]$. Usually pH is maintained at about 7.40 ($[H^+]$ = 40 nEq/L). The normal range of pH is 7.35 to 7.45 ($[H^+]$ = 45 to 35 nEq/L). The range of pH that is compatible with life is 6.8 to 7.7 ($[H^+]$ = 160 to 20 nEq/L).

Remember that a *nEq* is 10^{-9} equivalents, and when the concentration of other ions is measured, *mEq* (10^{-3}) are used. Thus compared to other ions, the concentration of H^+ is miniscule. The concentration of sodium (Na^+) is about 3,000,000 times the concentration of H^+. Another point worth repeating is that for monovalent ions (ions with a single charge), the number of equivalents is equal to the number of moles. Thus for these ions, the terms mmoles (millimoles) are interchangeable with mEq (milliequivalents).

At present, most hospital laboratories report the pH when evaluating acid-base status, whereas a few report $[H^+]$. There are good reasons to use either system. The reader is advised not only to be thoroughly familar with the system in use at his or her institution but also to have a general understanding of the other system.

Two types of systems defend the pH. First, is *buffering,* which is a chemical event, which is rapid in response. Second are *physiological responses* by the kidneys and lungs that *compensate* for the abnormal acid-base status. The respiratory system compensates for the pH changes in metabolic disorders, while the kidneys do the same in respiratory disorders. These physiological responses are slower but more effective than buffering in restoring pH to normal.

Buffers

An *acid* is a proton or an H^+ ion donor. A *base* is a proton or an H^+ ion acceptor.

$$\underset{\text{Acid}}{HA} \rightleftharpoons H^+ + \underset{\text{Base}}{A^-} \tag{1}$$

The above equation describes the relationship between an acid and a base. HA is the acid that can donate a hydrogen ion, while A^- is a base that can accept the hydrogen ion. HA is the *conjugate acid* of A^-, and A^- is the *conjugate base* of HA. Buffers are made up of a weak acid and its conjugate base, a *buffer pair*.

$$\underset{\substack{\text{Strong}\\\text{acid}}}{HCl} + \underset{\substack{\text{Conjugate}\\\text{base}}}{A^-} \longrightarrow \underset{\substack{\text{Weak}\\\text{acid}}}{HA} + \underset{\text{Anion}}{Cl^-} \tag{2}$$

Suppose we add a strong acid (like HCl) to a buffer pair; most of the H^+ of the strong acid (which dissociates easily) react with the conjugate base A^- to form HA, a weak acid which does not dissociate easily—thus, only a few H^+ ions remain free in solution. This minimizes changes in $[H^+]$. The formation of a weak acid from a strong acid is the way a buffer pair minimizes $[H^+]$ changes with an H^+ ion load.

Similarly when a strong base (e.g., OH^-) is added to a buffer pair, the change in $[H^+]$ is also minimized.

$$\underset{\substack{\text{Strong}\\\text{base}}}{OH^-} + \underset{\substack{\text{Weak}\\\text{acid}}}{HA} \rightleftharpoons \underset{\substack{\text{Conjugate}\\\text{base}}}{A^-} + \underset{\text{Water}}{H_2O} \tag{3}$$

The effectiveness of a buffer pair depends on the *pK*, which is the pH at which the buffer exists half as the weak acid and half as the conjugate base. Buffering is optimal at its pK. The effectiveness of a buffer pair also depends on the amount of buffer present; the greater the amount of buffer present, the greater is the capacity to defend against pH changes.

The equations that describe the relationship of a buffer pair to $[H^+]$ or pH are:

$$[H^+] = K\frac{[HA]}{[A^-]} = K\frac{[\text{weak acid}]}{[\text{conjugate base}]} \tag{4}$$

or

$$pH = pK' + \log\frac{[A^-]}{[HA]} = pK' + \log\frac{[\text{conjugate base}]}{[\text{weak acid}]} \tag{5}$$

Equation 4 is called the Henderson equation, while Equation 5 is called the Henderson-Hasselbalch equation.

There are several buffer pairs in the body. All these buffer pairs are in equilibrium with the same $[H^+]$. Thus, a detailed description of a single buffer pair suffices in assessing acid-base status. The bicarbonate buffer system (made up of the carbonic acid/bicarbonate buffer pair) is usually chosen to assess acid-base status (see below).

Acids in the Body

There are two types of acid produced by the body. The first type of acid is *carbonic acid* (H_2CO_3), which can dissociate into H^+ and HCO_3^-. Carbonic acid is in equilibrium with CO_2 and water by the following reaction:

$$\underset{\text{Produced by metabolism}}{CO_2 + H_2O} \rightleftharpoons \underset{\text{Carbonic acid}}{H_2CO_3} \rightleftharpoons H^+ + \underset{\text{Bicarbonate}}{HCO_3^-} \quad \textbf{(6)}$$

Carbon dioxide is continuously produced (about 13,000 mmoles/day) and is continuously excreted by the lungs and, hence, is a *volatile acid.* Because CO_2 is so soluble, it readily penetrates cell membranes and thus can alter intracellular $[H^+]$. H^+ ions do not cross cell membranes as readily as CO_2. Since carbonic acid is also one component of the carbonic acid/bicarbonate buffer pair, it cannot be buffered by this buffer pair and can only be buffered by the non-bicarbonate buffers that are described later.

The second group of acids are *fixed acids* (in contrast to volatile acid). These acids are produced by various metabolic reactions or are ingested. Examples of fixed acids are lactic acid, produced with anaerobic glycolysis; H_2SO_4, produced from protein catabolism; acetoacetic acid, produced during starvation or uncontrolled diabetes mellitus; and formic acid, produced after methanol ingestion. These acids do not penetrate cell membranes easily and, therefore, will cause severe intracellular acidosis in the cells that produced the acid. These strong acids are not parts of a buffer pair and thus can be buffered by all buffer pairs, including the bicarbonate and nonbicarbonate buffers.

Bicarbonate Buffer System

The bicarbonate buffer system is made of the carbonic acid/bicarbonate buffer pair.

$$\underset{\substack{\text{Carbonic acid}\\ \text{(weak acid)}}}{H_2CO_3} \rightleftharpoons \underset{\substack{\text{Bicarbonate}\\ \text{(conjugate base)}}}{HCO_3^-} + H^+$$

In fact, carbonic acid is also in equilibrium with dissolved CO_2:

$$CO_2 + H_2O \rightleftharpoons H_2CO_3 \rightleftharpoons HCO_3^- + H^+$$

Thus, in reality the amount of weak acid making up the weak acid component of the buffer pair is $CO_2 + H_2CO_3$. In other words, the carbonic acid pool that can be used for buffering is $CO_2 + H_2CO_3$. The equilibrium of the reaction $CO_2 + H_2O \rightleftharpoons H_2CO_3$ is far to the left, there being 600 parts of CO_2 in solution for every part of H_2CO_3. Thus, in practical terms, the carbonic acid pool is equal to the dissolved CO_2. Dissolved CO_2 in mmole = $.03 \times P_{CO_2}$. We may represent the weak acid component of the bicarbonate buffer system as $.03 \times P_{CO_2}$. If we now rewrite Equation 5:

$$\mathrm{pH} = \mathrm{pK}' + \log \frac{[\text{conjugate base}]}{[\text{weak acid}]} = 6.1 + \log \frac{[HCO_3^-]}{[.03 \times P_{CO_2}]} \quad \textbf{(7)}$$

The concentration of each is expressed in mmoles/liter.

Of the buffer pair, $[HCO_3^-]$ can be thought of as the metabolic component, being altered by metabolic processes, whereas $[.03 \times P_{CO_2}]$ can be thought of as the respiratory component, being altered by the level of alveolar ventilation. Thus:

$$\mathrm{pH} \propto \frac{\text{metabolic component}}{\text{respiratory component}}$$

One important advantage of the bicarbonate buffer system is that its weak acid is volatile; CO_2 is continuously excreted by the lungs and is maintained at about 40 mmHg. Suppose H^+ is added to bicarbonate; the following reaction would occur:

$$H^+ + HCO_3^- \longrightarrow H_2CO_3 \longrightarrow CO_2 + H_2O$$

For every mmole HCO_3^- used for buffering, one mmole of CO_2 is generated. The CO_2 generated is excreted, and P_{CO_2} is kept constant. This is called an *open buffering system.*

If this "blow off valve" were not present (i.e., a *closed system*) for every mmole drop in HCO_3^- there would occur an identical rise in CO_2 (in mmoles), which would offset the effectiveness of the buffer system. Remember that a 1 mmole rise in CO_2 causes P_{CO_2} to rise 33.3 mmHg! Thus when the system becomes "closed" and acid is produced (as occurs with cardiac arrest and apnea), an acute marked rise in both $[H^+]$ and P_{CO_2} occurs. Because usually the weak acid component of this buffer pair is "open" and can be regulated, the bicarbonate buffer system makes a powerful buffer. This is illustrated in Figure 12.1.

One aspect of the bicarbonate buffer system must be reemphasized and may be a source of confusion; a buffer pair cannot buffer one component of the pair. The bicarbonate buffer system does not function as an effective buffer when there occurs a rise in P_{CO_2}

When CO_2 increases the following reaction occurs:

$$CO_2 + H_2O \rightleftharpoons H_2CO_3 \rightleftharpoons H^+ + HCO_3^-$$

Another source of confusion has to do with the HCO_3^- formed in the above reaction. Why does this $[HCO_3^-]$ increase not offset the rise in P_{CO_2} and thus minimize pH changes when P_{CO_2} rises? Suppose P_{CO_2} doubles. This will dou-

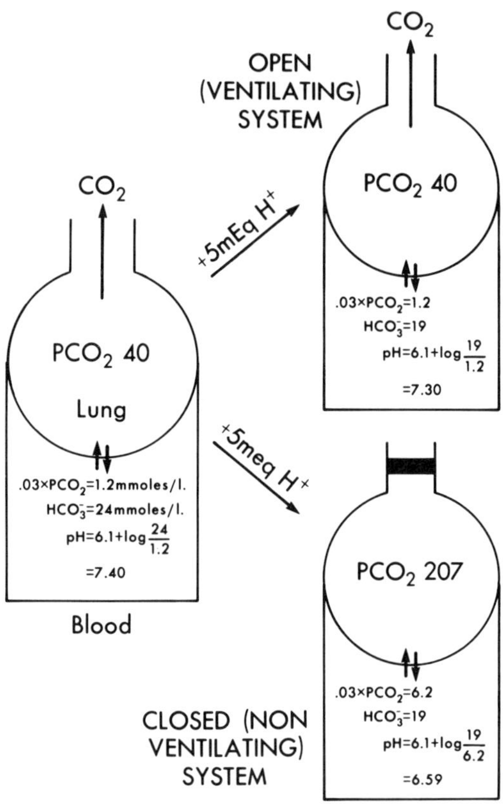

Figure 12.1. When H^+ is added to the bicarbonate buffer system, for every mEq drop in $[HCO_3^-]$ there would occur an identical rise in CO_2 (in mmoles), if the system were closed. In this situation, every 1 mmole rise in CO_2 causes P_{CO_2} to rise by 33.3 mmHg resulting in a marked drop in pH. Fortunately, this buffering system is usually open and P_{CO_2} is maintained by ventilation at about 40 mmHg.

ble $[H^+]$. For every mole $[H^+]$ rise, there will be an identical rise in $[HCO_3^-]$. Thus, $[HCO_3^-]$ will rise by only *40 mmole/L,* which is negligible compared to the 24 mmole/L usually present. Therefore, in the Henderson-Hasselbalch equation, the respiratory component doubles, while the metabolic component increases by only a small amount. The fact that rises in CO_2 are not buffered by the bicarbonate system is important, because some compartments in the body contain mainly the bicarbonate buffer system.

Nonbicarbonate Buffers

The *nonbicarbonate buffer* systems are very important in acid-base regulation, since only they can buffer changes in P_{CO_2}. The most important nonbicarbonate buffers are proteins (mainly hemoglobin) and the $H_2PO_4^-/HPO_4^=$ pair. In proteins it is the imadazole group of histidine that can accept H^+ ions. The nonbicarbonate buffers can be thought of as a buffer pair, the HBuf/Buf^- buffer pair. These buffers can buffer both carbonic acid and fixed acid.

$$H_2CO_3 + Buf^- \rightleftharpoons HBuf + HCO_3^- \text{ (Carbonic acid buffering)}$$

$$HCl + Buf^- \rightleftharpoons HBuf + Cl^- \text{ (Fixed acid buffering)}$$

Both the bicarbonate and nonbicarbonate systems buffer fixed acid. If we add an acid, HX, to the body we may write:

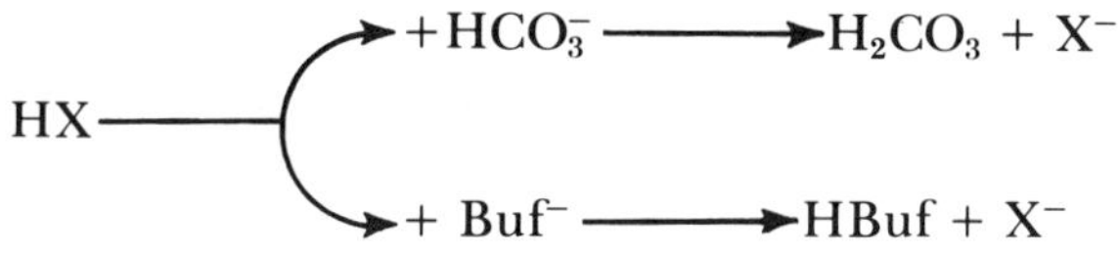

The change in the number of mmoles of HCO_3^- and Buf^- equals the number of mmoles of acid added. The term *whole blood buffer base* (BB) has been used to define the sum of the conjugate bases:

$$[BB] = [Buf^-] + [HCO_3^-]$$

Deviation from normal BB gives information about the total capacity to buffer fixed acid. When BB is elevated, there is an increase in $[Buf^-] + [HCO_3^-]$ and a *base excess (BE)* is present. When BB is reduced, a *base deficit* is present; the latter term is often abbreviated −BE.

Distribution of Buffers

Buffers are present throughout the body and are distributed in different concentrations in the different compartments (Table 12.1).

Table 12.1. Distribution of Buffers

	Major Buffers	*Major Buffering of* Carbonic Acid	*Major Buffering of* Fixed Acid
Plasma		No	Yes
	Proteins		
	HCO_3^- and H_2CO_3 pair		
	$H_2PO_4^-$ and $HPO_4^=$ pair		
Red cells		Yes	Yes
	HCO_3^- and H_2CO_3 pair		
	Hemoglobin		
Interstitial fluid		No	Yes
	HCO_3^- and H_2CO_3 pair		
Intracellular fluid		Yes	Yes
	Proteins		
	HCO_3^- and H_2CO_3 pair		

Blood is made up of red blood cells (about 45%) and plasma (55%). *Red blood cells* contain both bicarbonate buffers and nonbicarbonate buffers, the latter mainly in the form of hemoglobin. The bicarbonate is produced in a reaction catalyzed by carbonic anhydrase as described on p. 206. Each hemoglobin molecule has 36 histidine residues and thus is a very effective buffer. When fixed acid is added to red cells, hemoglobin buffers about 60% and HCO_3^- about 30% of the acid load. As mentioned above, when carbonic acid is added, it is buffered almost entirely by the hemoglobin. Unoxygenated hemoglobin is a better buffer than oxygenated hemoglobin.

Plasma contains bicarbonate, phosphate, and protein buffers. Because bicarbonate is the main plasma buffer, plasma can effectively buffer the fixed acid but not CO_2.

The bicarbonate buffer system is virtually the only one in the protein poor *interstitial fluid compartment* (including the cerebrospinal fluid). This compartment is an important buffer of fixed acid, being 4 times as large as blood volume.

Intracellular fluid is rich in proteins and phosphates and thus can buffer carbonic and fixed acid. Because intracellular fluid makes up about two-thirds of total body water, this compartment is probably the most important. Unfortunately, much less is known about intracellular buffering than buffering in the blood and interstitial fluid.

Ion Shifts

Ion shifts in and out of cells can also minimize deviations in pH. When H^+ is added to extracellular fluid, many of these ions diffuse into intracellular fluid and are buffered by the mechanisms mentioned above. Since H^+ is positively charged, this movement must be accompanied by either a negative ion entering the cell or a positive ion leaving the cell. Intracellular fluid is rich in potassium; thus potassium participates in these ion shifts. During acidemia, the concentration of potassium in blood may increase markedly. Similarly during alkalosis, the potassium concentration in blood may be very low.

Physiological Responses

When an acid-base disorder is present, chemical buffering, although helping to prevent deviations in pH, is far from perfect and pH is still abnormal.

Let us examine the Henderson-Hasselbalch equation again:

$$pH = 6.1 + \log \frac{[HCO_3^-]}{[.03 \times P_{CO_2}]}$$

When an acid-base disorder is present, the ratio $[HCO_3^-]/[.03 \times P_{CO_2}]$ is abnormal. Physiological responses attempt to reestablish a normal ratio and thus restore pH to normal. It is intuitively obvious that if $[HCO_3^-]$ were reduced to half, that reducing $[.03 \times P_{CO_2}]$ by half would restore pH to normal.

The numerator of the ratio [HCO_3^-] is controlled by the kidney, whereas the denominator [.03 × P_{CO_2}] is regulated by the respiratory system. These physiological responses to alterations in acid-base status are compensatory responses. With *full compensation,* pH is restored to normal; with *partial compensation,* the pH has not been restored to normal; when no physiological response is present, the acid-base disturbance is *uncompensated.*

Respiratory Compensation

The denominator [.03 × P_{CO_2}] of the above equation is controlled by the respiratory system. Changes in alveolar ventilation will change P_{CO_2}; an increase in ventilation lowers P_{CO_2}, while a reduction raises P_{CO_2}. Changes in [H^+] are sensed both in the carotid body and the central chemoreceptor in the medulla. It is possible that these two sensors may give different information about acid-base status. This is because the carotid body directly samples arterial blood, while the central chemoreceptor samples cerebral interstitial fluid.

Because of the blood-brain barrier, [HCO_3^-] and [H^+] change less rapidly in the brain interstitial fluid than in blood when an acid-base disturbance is present. This is because the movement of ions is affected not only by concentration gradients but also by electrical charges. HCO_3^- ions are not freely permeable through the blood-brain barrier. For example, in an acute metabolic acidosis, [HCO_3^-] and pH drop rapidly in the blood. While this is occurring, brain interstitial fluid [HCO_3^-] and thus pH will not drop as much. Therefore, the central (more powerful) chemoreceptor "sees" less [H^+] change and thus "underestimates" the compensation necessary to correct blood pH to normal (Figure 12.2).

Because of these reasons, usually the respiratory system never fully compensates for a metabolic disorder, although it is perfectly capable of doing so. Although respiratory compensation begins within minutes, the maximal response may require 5 to 6 hours.

Renal Compensation

The kidney regulates the numerator [HCO_3^-], the metabolic component in the above version of the Henderson-Hasselbalch equation. In essence, the kidney accomplishes this by producing either an acid or an alkaline urine. When urine is acidified (H^+ ions excreted), this causes the [HCO_3^-] concentration of blood to be increased. When urine is made alkaline (HCO_3^- ions excreted), the blood [HCO_3^-] decreases. Renal compensation begins hours after onset of an abnormality but is not complete until several days later (often 5 to 7 days).

Increasing Blood [HCO_3^-]. Normally, the kidney reclaims virtually all the HCO_3^- in the glomerular filtrate. The process is a bit circuitous, since it involves secretion of H^+ into the glomerular filtrate in the proximal tubule. This mechanism is shown in Figure 12.3. In the presence of acidosis, the proximal tubule cells increase H^+ secretion over and above the amount needed to

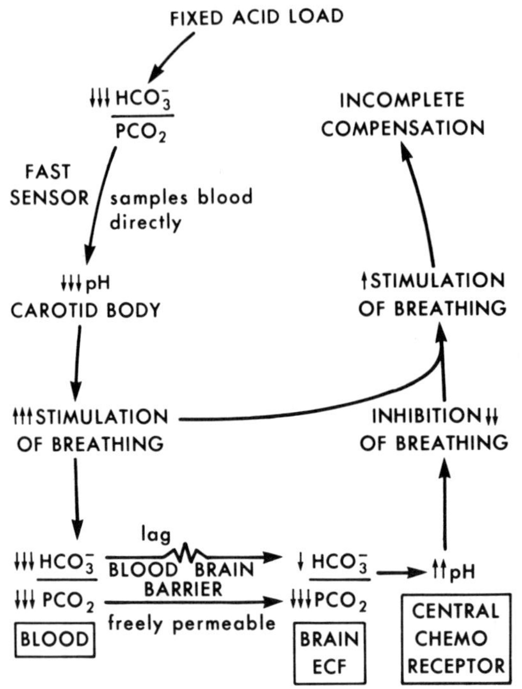

Figure 12.2. Because of the blood-brain barrier, the change in brain ECF [HCO_3^-] lags behind the change in blood [HCO_3^-]. CO_2 is freely diffusible. This causes the central chemoreceptor to "see" a different pH than the carotid body. Thus, respiratory compensation seldom returns blood pH to normal with a metabolic disorder.

reclaim filtered HCO_3^-, a process that generates *new* HCO_3^-. This process is more complex than reclamation of filtered bicarbonate, because the secreted H^+ must be "trapped" in the tubular fluid by an ion other than HCO_3^- (Figure 12.4).

The secreted H^+ remains in the urine in one of three forms. Most H^+ ions combine with ammonia to form the charged ammonium ions, NH_4^+, which are then trapped in the tubular fluid. A smaller quantity of H^+ ions are buffered by filtered $HPO_4^=$, and a tiny quantity of H^+ ions remain free in the urine.

Reducing Blood [HCO_3^-]. This can usually be accomplished quite easily by simply allowing filtered HCO_3^- to escape in the urine. However, in some circumstances other processes interfere with this. When Na^+ is resorbed in the proximal tubule, it is usually accompanied by Cl^-. When Cl^- depletion is present, HCO_3^- from the tubular fluid will accompany the Na^+ instead. Thus, chloride depletion offsets HCO_3^- excretion.

Intravascular volume contraction initiates enhanced Na^+ resorption in the proximal nephron that is accompanied by a negatively charged ion, often an HCO_3^- ion. The same volume contraction also initiates mineralocorticoid

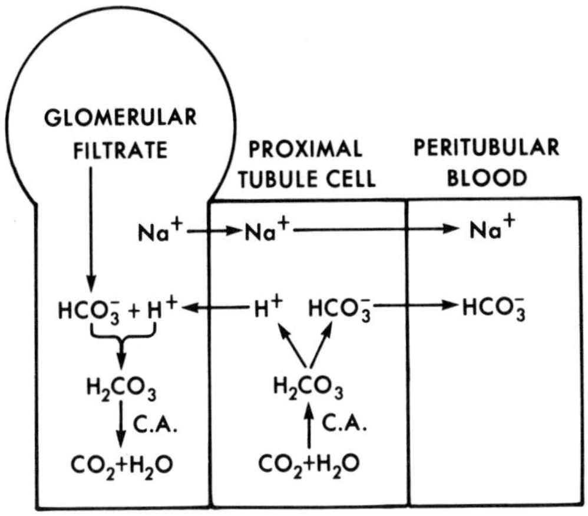

Figure 12.3. Bicarbonate reclamation from the glomerular filtrate is indirect. H^+ is secreted into the glomerular filtrate leaving behind in the tubule cell an HCO_3^- ion, which enters the peritubular blood. Meanwhile, the secreted H^+ ion has combined with the HCO_3^- in the filtrate. This circuitous HCO_3^- resorption requires the enzyme carbonic anhydrase (C.A.). To maintain electroneutrality H^+ secretion is linked to N^+ resorption.

enhanced Na^+ resorption from the distal tubule, a process linked to H^+ or K^+ secretion. If H^+ secretion occurs, new HCO_3^- is generated. This is particularly true if potassium depletion is present causing H^+ to be preferentially exchanged for Na^+. Thus, reduction of blood $[HCO_3^-]$ is easy; but this process can be sabotaged by low chloride, low blood volume, or low potassium. These three factors can perpetuate or maintain a metabolic alkalosis, even though the primary event (e.g., vomiting) may have stopped.

Time Course of Defense of pH

Extracellular buffering is instantaneous. *Intracellular buffering* that is accompanied by ion shifts takes 2 to 4 hours. *Respiratory compensation* begins within minutes but requires about 5 to 6 hours to be maximal. *Renal compensation* is slow, beginning within hours and taking up to about 5 to 7 days to be complete.

ACID-BASE DISORDERS

The Language of Acid-Base Disorders

A physiological process must not be confused with a laboratory measurement. *Acidosis* is a physiological process caused by accumulation of acid or loss of base. Acidosis may be associated with a low measured pH (*acidemia*) or a normal pH if compensatory mechanisms are adequate. The suffix *emia* refers

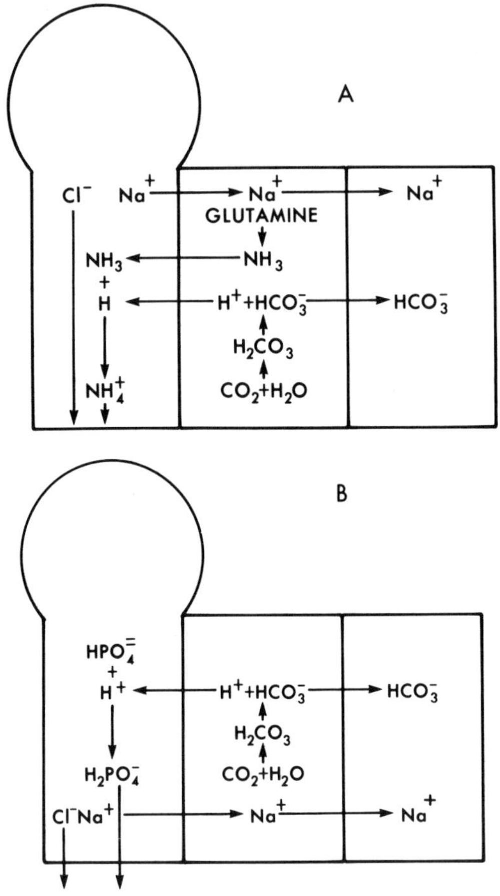

Figure 12.4. Generation of new HCO_3^- is linked to secretion of H^+ into glomerular filtrate. The secreted H^+ must be trapped in the filtrate by an ion other than HCO_3^-. In (*a*) the H^+ is trapped by NH_3 and in (*b*) by $HPO_4^=$. Note that H^+ secretion is accompanied by Na^+ resorption, which maintains electroneutrality. This leaves Cl^- behind in the glomerular filtrate.

to a laboratory measurement; the suffix *osis* refers to the physiological process. A person may have an "osis" without an "emia."

In sorting out an acid-base disorder, the *primary* physiological disturbance must be ascertained. In other words, what caused the physiological disorder? Was it a respiratory or a metabolic problem? Sometimes the problem is *mixed,* a combination of the two. In this terminology, there are four possible *primary physiological acid-base disturbances;* metabolic acidosis, metabolic alkalosis, respiratory acidosis, and respiratory alkalosis (Table 12.2).

Also, if two processes are causing the abnormality, the terms are combined; for example, *mixed metabolic alkalosis and respiratory acidosis.*

Table 12.2. Approach to Diagnosis of Acid-Base Disorders

$$pH \propto \frac{[HCO_3^-]}{[Pco_2]}$$

High pH	$\frac{[HCO_3^-]}{\text{low }[Pco_2]}$	Respiratory alkalosis
High pH	$\frac{\text{high }[HCO_3^-]}{[Pco_2]}$	Metabolic alkalosis
Low pH	$\frac{[HCO_3^-]}{\text{high }[Pco_2]}$	Respiratory acidosis
Low pH	$\frac{\text{low }[HCO_3^-]}{[Pco_2]}$	Metabolic acidosis

In trying to sort out acid-base disorders, we must consider the adequacy of measures to defend the pH, chemical buffers and the physiological responses. Physiological responses were discussed previously, and depending on the degree of physiological compensation, a primary process could be uncompensated, partially compensated, or fully compensated. For example, a disorder may be more accurately described as an *uncompensated metabolic acidosis,* indicating that there is no respiratory compensation for the metabolic acidosis.

Laboratory tests are used to ascertain the cause of the primary disorder and the adequacy of physiological response. All the necessary information can be obtained by knowing blood pH, Pco_2, and $[HCO_3^-]$. The last variable is not usually measured but calculated from the other two using the Henderson-Hasselbalch equation.

The final variable to be considered in the sorting of these disorders is correction, the way in which a primary disorder is fully corrected. For example, correction of respiratory acidosis to normal involves increasing alveolar ventilation back to normal. If an acid load is added to the body, the acid must be excreted. This is different from compensation; compensation may restore the pH to normal but does not stop the primary disturbance.

In the remainder of this chapter, we will integrate what we have mentioned above and review the major acid-base disorders. An approach to diagnosis is outlined in Table 12.2.

Metabolic Acidosis

Definition

A metabolic acidosis is a disorder caused by a physiological process that reduces pH (increases $[H^+]$) by decreasing $[HCO_3^-]$.

Causes

A lowered $[HCO_3^-]$ can be caused by gain of strong acid that is buffered by HCO_3^- or by loss of HCO_3^- from the body.

Gain of Strong Acid. Strong acid can be gained by either ingestion or abnormal metabolism. Examples of ingested substances causing metabolic acidosis are *salicylates* (aspirin), *methyl alcohol* (wood alcohol), and *ethylene glycol* (antifreeze). Salicylate poisoning can also cause respiratory alkalosis, but in children the metabolic acidosis predominates. Examples of abnormal metabolism causing acidosis are *diabetic ketoacidosis* (acetoacetic and β-hydroxybutyric being the added acids), *lactic acidosis* (most often caused by inadequate O_2 delivery to tissues or failure of O_2 utilization), and *starvation* (same strong acids as diabetic ketoacidosis). *Alcoholics* may also develop ketoacidosis. Inability to excrete H_2SO_4 and other acids in *renal failure* (uremia) is equivalent to the addition of strong acids to the body. With the gain of strong acid for every HCO_3^- used in buffering, there would remain the anion of the strong base. These anions are unmeasured and cause the *anion gap* discussed below.

Loss of HCO_3^- from the Body. The most common sources of HCO_3^- loss from the body are from the gastrointestinal tract (usually caused by diarrhea or loss of fluid from the upper GI tract) or via the kidneys (usually a tubular defect of bicarbonate absorption or acid secretion). This latter problem is called *renal tubular acidosis,* which is dealt with in detail in textbooks of renal physiology. In these abnormalities, no new acid and hence no new anion is added to the body; there is no anion gap. The reduction in $[HCO_3^-]$ is offset by an increase in $[Cl^-]$. These types of disorders are sometimes called *hyperchloremic metabolic acidosis* or *normal anion gap acidosis* (Table 12.3).

Buffers

If we examine the situation for the addition of an acid H^+X^- the following occurs:

$$H^+X^- + HCO_3^- \rightarrow X^- + H_2CO_3$$

For every ion of HCO_3^- consumed, one ion of X^- is generated. X^- is not usually measured. Thus, if we add up all the usually measured anions, some anions are unaccounted for. The *anion gap* is calculated by subtracting all the measured anions from the measured cation Na^+. Thus:

$$\text{Anion gap} = \underbrace{[Na^+]}_{\text{Cation}} - \underbrace{([Cl^-] + [HCO_3^-])}_{\text{Anions}}$$

Normally this gap is 10 to 14 mEq/L (being accounted for mainly by plasma proteins). In most situations of acid addition, this gap is increased.

Respiratory Compensation

Since the numerator of the Henderson-Hasselbalch equation is reduced, reduction of the denominator P_{CO_2} can return the pH toward normal. Thus, there occurs an increase in alveolar ventilation that reduces P_{CO_2}. As men-

Table 12.3. Causes of Metabolic Acidosis

Increased Anion Gap[a]	*Normal Anion Gap*[b]
Increased production of acid	GI loss
Ketoacidosis	Diarrhea
Diabetes	Loss of small bowel fluid
Alcoholism	Loss of pancreatic fluid
Starvation	Uterosigmoidostomy
Lactic acidosis	Renal loss
Inadequate O_2 delivery	Renal tubular acidosis
Hypoxemia	Drugs inhibiting carbonic anhydrase
Reduced cardiac output	
Severe anemia	
Inadequate O_2 Utilization	
Drugs (phenformin, isoniazid)	
Diabetes mellitus	
Leukemia	
Unknown causes (common)	
Ingestion	
Salicylate	
Paraldehyde	
Methyl alcohol	
Ethylene glycol	
Inability to excrete fixed acid	
Renal failure	

[a]Addition of acid to body.

[b]Loss of HCO_3^- from body.

tioned on page 239, this compensation is seldom complete, because the central chemoreceptor, which is the slower but more powerful [H^+] sensor, "sees" less of an acidosis than the carotid body chemoreceptor. Roughly, the Pco_2 will decrease by 1 to 1.5 mmHg for every mEq drop in HCO_3^-. Expected respiratory compensation is shown in Figure 12.5. Notice that respiratory compensation does not restore pH to normal.

The pattern of breathing (Kussmaul's breathing) observed in metabolic acidosis is a regular deep sighlike pattern (see p. 120), usually without an increase in breathing frequency. Physicians are often amazed to find a Pco_2 of 20 mmHg in such patients, not realizing that hyperventilation and rapid breathing pattern are not synonymous terms.

If a reduced [HCO_3^-] is abruptly returned to normal, pH of the blood may return to normal, but because there is a lag in movement of HCO_3^- ions across the blood-brain barrier, [HCO_3^-] will be lower in the brain interstitium. Since Pco_2 will be the same in blood and the brain interstitium, that means that brain interstitium and thus the central chemoreceptor will "see" a lower pH. Indeed, inappropriately high ventilation is common for about a day after correction of metabolic acidosis.

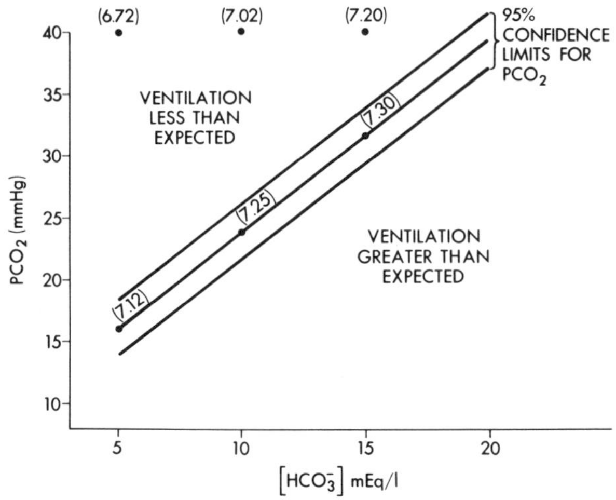

Figure 12.5. The expected change in P_{CO_2} with metabolic acidosis. As $[HCO_3^-]$ falls, alveolar ventilation increases which lowers P_{CO_2}. The numbers in the confidence limits are the expected pH's. Notice that respiratory compensation does not correct pH to normal. The numbers at the top of the figure are the pH's which would be present without any respiratory compensation. Points falling above the limit indicate less than expected ventilation, while those below indicate more than expected ventilation. Notice that in Figure 12.10, the same data is presented but the axes have been switched. (Modified, with permission, from Albert MS, Dell RB, Winters RW Jr: Quantitative Displacement of Acid-Base Equilibrium in Metabolic Acidosis. *Ann Intern Med* 66:312, 1967.)

Correction

Treatment of the underlying condition is paramount. For example, if lactic acidosis is caused by tissue hypoxia, this must be corrected. Diabetic acidosis is treated with insulin and fluids. Often the offending acid can then be metabolized. For example, when the metabolic derangement has been corrected, both lactic acid and β-hydroxybutyric acid can be metabolized into less acidic substances. If the acid cannot be changed into a "less acid" form, it must be excreted. Only the kidney can excrete fixed acid; this involves H^+ secretion into the tubular lumen with generation of new HCO_3^-. If the acid cannot be excreted by the kidney, as may occur in renal failure, hemodialysis may have to be used.

Metabolic Alkalosis

Definition

Metabolic alkalosis is a disorder caused by a physiological process that increases pH (lowers $[H^+]$) by increasing $[HCO_3^-]$.

Causes

An increased [HCO_3^-] can be caused by gain of [HCO_3^-] by the body, loss of H^+ from the body, or loss of another anion (chloride) from the body.

Gain of HCO_3^-. This is a rare cause of metabolic alkalosis and occurs mainly when HCO_3^- or substances that are metabolized into HCO_3^- are administered in excessive amounts. An example of such a substance is lactate, which can be metabolized into bicarbonate by the liver. Usually the kidney can excrete the HCO_3^- about as fast as it is administered or produced.

Loss of H^+. This is an important cause of metabolic alkalosis. H^+ can be lost via the gastrointestinal tract or via the kidney. When the acid-producing parietal cells secrete H^+ into the stomach, an equal number of HCO_3^- are generated and returned to the blood. In addition, H^+ secretion is coupled to Cl^- secretion. Thus, loss of stomach contents (vomiting or aspiration) will result in loss of H^+ and Cl^- from the body and in an increase in [HCO_3^-]. The loss of chloride is also important in maintaining the alkalosis, as will be discussed below. Villous adenoma of the colon may also secrete H^+ and cause alkalosis.

The kidney can, of course, secrete H^+, and for every H^+ secreted, HCO_3^- is generated. When H^+ secretion is excessive, [HCO_3^-] will rise. Causes of increased H^+ loss in the urine include the mineralocorticoid effect of adrenal hormones, K^+ depletion, with or without intravascular volume contraction. The mineralocorticoid effect enhances distal tubule resorption of Na^+ in exchange for either H^+ or K^+, thus causing K^+ depletion and alkalosis. *Oat cell carcinoma* producing ectopic ACTH presents with this type of metabolic alkalosis. With K^+ depletion, K^+ ions leave cells and H^+ enter cells, so that when Na^+ is now resorbed in the distal tubule, H^+ is preferentially exchanged for it. As mentioned on p. 240, severe intravascular volume contraction also causes an excess loss of H^+ in the urine.

A patient with a chronic respiratory acidosis has an elevated [HCO_3^-] due to renal compensation and a pH that is close to normal. If such a patient suddenly increases alveolar ventilation to normal levels, P_{CO_2} will fall to normal. The kidney cannot excrete HCO_3^- fast enough to drop [HCO_3^-] in proportion to the drop in P_{CO_2}. In essence, this represents an acute loss of H^+ (in a volatile form) from the body, a metabolic alkalosis. This serious condition can occur when a patient with chronic hypercapnia is mechanically ventilated.

Chloride Depletion. Na^+ resorption in the proximal tubule is usually accompanied by Cl^- to maintain electroneutrality. When the body is chloride depleted (by diuretic drugs, loss of stomach contents), and the concentration of Cl^- in the tubular fluid is low, the Na^+ resorption must be accompanied by other mechanisms to maintain electroneutrality. These are enhanced HCO_3^-

Table 12.4 Factors Maintaining Metabolic Alkalosis

Volume contraction
K^+ depletion
Cl^- depletion

resorption or H^+ and K^+ secretion. These mechanisms can cause $[HCO_3^-]$ to be elevated. A loss from the body of a large volume of fluid containing a high concentration of NaCl (as occurs with diuretics) causes the $[HCO_3^-]$ of blood to increase, because the remaining HCO_3^- is distributed over a smaller volume. This has been called *contraction alkalosis.* The most common causes of chloride depletion are diuretic drugs (that cause NaCl loss), loss of HCl from the stomach, and chloride diarrhea, which is caused by an impaired ability to resorb H^+ and Cl^- ions from the GI tract.

Two threads have emerged from our discussion of causes of metabolic alkalosis. First is that certain processes primarily increase $[HCO_3^-]$ and thus cause the alkalosis. Second is that certain variables, which may emerge in the development of the alkalosis, may then *maintain or perpetuate the alkalosis* (Table 12.4). These variables include low Cl^-, low K^+, and low blood volume. Understanding this is critical to understanding of therapy.

In terms of therapy, it is useful to classify metabolic alkalosis on the basis of its response to NaCl fluid therapy (Table 12.5). The forms of alkalosis *responding to NaCl* therapy are those in which Cl^- or volume depletion is present, mainly loss of stomach contents, villous adenoma, diuretic therapy, intravascular contraction, or chloride diarrhea. The forms of alkalosis *not responding to NaCl* are those in which H^+ is preferentially secreted into tubular fluid, mainly excess mineralocorticoid activity or K^+ depletion. One test that is useful in predicting the presence of an NaCl responsive alkalosis is simply to

Table 12.5. Disorders Causing Metabolic Alkalosis

Responsive to sodium chloride (urine $[Cl^-] < 10$ mEq/L)	*Not responsive to sodium chloride (urine $[Cl^-] > 20$ mEq/L)*
H^+ loss from GI tract	H^+ loss via kidney
Loss of acid stomach contents (vomiting, drainage)	Excessive mineralocorticoid effect
Villous adenoma	Cushing's syndrome (incl. ectopic ACTH)
Chloride diarrhea	Hyperaldosteronism
Excess HCO_3^- resorption or generation by kidney	Licorice
Volume contraction (e.g., diuretics[a])	Potassium depletion
Cl^- depletion (diuretics, GI H^+ loss)	
Acute correction chronic hypercapnia	

[a]Urine $[Cl^-]$ may be high soon after diuresis.

measure urinary Cl^- concentration. A very low urinary $[Cl^-]$ (< 10 mEq/L) suggests avid NaCl resorption caused by volume contraction and/or Cl^- depletion. A high urinary $[Cl^-]$ suggests that alkalosis will be resistant to NaCl. This test is valid only if the patient has not received diuretics within a day of the test.

Respiratory Compensation

Since the numerator $[HCO_3^-]$ of the Henderson-Hasselbalch equation is increased in metabolic alkalosis, an increase in the denominator P_{CO_2} should restore pH to normal. In fact, respiratory compensation is unpredictable and, when present, is incomplete (Figure 12.6). Several variables appear to play a role in this unpredictable response. First, alkalosis can blunt chemical drives to breathe, and patients who hypoventilate with alkalosis have blunted hypercapnic drives. On the other hand, hypoventilation always causes hypoxemia, and if the hypoxemia is severe enough, it will stimulate ventilation thus offsetting the inhibition of breathing caused by the alkalosis.

Where there is respiratory compensation for metabolic alkalosis, P_{CO_2} will go up by about .5 to 1 mmHg for every mEq/L rise in $[HCO_3^-]$. But it must be emphasized that the response is often unpredictable and even when present will not restore pH to normal.

Correction

It has been mentioned that in certain instances, other factors that are often associated with a metabolic alkalosis may maintain the alkalosis. Volume

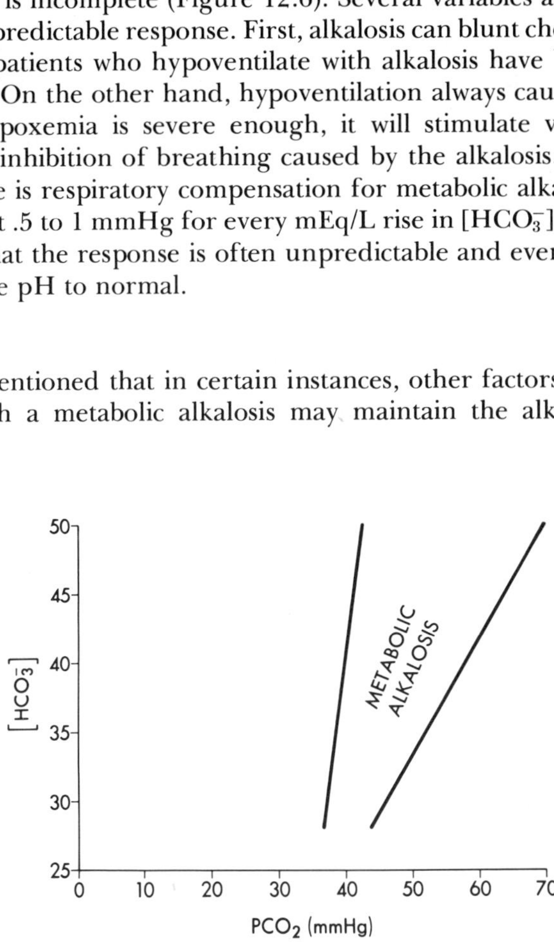

Figure 12.6. With metabolic alkalosis, there occurs a primary rise in $[HCO_3^-]$ (mEq/L). Notice that respiratory compensation is unpredictable. An $[HCO_3^-]$ of 45 mEq/L can be associated with P_{CO_2} ranging from 40 to 65 mmHg. This is actually a segment of Figure 12.10. (Modified, with permission, from Arbus GS: An in vivo acid-base nomogram for clinical use. *Can Med Assoc J* 109:291, 1973.)

depletion, chloride depletion, or potassium depletion can perpetuate an alkalosis.

Reversal of the primary abnormality is often not sufficient to restore acid-base balance. After the cause has been eliminated (e.g., loss of acid stomach contents), in order for the kidney to excrete HCO_3^-, volume depletion, Cl^- depletion, and K^+ depletion must be corrected first. Simple administration of NaCl solutions will correct volume and chloride depletion, when these are present, and allow the kidney to eliminate excess HCO_3^-. These are the NaCl responsive diseases. K^+ depletion can be treated by K^+Cl^- administration. Excess mineralocorticoid effect can be blocked by a mineralocorticoid antagonist, spironolactone, or by surgical removal of hormone-secreting tissue.

Respiratory Acidosis

What follows is a review. See also Chapter 10 for a more detailed discussion.

Definition

Respiratory acidosis is a disorder that reduces pH (increases $[H^+]$) due to a primary increase in P_{CO_2} (hypercapnia).

Causes

Respiratory acidosis occurs when there is a primary increase in P_{CO_2} (hypercapnia). The causes of hypercapnia have already been reviewed in Chapter 10. Briefly, they are hypoventilation and ventilation-perfusion mismatching.

Hypoventilation is caused by reduced drive to breathe, respiratory muscle weakness, or the combination of reduced drive and abnormal lungs or chest wall. Ventilation-perfusion mismatching results in hypercapnia if reduced hypercapnic drive to breathe is present, which allows the elevated P_{CO_2} to persist.

Alveolar CO_2 is in equilibrium with CO_2 in aqueous solution, which is in turn in equilibrium with carbonic acid, H_2CO_3, which in turn dissociates into H^+ and HCO_3^-. With an increase in alveolar P_{CO_2}, $[H^+]$ will therefore increase:

$$\text{alveolar } CO_2 \rightleftharpoons CO_2 + H_2O \rightleftharpoons H_2CO_3 \rightleftharpoons H^+ + HCO_3^-$$

To calculate the effect of hypercapnia on pH, we may use the Henderson-Hasselbalch equation:

$$pH = 6.1 + \log \frac{[HCO_3^-]}{[.03 \times P_{CO_2}]}$$

CO_2 is a very diffusible molecule, and an increase in alveolar P_{CO_2} is soon followed by an increase in P_{CO_2} (and hence $[H^+]$) throughout the body including intracellular fluid. Thus CO_2 is, in a sense, a diffusible acid capable of altering intracellular and extracellular pH.

Buffers

As previously mentioned, a rise in P_{CO_2} can only be buffered by the nonbicarbonate buffers.

Renal Compensation

Since the denominator, P_{CO_2}, of the Henderson-Hasselbalch equation is increased, an increase in the numerator $[HCO_3^-]$ will increase pH toward normal. The kidney has several ways available to increase $[HCO_3^-]$. First, the kidney reclaims all filtered HCO_3^-, a process involving H^+ secretion by the proximal tubule cells. Second, the kidney generates *new* HCO_3^-, a process also requiring H^+ secretion. With complete compensation that may require up to 5 to 7 days, $[HCO_3^-]$ will usually have increased by about 4 mEq/L for every 10 mmHg rise in P_{CO_2}.

Figure 12.7 shows the 95% confidence bands for acute (uncompensated) and fully compensated respiratory acidosis. See also Figure 10.7 of Chapter 10, which shows that acute respiratory acidosis does not cause pH to drop lower than about 7.10, and then when compensation is complete, pH is maintained above 7.20. If the pH is lower than these values in the appropriate clinical settings, a metabolic acidosis is also likely to be present.

Patients with chronic hypercapnia may develop acute exacerbation of the underlying disease with the development of *acute respiratory acidosis superim-*

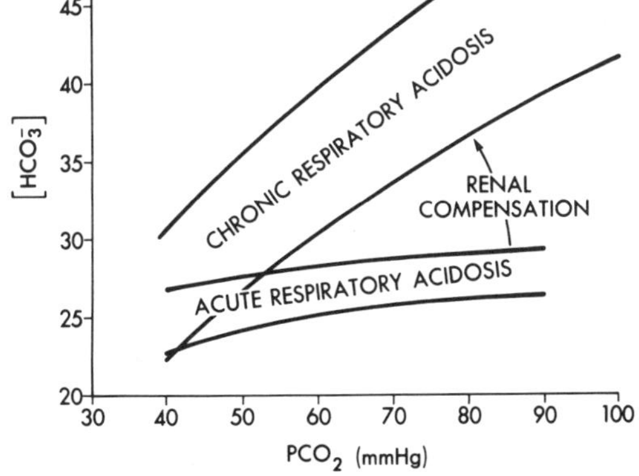

Figure 12.7. With acute respiratory acidosis there occurs only a small increase in $[HCO_3^-]$ (mEq/L). Renal compensation raises $[HCO_3^-]$, a process which may require 5 to 7 days. (Adapted, with permission, from Brackett NC Jr, Cohen JJ, Schwartz WB: Carbon Dioxide Titration Curve of Normal Man—Effect of Increasing Degrees of Acute Hypercapnia on Acid-Base Equilibrium. *New Engl J Med* 272:6, 1965, and from Brackett NC Jr, Charles MD, Wingo F, et al: Acid-Base Response to Chronic Hypercapnia in Man. *New Engl J Med* 280:124, 1969.)

posed on chronic respiratory acidosis. This causes a shift of the patient's data on a line that is roughly parallel to the "acute" line, so that at a given P_{CO_2}, $[HCO_3^-]$ is higher (and therefore pH is higher) with acute on chronic acidosis than with acute acidosis alone. If then $[HCO_3^-]$ exceeds that expected with full compensation, then in addition, a metabolic alkalosis is present. If $[HCO_3^-]$ is less than that expected without any compensation then, in addition, a metabolic acidosis is present. It must be borne in mind that the 95% confidence bands are for simple respiratory acidosis. The fact that a patient's data falls in or between the bands does not mean that a simple disorder is present. This will be discussed below under mixed disorders.

Correction

The respiratory control system, when normal, will increase ventilation briskly when confronted by increased P_{CO_2}, as during a CO_2 rebreathing test. However, when hypercapnia is present in a patient, the system has failed. Hypercapnia is caused by hypoventilation or ventilation-perfusion mismatching. Correction of respiratory acidosis would therefore require reversal of the cause of the hypoventilation. In some patients, the lesions are not reversible and chronic hypercapnia remains. Some patients with chronic hypercapnia treated with chronic oxygen therapy do remarkably well with a P_{CO_2} approaching 100 mmHg.

When alveolar ventilation is abruptly increased in a patient with chronic hypercapnia, for example, with mechanical ventilation, the P_{CO_2} drops at a rate greatly in excess of the kidneys' ability to excrete HCO_3^-. This causes an acute drop in P_{CO_2} with little acute change in $[HCO_3^-]$ causing an acute alkalosis. This alkalosis is particularly severe in the nervous system for two reasons. First, there is a lag in the HCO_3^- ions crossing from the nervous system to systemic blood, due to the blood-brain barrier, so that even though HCO_3^- may fall slowly in the blood, it will fall even more slowly in the nervous system. Second, the interstitial space of the brain is protein poor and has for all intents and purposes only the bicarbonate buffer system. This system cannot buffer one of its pair (CO_2); therefore, the acute change in CO_2 is not as well buffered in the CNS as in the rest of the body. Because of these reasons, a very severe increase in pH occurs that may cause nervous system irritability and seizures.

Respiratory Alkalosis

Definition

Respiratory alkalosis is a disorder that increases pH (reduces $[H^+]$), due to a primary decrease in P_{CO_2} caused by alveolar hyperventilation.

Causes

Alveolar hyperventilation is present when ventilation exceeds that required for CO_2 elimination, resulting in a reduced P_{CO_2}.

Hyperventilation occurs when the drive to breathe is increased. As we have shown (Chapter 6), the output of the respiratory center is modulated by three different kinds of inputs; information about higher brain centers, information about the chemical state of blood mediated by chemoreceptors, and information about the lung mediated by reflexes whose afferent arc is the vagus nerve. A useful classification of hyperventilation can thus be made (Table 12.6).

Inputs from higher centers can increase the output of the respiratory center. The best example of this is the syndrome of psychogenic hyperventilation in which anxiety results in severe hyperventilation. Cerebral dysfunction caused by vascular lesions, abnormal accumulation of chemicals (hepatic encephalopathy), or infections (encephalitis) may also cause severe hyperventilation. Drugs such as progesterone also cause hyperventilation and are responsible for the "normal" P_{CO_2} of about 30 mmHg observed in pregnancy.

Surprisingly, abnormal blood chemistry (hypoxemia or acidemia) is *not* an important cause of chronic hyperventilation. Hypoxemia caused by high altitude or right to left shunts is usually associated with hyperventilation; however because hypoxemia itself blunts hypoxic drive to breathe (p. 109), hyperventilation may not be brisk or may even be absent.

Vagal efferents are an important cause of hyperventilation. Reflexes arising in the lungs travel via the vagus nerve to the medulla and change the output of the respiratory center, resulting in a rapid shallow breathing pattern.

Table 12.6. Causes of Respiratory Alkalosis

Increase in Respiratory Center Output Acts in Response to
Information from higher cortical centers
Psychogenic hyperventilation
Cerebrovascular accidents
Diffuse cerebral dysfunction, hepatic encephalopathy
Drugs
Progesterone
Salicylates
Pregnancy (progesterone effect)
Sepsis
Information about chemical state of the blood
Hypoxemia
High altitude
Right to left shunts (early)
Information about state of the lung (vagally mediated reflexes)
Interstitial diseases
Pulmonary edema
Pneumonia
Atelectasis

This explains the often intense respiratory alkalosis seen in interstitial disease, pulmonary edema, pulmonary embolism, pneumonia, and atelectasis. Another common cause of hyperventilation occurs when a patient is being overventilated by a mechanical ventilator.

Buffers

Again only the nonbicarbonate systems buffer changes in CO_2.

$$CO_2 + H_2O \rightleftharpoons H_2CO_3 + Buf^- \rightleftharpoons HCO_3^- + HBuf$$

For respiratory alkalosis, alveolar CO_2 is reduced and the above reaction is forced to the left. An H^+ from HBuf combines with HCO_3^- to produce carbonic acid. This reduces $[HCO_3^-]$ and thus corrects pH toward normal. Most of the H^+ donated from HBuf comes from intracellular protein buffers. With respiratory alkalosis, another source of H^+ ions is lactic acid, which may be caused by reduced O_2 delivery caused by vasoconstriction and the fact that alkalemia increases O_2-hemoglobin affinity. The body is not really well prepared to deal with an acute respiratory alkalosis, and pH may rise to very high levels (Figure 12.8).

Because of the lack of nonbicarbonate buffers in the interstitial fluid of the brain and the lag in HCO_3^- movements across the blood-brain barrier, $[HCO_3^-]$ drops much more slowly than the drop in P_{CO_2} (which equilibrates with all tissues). This causes a severe alkalosis in the nervous system, which reduces levels of ionized calcium, which causes neuromuscular irritability. This leads to a "pins and needles" feeling (paresthesias) of the fingers, numbness around the mouth, cramps, tetany, and seizures. Some of these symptoms may also be caused by the reduction in cerebral blood flow, which regularly accompanies hypocapnia.

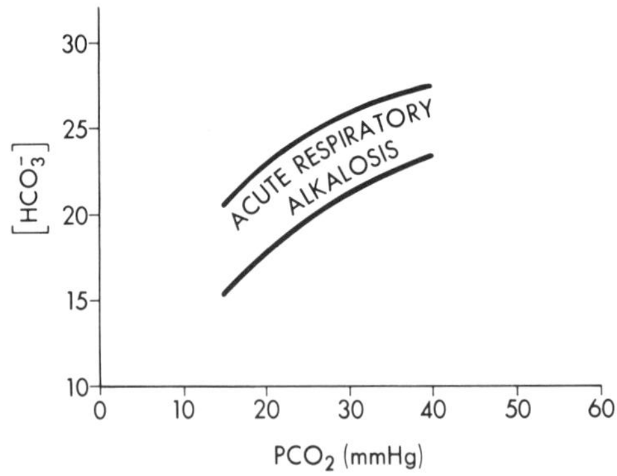

Figure 12.8. Expected changes in P_{CO_2} and $[HCO_3^-]$ (mEq/L) with acute respiratory alkalosis. (Adapted, with permission, from Arbus GS, Lee MD, Hebert A, et al: Characterization and clinical application of the "Significance Band" for Acute Respiratory Alkalosis. *New Engl J Med* 280:117, 1969.)

Renal Compensation

Since the denominator [.03 × P_{CO_2}] of the Henderson-Hasselbalch equation is reduced, a reduction in the numerator [HCO_3^-] will reduce pH toward normal. The kidney is capable of reducing [HCO_3^-] by simply allowing filtered HCO_3^- ions to be lost in the urine. Since more anion (HCO_3^-) will be excreted, it will be accompanied by cations, Na^+ or K^+. Thus, a depletion of these can inhibit this response. Complete renal compensation may restore pH to normal in chronic respiratory alkalosis.

Correction

Respiratory alkalosis, as Table 12.6 shows, often occurs in severe dysfunction of nonrespiratory organ systems, and some of these disorders may not be reversible (e.g., cerebrovascular accidents). The hyperventilation of interstitial lung disease also is often not reversible. When the disorder or drug effect is reversible (pregnancy, pneumonia, atelectasis, sepsis, hepatic encephalopathy, pulmonary edema), the hyperventilation usually resolves spontaneously. The syndrome of psychogenic hyperventilation is often treated by having the patient rebreathe from a bag, which raises the P_{CO_2} and promptly relieves most of the symptoms caused by the low P_{CO_2}.

Mixed Acid-Base Disorders

In order to understand mixed acid-base disorders, it is necessary to be able to recognize simple disorders. One way to do this is to use an acid-base nomogram. There are many different nomograms available. We prefer to plot acid-base data as shown in Figure 12.9. The horizontal axis represents the

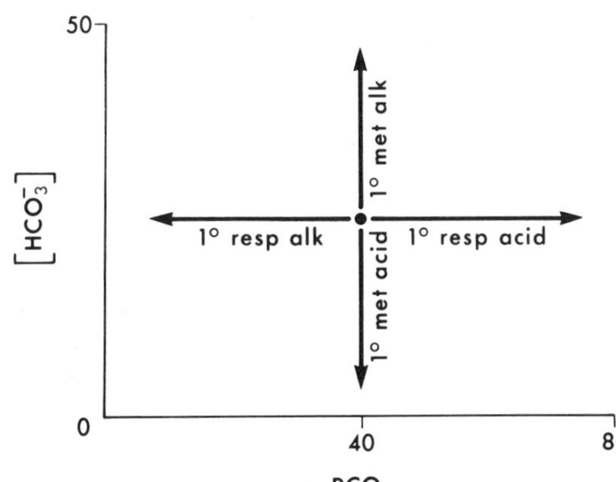

Figure 12.9. Development of an acid-base nomogram. The horizontal axis represents the respiratory component, while the vertical represents the metabolic component. The arrows indicate the direction of changes of the primary uncompensated acid-base disorders.

respiratory component, P_{CO_2}, while the vertical axis represents the metabolic component. This means that a rightward displacement of a point represents an uncompensated and unbuffered rise in P_{CO_2}; similarly a downward displacement in a point represents a reduction in $[HCO_3^-]$. Using a graph with such axes means that if a patient develops a metabolic acidosis, the data point will be displaced downward, whereas a respiratory acidosis will be represented by rightward displacement.

In Figure 12.10 we have consolidated several of the figures previously shown in this chapter. The bands represent 95% confidence limits for a single respiratory or metabolic acid-base disorder. That means, for example, if a person develops an acute metabolic acidosis that 95 times out of a hundred the point determined by $[HCO_3^-]$ and P_{CO_2} will fall within the confidence band

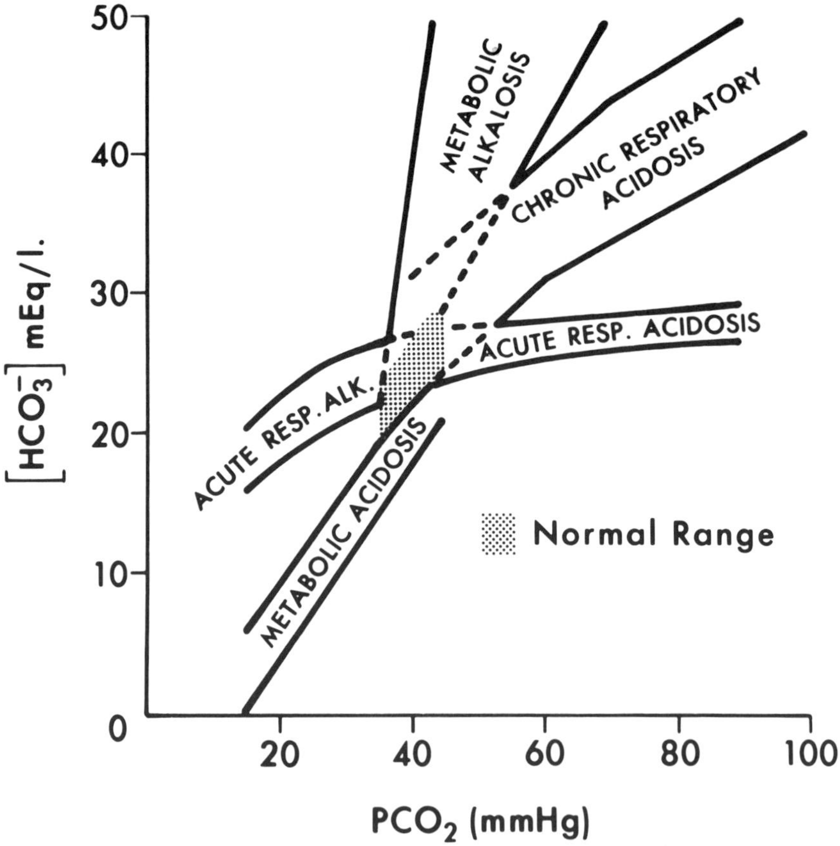

Figure 12.10. Confidence bands for acid-base disorders. (Adapted, with permission, from Arbus GS: An in vivo acid-base nomogram for clinical use. *Can Med Assoc J* 109:291, 1973.)

shown. However, the fact that a point falls into a band does not mean a simple disorder is present. There are many ways a data point can be obtained. For example, a patient may have a primary metabolic alkalosis followed by an episode of acute hypoventilation, which would fall into the confidence band for chronic respiratory acidosis. Similarly, a patient's data point shown between 2 bands may have gotten there in different ways. Consider a data point between the chronic and the acute respiratory acidosis bands. This could represent upward displacement (incomplete renal compensation of acute respiratory acidosis), rightward displacement (acute on chronic respiratory acidosis), or downward displacement (metabolic acidosis in a patient with chronic hypercapnia).

Because the laboratory data may be inconclusive, *the most reliable information is obtained from the history and physical examination, still the physician's secret weapon.* These will usually provide the important clues for accurate diagnosis in the more complex mixed disorders. For example, a history of methanol ingestion or untreated diabetes mellitus suggests that metabolic acidosis is contributing to the problem.

Metabolic Acidosis and Respiratory Alkalosis

This combination is common in hepatic failure and salicylate poisoning. Both these conditions increase the drive to breathe and can also cause a metabolic acidosis. The clue is the P_{CO_2} which is lower than the confidence band would predict for metabolic acidosis alone. This combination may result in a normal pH, in spite of the fact that such disorders may be lethal.

Metabolic Alkalosis and Respiratory Acidosis

This combination is very common in patients with chronic respiratory acidosis who are treated with diuretic agents, which can induce metabolic alkalosis. The clue here is that $[HCO_3^-]$ is much greater than expected in a patient with chronic hypercapnia.

Metabolic and Respiratory Acidosis

Cardiac arrest or acute heart failure may lead to metabolic and respiratory acidosis. The metabolic acidosis is lactic acidosis caused by the tissue hypoxia due to the circulatory arrest. When the H^+ is buffered by the reaction, $H^+ + HCO_3^- \rightarrow H_2CO_3 \rightarrow CO_2 + H_2O$, excess CO_2 is produced. This together with the fact that the patient usually stops breathing (i.e., a "closed buffer system") leads to a rapid rise in P_{CO_2}. The clue is the clinical setting and a low $[HCO_3^-]$ and an inappropriately high P_{CO_2}.

Acute on Chronic Respiratory Acidosis

Although not a true mixed disorder, acute on chronic respiratory acidosis is common and is almost always suggested by the patient's clinical setting. The patient's data falls between the confidence bands for acute and chronic respiratory acidosis.

BIBLIOGRAPHY

Davenport HW: *ABC of Acid-Base Chemistry: The Elements of Physiological Blood-Gas Chemistry for Medical Students and Physicians*, ed 6. Chicago, University of Chicago Press, 1974.

Dell RB: Normal Acid-Base Regulation, in Winters RW (ed): *The Body Fluids in Pediatrics.* Boston, Little, Brown & Co, 1973, p 23.

Goldberger E: *A Primer of Water, Electrolyte & Acid-Base Syndromes*, ed 6. Philadelphia, Lea & Febiger, 1980.

Kaehny WD: Pathogenesis and Management of Metabolic Acidosis and Alkalosis, in Schrier RW (ed): *Renal and Electrolyte Disorders.* Boston, Little, Brown & Co, 1976, p 79.

Kaehny WD: Pathogenesis and Management of Respiratory and Mixed Acid-Base Disorders, in Schrier RW (ed): *Renal and Electrolyte Disorders.* Boston, Little, Brown & Co, 1976, p 121.

Masoro EJ, Siegel PD: *Acid-Base Regulation: Its Physiology, Pathophysiology and the Interpretation of Blood-Gas Analysis*, ed 2. Philadelphia, WB Saunders Co, 1977.

Winters RW: Physiology of Acid-Base Disorders, in Winters RW (ed): *The Body Fluids in Pediatrics.* Boston, Little, Brown & Co, 1973, p 23.

13

Pediatric Lung Disease

Victor Chernick
Meir H. Kryger

THE NEWBORN

The fetus in its mother's uterus depends on the placenta for oxygen delivery and carbon dioxide excretion. With birth, a dramatic change occurs and the lungs must quickly become the organ of gas exchange. The major respiratory problems in this period of life are related to immaturity of the lungs, *the respiratory distress syndrome of the newborn* (or hyaline membrane disease), and abnormality in respiratory control, which can cause *apnea* and *periodic breathing.*

Fetal gas exchange occurs in the placenta. P_{O_2} and P_{CO_2} of *umbilical vein* blood has equilibrated with the maternal blood in the placenta. The P_{O_2} at which oxygen loading of fetal blood occurs in the placenta is only about 30 mmHg. Fetal hemoglobin has increased oxygen affinity facilitating O_2 uptake at such low P_{O_2} (see p. 172). The oxygenated blood travels in the umbilical vein, bypasses the liver via the ductus venosus, and joins the inferior vena cava mixing with the venous blood returning from the fetal extremities. On reaching the right atrium, about 85% of this blood traverses the foramen ovale, the left atrium, and the left ventricle and is pumped into the aorta to perfuse the peripheral tissues including the upper body and brain. The blood that did not traverse the foramen ovale mixes with superior vena caval blood and enters the right ventricle to be pumped into the pulmonary artery. The pulmonary artery is connected to the aorta by the ductus arteriosus, and because pulmonary vascular resistance is high, more than 90% of the blood pumped into the pulmonary artery bypasses the lung and perfuses the lower body.

In summary, most of the output of both ventricles goes into the aorta, and less than 10% of the combined ventricular output passes through the lungs. The major changes in the circulation after birth are reduction of pulmonary vascular resistance caused by aeration of the lung, closure of the foramen ovale, and constriction of the ductus arteriosus. Pulmonary vascular resistance is reduced by a combination of factors including the reversal of hypoxic vasoconstriction, since there is no longer airway hypoxia, and the effect of lung inflation itself. The foramen ovale closes, because left atrial pressure exceeds right atrial pressure. Right atrial pressure is reduced with obliteration of umbilical vein blood flow; left atrial pressure increases as pulmonary flow increases. The ductus arteriosus has the unusual property of constricting when Po_2 is high and dilating when Po_2 is low; it thus constricts at birth. This results in the "adult" circulation, the right ventricle pumping blood into the pulmonary circulation to take part in gas exchange and the left ventricle pumping oxygenated blood into the aorta. Occasionally the ductus fails to constrict; and this is found most often in prematurely born infants. It is known that prostaglandin E will dilate the ductus and prostaglandin F will constrict the ductus. Patent ductus arteriosus can be closed with indomethacin, a prostaglandin synthetase inhibitor, or may require surgical ligation.

After birth, the pressures required for the first breath, to fill the airless lung, are very high (reaching peak pressure of -60 cmH_2O and occasionally up to -100 cmH_2O, lasting less than a second) and require marked respiratory muscular effort. The volume of the fetal thorax is low (about 2/3 of FRC) and is reduced even further by compression during passage through the vagina; thus there is a tendency for outward recoil of the chest wall. In addition, the muscles of inspiration, including diaphragm and intercostals, have a mechanical advantage that allows the generation of high inspiratory pressures at the time of birth. These are only applied for a brief time, and ordinarily the lung does not rupture. However, spontaneous pneumothorax does occur in about .5 to 1% of normal newborn infants. The first breath seems to resemble a gasp, perhaps caused by severe hypoxia of the nervous system. In any case, after breathing has started, the lungs are rapidly inflated with air and breathing becomes rhythmic. Alveolar stability is enhanced by the remarkable characteristics of pulmonary surfactant.

Pulmonary Surfactant

The elastic recoil of the lung is determined by the characteristics of its structure, including collagen and elastin. Once aerated, however, it is the contribution of surface tension that accounts for about two-thirds of the elastic recoil force of the lung.

Molecules exert attractive forces on each other (van der Waals forces). Inner molecules are attracted in all directions by their neighbors and thus experience no net force. Molecules on a surface are attracted inward, and it is because of this inward pull that the surface of a liquid tends to contract to the smallest possible surface area, a sphere. As a result of this tendency to contract, the surface behaves as if it were in a state of tension, rather like a stretched sheet of rubber. When pressure is applied to inflate the lung, the pressure is used to stretch the tissues of the lung itself and the sheet of surfactant, which is under tension.

To understand the role of surface tension in the lung, it helps to understand the effect of surface tension on bubbles, such as soap bubbles (Figure 13.1). Because of surface tension, the wall of a bubble behaves as though it were stretched, and thus it compresses the gas in the bubble and increases the pressure of this gas. The relationship between the bubble gas pressure (P) and the wall surface tension (t) is:

$$P = \frac{2t}{r} \qquad \text{Laplace equation for a sphere}$$

where t is a measure of surface tension (dynes/cm^2), P is the bubble pressure, and r is the radius of the bubble. This very important equation says that the smaller the radius of a bubble, the greater the pressure inside, if surface tension is constant. If the alveoli can be thought of as bubbles, this means that pressure in a small alveolus will be greater than the pressure in a large alveolus if surface tension were the same. Because of this pressure difference, gas will flow from the small alveolus into the large alveolus; because the small alveolus becomes smaller and smaller, its pressure becomes larger and larger. Eventually the small alveolus will empty entirely and collapse. During normal expiration, if surface tension were constant, as alveoli decrease in size, the

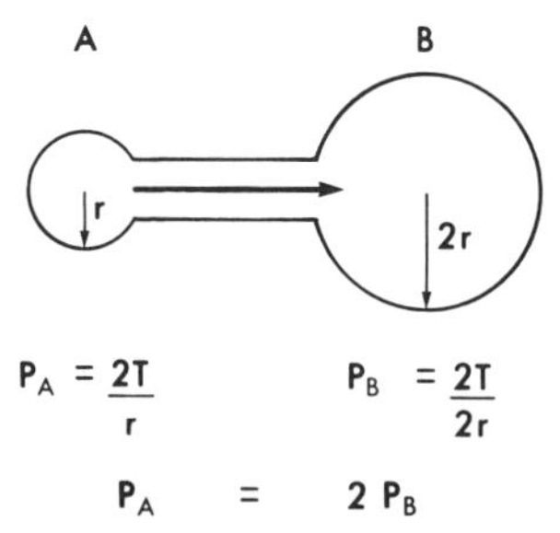

Figure 13.1. Two bubbles connected by an airway. If the surface tension were the same in units A and B, since the radius of A is half that of B, by the Laplace equation the pressure inside A is twice that inside B. This pressure difference causes air to flow from A to B, and eventually A will empty.

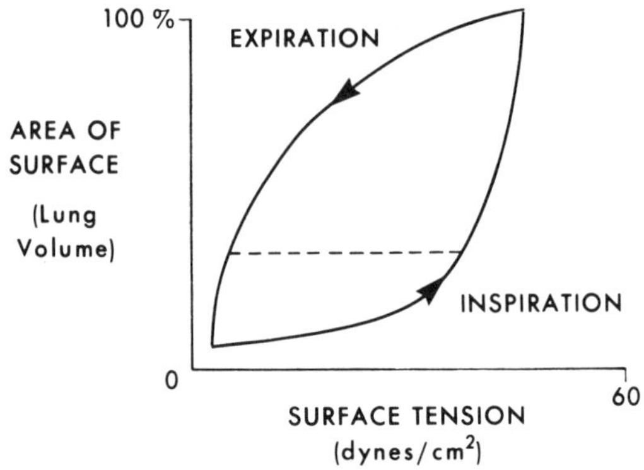

Figure 13.2. The change in surface tension as the area of film of surfactant is increased. This is equivalent to an increase in lung volume. At a given surface area (dashed line), surface tension is much less during the expiratory phase than the inspiratory phase.

pressure in them would progressively increase, and they would empty entirely, that is, become atelectatic. Obviously these events do not occur. The surface tension of the lining of alveoli is not constant but depends on phase of respiration being higher during inspiration and falling close to zero at low lung volumes (Figure 13.2).

This remarkable and unique property of the pulmonary surfactant allows different size alveoli to exist and prevents the lung from becoming airless with each expiration.

Surfactant is synthesized and secreted by alveolar type II cells. The lamellar bodies of these cells are storage sites for the lipoprotein which constitutes surfactant (Figure 13.3). Surfactant is probably made up of many constituents, the major lipid being dipalmitoyl phosphatidylcholine (dipalmitoyl lecithin or DPL) and a protein that helps stabilize DPL at the air-liquid interface. The fetal lung contains glucocorticoid receptors that, when stimulated by endogenous or administered corticosteroids, accelerate the production of surfactant, probably by accelerating the maturation of enzymes necessary for DPL synthesis.

Respiratory Distress Syndrome of the Newborn

The lungs must be capable of function before extrauterine life is possible. The development of airways and capillaries is not usually sufficiently advanced to be able to take part in gas exchange until about 26 to 28 weeks of gestation, when alveoli begin to appear. Usually, at roughly the same time, alveolar type II cells and surfactant begin to appear. It must be emphasized, however, that maturation of the lung and the production of surfactant vary widely. In some instances, a 30-week gestational age fetus may have the "machinery" necessary to sustain life, whereas a 34-week-old fetus may not.

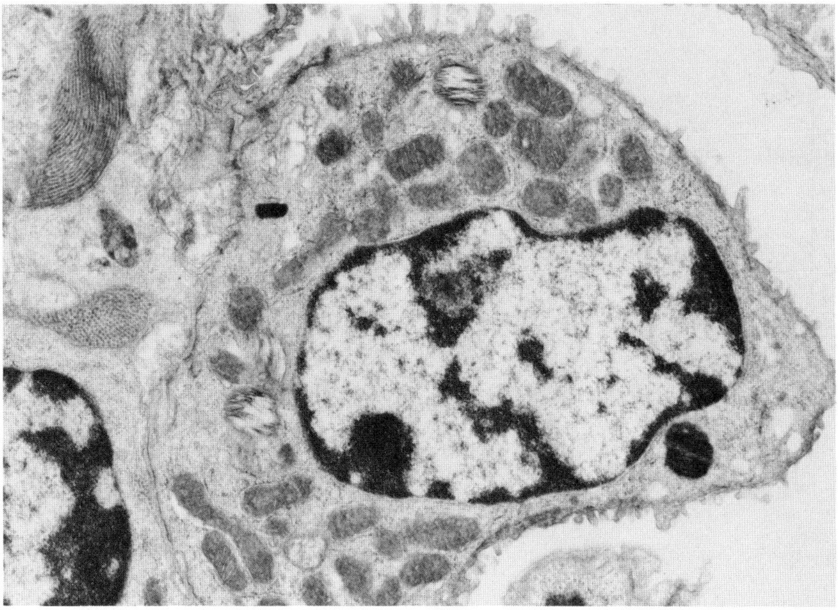

Figure 13.3. An electronmicrograph of an alveolar type II cell (magnification ×17,000). (The author acknowledges the work of Dr. J.M. Papadimitriou, Pathologist, Sir Charles Gairdner Hospital, The Queen Elizabeth II Medical Centre, Nedlands, Western Australia, 6009.)

What then happens when birth occurs before the respiratory system has matured sufficiently for gas exchange? When such a child is born, it tries to breathe but develops the *respiratory distress syndrome of the newborn,* also called *hyaline membrane disease.*

This disease is caused by the interaction of deficient surfactant and immature gas-exchanging units, which then cause reduced compliance (stiff lungs) and a tendency for lung units to collapse (Figure 13.4). There then occurs ventilation-perfusion mismatching and right to left shunting of blood through the lung leading to severe hypoxemia and pulmonary hypertension. This may result in opening of the foramen ovale with worsening of hypoxemia. The hypoxemia may lead to a marked reduction in oxygen delivery, with the resultant anaerobic metabolism causing metabolic acidosis. The infant tries to expand the stiff lungs by generating very negative pleural pressures. This results in a marked increase in the work of breathing, which may then lead to respiratory muscle fatigue, hypercapnia, and apnea. The very high negative pressure also facilitates movement of fluid into the alveoli.

It is the protein from this fluid (fibrin and other blood constituents), which causes the hyaline membranes seen on microscopy. The examination of the infant reveals cyanosis and a rapid respiratory rate. Because of the very negative pressures required to ventilate the stiff lungs, and because the chest wall

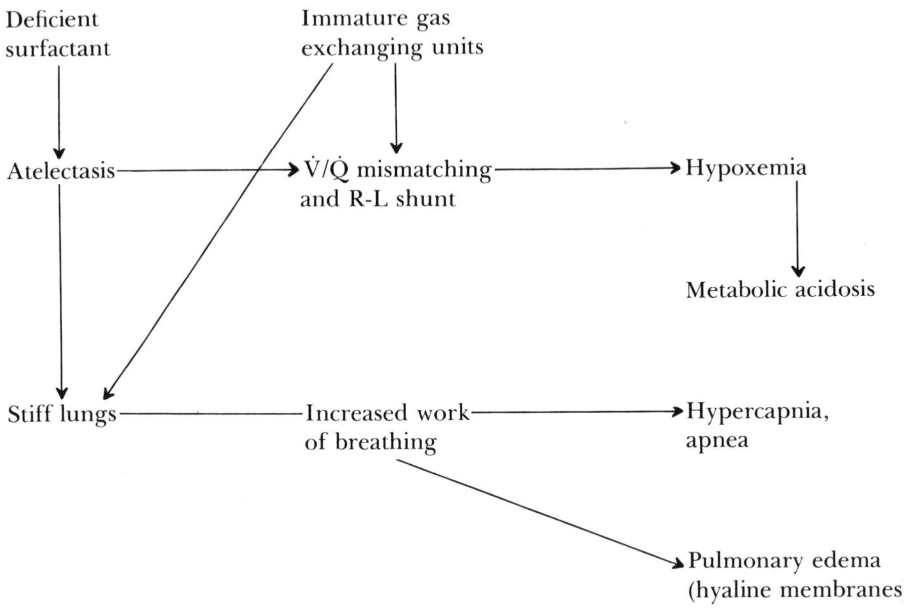

Figure 13.4. The pathophysiology of the respiratory distress syndrome of the newborn.

in neonates is very compliant, respiratory efforts are accompanied by severe retraction of segments of the chest wall. These infants may also grunt on expiration. It is thought that these grunts represent laryngeal closure, which has the effect of maintaining positive airway pressure at the end of expiration and preventing collapse.

Treatment of this disorder includes oxygen administration and maneuvers to prevent atelectasis, such as continuous positive airway pressure. If the work of breathing required to maintain ventilation is too high for the neonate, mechanical ventilation is required.

The most exciting development in this field concerns the development of methods that indicate the state of lung maturity before birth and the use of glucocorticoids to hasten lung development.

Amniotic fluid contains liquid that is actively secreted from the fetal lung. Chemical analysis of amniotic fluid can be used to accurately predict whether the fetal lung is producing sufficient surfactant to avoid alveolar instability at birth. In general, amniotic fluid that contains a lecithin/sphingomyelin ratio of $\geq 2:1$ indicates mature fetal lungs.

Lungs contain specific glucocorticoid receptors, which are proteins found in cytoplasm. The binding of corticosteroids modifies these receptors, which then migrate to the nucleus and influence the synthetic rates of mRNA for various proteins including enzymes used in synthesis of surfactant. Thus, glucocorticoids accelerate the normal pattern of lung development including the production of surfactant. This is true whether the glucocorticoid is endogenous or administered as treatment. Glucocorticosteroids can be administered to mothers in premature labor, and if delivery can be delayed for 24 hours, the incidence of hyaline membrane disease decreases dramatically and the survival rate of premature infants has been shown to increase.

Abnormal Breathing Patterns

Prior to birth, the fetus makes episodic respiratory movements consisting of rapid, irregular breaths associated with the rapid eye movement (REM) stage of sleep. The movements are not increased as in the adult by hypoxemia and hypercapnia; indeed, mild hypoxemia may inhibit fetal breathing. When the mother smokes cigarettes, uterine vasoconstriction occurs causing a low fetal Po_2, which then inhibits fetal breathing. Fetal breathing pattern becomes grossly abnormal, either totally absent or gasping in type, in fetuses who die in utero. Caffeine is known to stimulate fetal breathing activity.

Unlike the adult, when a newborn baby is made hypoxemic, there occurs a temporary increase in ventilation that is then followed by a sustained reduction in ventilation. The hypoxemia may also induce a periodic breathing pattern, a waxing and waning of tidal volume that may be followed by short episodes of apnea lasting 10 to 20 seconds. In other words, hypoxemia depresses breathing in neonates, In addition, hypoxemia reduces CO_2 drive in neonates.

Another factor that may contribute to abnormal breathing patterns is the compliant chest wall of neonates. During dreaming (REM) sleep (making up 50 to 80% of sleep time in neonates), there occurs a loss of tone of various muscles including the intercostals. When the diaphragm contracts, the chest wall, unstabilized by loss of intercostal tone, may retract causing paradoxical chest wall motion. Thus, in spite of respiratory efforts there may be little or no airflow.

Factors that induce periodic breathing and apnea are factors that depress the drive to breathe in the neonate: narcotics, hypoxia, sleep, and an abnormal or immature respiratory center. Episodes of periodic breathing and apnea are most severe in the prematurely born infant and occur primarily during sleep.

Some children have prolonged episodes of apnea during sleep requiring resuscitation. Such children have been found to have abnormal chemical drive to breathe and presumably an abnormal respiratory center. It is thought that apnea during sleep is one cause of *crib death*, the *sudden infant death syndrome*.

Periodic breathing and apnea are treated by oxygen therapy (since in neonates hypoxemia depresses breathing), stimulating or waking the child, or using aminophylline or caffeine, which have respiratory stimulant properties.

Periodic breathing and apnea may be manifestations of other diseases and may occur in infections, congenital heart disease, the respiratory distress syndrome, in association with intracranial hemorrhage, or during metabolic disturbances such as hypoglycemia or hypocalcemia.

THE OLDER CHILD

In the newborn infant one of the major diseases affecting the lung is respiratory distress syndrome, a restrictive disorder that is associated with stiff lungs and difficulty in lung expansion. In contrast, the older child is largely affected by diseases that cause airway obstruction and consequently difficulty in moving air in and out of the lung. Airways and alveoli grow as the child grows, and compared to adults, children have small diameter airways. Thus, a disease that may have little effect in adults may have devastating effects in children if airway diameter is compromised. Croup and bronchiolitis are examples of inflamed airways that cause clinical problems in children but not usually in adults.

Croup

Croup (laryngotracheobronchitis) is a disorder that usually affects children under 3 years of age. It is caused by a viral infection of the larger airways (usually parainfluenza virus), which causes mucosal edema and inflammation in the subglottic region and may extend to the trachea and large bronchi. Because the major obstruction to airflow is outside the thorax in the subglottic area, the child has difficulty getting air in, while during expiration, the positive pressure inside the lumen of the airway tends to expand the airway and allow an easier expiration (see p. 40). Clinically, these children have a raspy or croupy inspiratory sound and may have a barking or "brassy" cough. Therapy includes the use of mist to avoid local mucosal drying, epinephrine inhalation to decongest and reduce mucosal swelling, and, rarely, endotracheal intubation for a few days to provide an adequate airway. A more serious form of this disease is caused by a bacterial infection, *H influenza,* and tends to afflict older children. The swelling in this case involves the epiglottis as well as the subglottic area, and emergency tracheotomy or endotracheal intubation is often necessary to provide an adequate airway.

Bronchiolitis

Bronchiolitis is caused by a viral infection, most often respiratory syncitial virus (RSV), which results in swelling and inflammation of the mucosa of small airways (bronchioles) leading to small airway obstruction. The disease usually affects children under the age of 2 years. Although inspiratory airway resistance is increased, the major problem is during expiration. Because of expiratory airway obstruction, lung volume increases causing an increase in the arteroposterior diameter of the chest. There is ventilation-perfusion mismatching leading to hypoxemia, and in severe cases, respiratory failure may occur leading to respiratory acidosis and occasionally sudden apnea, when respiratory muscles fatigue. Clinically, these children present with rapid respiratory rates, wheezing, and when severe, cyanosis. Therapy includes oxygen, hydration to reduce viscosity of respiratory secretions, and bronchodilators, which have both decongestant and bronchodilating properties (α- and β-adrenergic agonists).

Asthma is a disorder, which commonly begins in childhood, and is discussed elsewhere (p. 142). Other disorders that appear during childhood are the following.

Cystic Fibrosis

Cystic fibrosis (mucoviscidosis) is a disorder of exocrine function, which is inherited as an autosomal recessive, and results in pancreatic insufficiency, chronic airflow obstruction, and elevated sweat sodium and chloride concentrations. Respiratory difficulty may present for the first time in the infant, the older child, or even in adults. Impaction of viscid airway secretions leads to air trapping, atelectasis, and recurrent infections. The airway secretions also become colonized by *pseudomonas aeruginosa.* These children develop severe chronic airflow obstruction, bronchiectasis, and eventually respiratory failure.

Immotile Cilia Syndrome (see p. 286)

Cilia in the respiratory tract are abnormal causing recurrent ear, nasal sinus, and respiratory tract infections. The recurrent infections may result in bronchiectasis and airflow obstruction. The disorder is frequently associated with situs inversus (Kartagener's syndrome).

BIBLIOGRAPHY

Avery ML, Fletcher BD: *The Lung and its Disorders in the Newborn Infant*, ed 3. Philadelphia, WB Saunders, 1977.

Chernick V, ed: *Onset and Control of Fetal and Neonatal Respiration.* New York, Grune and Stratton, 1977. (Seminars in Perinatology, Vol 1, No 4)

Chernick V, ed: *Respiratory Problems in Children.* South New York, New York, Stratton Intercontinental Medical Book Corp, 1979. (Seminars in Respiratory Medicine, Vol 1, No 2)

Kendig EL, Chernick V: *Disorders of the Respiratory Tract in Children.* Philadelphia, WB Saunders, 1977.

Levison H, ed: *The Chest.* Philadelphia, WB Saunders, 1979. (The Pediatric Clinics of North America, Vol 26, No 3)

14

Lung Cancer

Meir H. Kryger

PRIMARY LUNG CANCER
Etiology
Cell Types
Abnormal Function Due to Local Growth of the Tumor
- Airways
- Blood vessels
- Lymphatics
- Nerves
- Pleura

Abnormal Function Due to Extrathoracic Spread
Abnormal Function Due to Ectopic Hormone Production
Abnormal Function Due to Unknown Effects of Lung Cancer
- Neuromuscular abnormalities
- Bone and connective tissue

Is the Patient Operable?

METASTATIC DISEASE IN THE THORAX

Lung cancer is the most common form of malignancy in North American and European men and is the cause of death in about one third of all male patients with cancer (Figure 14.1). It must be remembered that a malignant lesion in the lung may not disturb lung function at all; the first adverse effect of a malignant lung lesion may be on another organ system. The major factor determining abnormality in lung function is the *location* of the malignancy. The major factor determining the survival of the patient is the *biological activity* of the malignancy, which depends on the cell type and the propensity of the tumor to spread in the lungs and elsewhere.

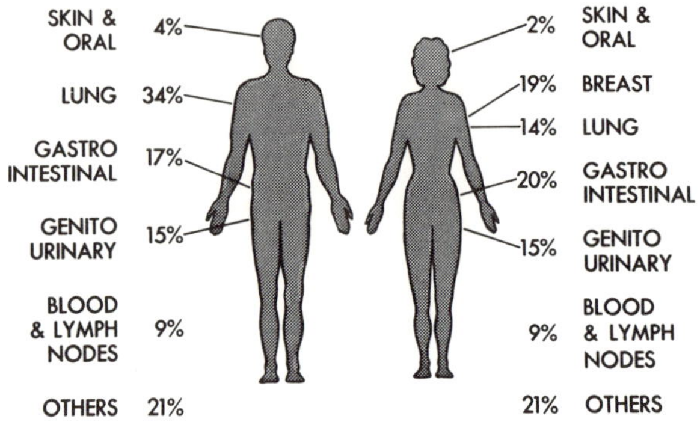

Figure 14.1. Deaths from cancer in men and women, 1979.

PRIMARY LUNG CANCER

Etiology

The major cause of lung cancer is cigarette smoking. People who smoke 40 or more cigarettes daily have a death rate from lung cancer that is 65 times greater than in nonsmokers. Exposure to asbestos, ionizing radiation, beryllium, nickel, and chromates increase the risk of developing lung cancer. A cigarette smoker also exposed to the above factors has a much greater risk of developing cancer.

Cell Types

Squamous cell carcinoma (called epidermoid when well differentiated) is the most common lung cancer accounting for about 60% of the total and is found almost exclusively in cigarette smokers. This type of tumor most often arises from the larger airways and, therefore, produces symptoms early. This tumor often outgrows its blood supply; therefore its core may necrose and result in *cavitation*.

Adenocarcinoma, making up about 15% of the total, usually arises from more peripheral locations of the lung and is often asymptomatic until it has metastasized widely. This type of malignancy may arise from fibrotic tissue, scars or fibrosis in the interstitial space.

Undifferentiated (anaplastic) carcinoma, further subdivided into small (oat cell) and large cell undifferentiated cell types, makes up about 20% of the total. The *oat cell* variety is associated with the production of *ectopic hormones* and has usually metastasized to bone marrow when the diagnosis is made.

Alveolar cell (or bronchiolar-alveolar cell) carcinoma, which makes up less than 5% of lung cancers, may arise simultaneously in several locations and may fill up alveoli in a large region or spread in the lymphatics. This type of malignancy can result in the production of copious quantities of sputum, bronchorrhea.

Atypical cells may be present in the respiratory tract of persons exposed to carcinogens. These changes may be reversible if the carcinogenic stimulus is eliminated. In patients with established squamous cell carcinoma, other parts of the bronchial tree almost always contain atypical cells and occasionally *carcinoma in situ.* Tumor cells have decreased cohesiveness and are easily separated from the main tumor mass, thus explaining the usefulness of exfoliative cytology in diagnosis.

Lung cancer will invade local tissues and may spread to other parts of the body in vascular or lymphatic vessels. Lung cancer can disturb function because of *local growth, metastatic growth, and ectopic hormone production;* some of the effects of lung cancer are unknown (Table 14.1).

Table 14.1. Disturbance of Function in Lung Cancer

Due to local growth	
In airways	Localized obstruction, recurrent pneumonia, hemoptysis.
In blood vessels	Vascular compression, hemoptysis, tumor embolization.
In lymphatics	Lymphatic obstruction, exudative effusion, lymphangitic carcinomatosis.
In pleura	Exudative or bloody effusion.
In nervous tissue	Invasion of inferior cervical ganglion, brachial plexus, recurrent laryngeal nerve, phrenic nerve.
Due to extrathoracic spread	
Brain	Seizures, cerebral edema, focal defects.
Bone marrow	Anemia, fractures, hypercalcemia.
Due to ectopic hormone production	
ACTH: Cushing's syndrome	Hypokalemia, metabolic alkalosis, hyperglycemia, muscular weakness.
ADH: Inappropriate ADH	Hyponatremia, concentrated urine, cerebral edema.
PTH: Hyperparathyroidism	Hypercalcemia, hypophosphatemia, confusion, weakness, constipation, polyuria.
Gonadotropin	Gynecomastia.
5-Hydroxytryptamine: Carcinoid syndrome	Episodic diarrhea, flushing, bronchoconstriction.
Due to unknown effects	
Neural tissue	Leukoencephalopathy, peripheral neuropathy.
Neuromuscular junction	"Myasthenic" syndrome.
Muscle	Polymyositis.
Bone	Osteoarthropathy.

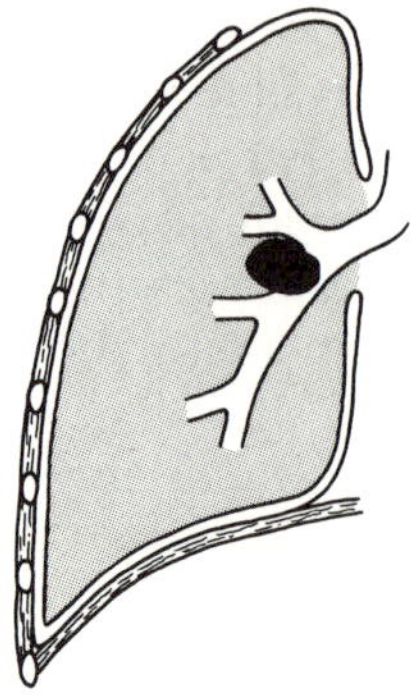

Figure 14.2. Sequelae of tumor obstruction of bronchi.

Abnormal Function Due to Local Growth of the Tumor

Airways

Since lung cancer often develops in airways, it is not surprising that cough and localized bronchial obstruction are common manifestations (Figure 14.2). With partial obstruction, there will be a reduction in airflow, which may be heard as a *localized* audible wheeze. With obstruction, there may be a breakdown of local antibacterial mechanisms with the development of infection. With complete obstruction, the gas in the lung distal to the obstruction will be absorbed and will become atelectatic (gas-free). If the tumor invades blood vessels, the patient may cough up blood (*hemoptysis*), an important symptom.

Blood vessels

Tumor emboli may be carried to many parts of the body to cause metastatic disease. Malignant tissue will compress low pressure vessels (veins) more easily than high pressure vessels (arteries). An important syndrome occurs when tumor causes superior vena caval obstruction (Figure 14.3). Flow into the right atrium is impeded causing a marked increase in pressure in the superior vena cava; since the cerebral circulation empties into this vein, there will occur an increase in intracranial pressure, which causes severe headaches. In addition, there will be marked swelling of the face and neck.

Lymphatics

Cancer cells may invade lymphatic vessels and then multiply in hilar or mediastinal lymph nodes (Figure 14.4). This may impede lymphatic flow and cause a protein-rich exudative pleural effusion. Tumor cells may also grow in the lymphatic channels of the lung causing *lymphangitic carcinomatosis.* Growth of the tumor may be so extensive as to fill virtually all the lymphatic channels and the interstitial space of the lung and cause a severe restrictive disorder, with hypoxemic respiratory failure. Activation of lung reflexes leads to dyspnea and a rapid shallow breathing pattern.

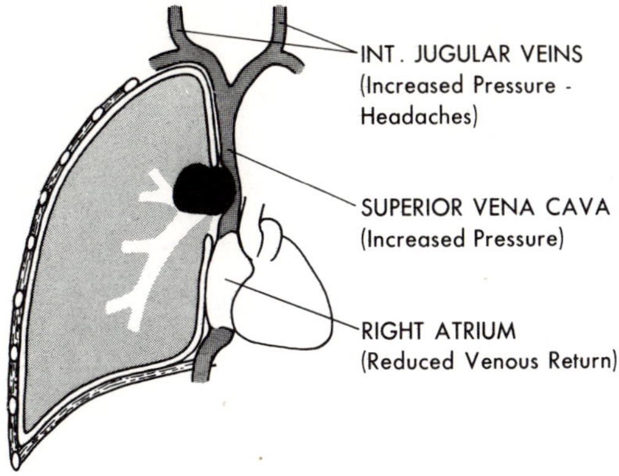

Figure 14.3. Malignant tissue can compress or invade the superior vena cava. This causes a reduction in venous return and consequently a reduced or fixed cardiac output. The resultant increase in internal jugular venous pressure causes increased intracranial pressure and headaches.

Nerves

Malignant tissue may invade the phrenic nerve and cause paralysis of a diaphragm. Tumors growing in the apex of the lung (Pancoast tumor) can encounter several different neural structures and cause several problems (Figure 14.5). These tumors can invade the recurrent laryngeal nerve, which innervates a vocal cord, and cause hoarseness. Another neural structure in this region is the inferior cervical ganglion, which is part of the sympathetic chain. Invasion of this ganglion causes *Horner's syndrome.* An apical tumor may also invade the lower nerves of the brachial plexus and cause pain and

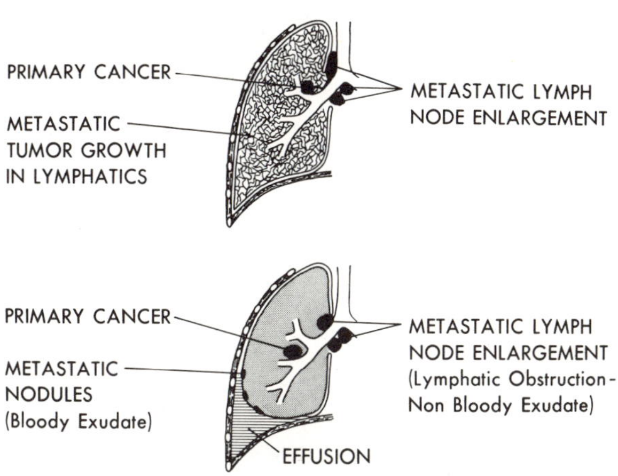

Figure 14.4. Invasion and metastatic disease in the lymphatics causes lymphangitic carcinomatosis (top) or pleural effusion (bottom).

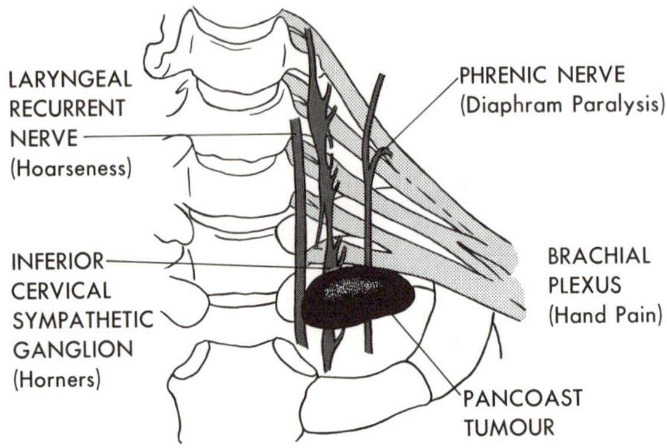

Figure 14.5. Neural structures encountered in the lung apex. Shown are the top of the sternum and the first rib joining the sternum and the spine. A tumor in this region ("Pancoast" tumor) can cause a paralyzed diaphragm, hoarseness, hand pain, and Horner's syndrome.

paralysis in the distribution of the C8 and T1 nerve roots. In some patients with Pancoast tumors, all the above neural problems are present.

Pleura

Lung cancer may seed the pleura and cause effusion. These effusions are usually exudates and are often bloody. Because the pleural fluid is protein rich, there is a reduction in the forces driving fluid into the visceral pleura (see Chapter 7), and such effusions may become chronic.

Abnormal Function Due to Extrathoracic Spread

Metastases to other parts of the body spread via lymphatic and vascular channels. The tissues commonly involved are the brain, liver, bone marrow, lymph nodes, and adrenals.

Symptoms of brain involvement are common and may predate diagnosis of the primary lung tumor by years. The neurological defect may be focal due to local invasion of the metastatic lesion. Focal seizures are an example of such a lesion. Occasionally, the major effect of a cerebral metastatic lesion is to increase intracranial pressure and cause headaches.

When lung cancer spreads to bone, most of the lesions are osteolytic, which may cause hypercalcemia from breakdown of bone. Metastatic tumor in the liver and the adrenals does not usually cause failure of these organs.

Abnormal Function Due to Ectopic Hormone Production

Lung cancer cells may synthesize polypeptide hormones. The clinical manifestations of this polypeptide secretion may precede the recognition of the primary tumor. Besides synthesizing intact hormones, neoplastic cells may also produce hormonal subunits, precursors, and fragments, which may have biological activity. Ectopic hormone is defined as a hormone produced by a tissue not normally producing that hormone. There are two mechanisms that may explain ectopic hormone synthesis. First, since all cells with nuclear material contain all the genetic information (most of which is repressed), malignant transformation may result in genetic derepression and hence synthesis of polypeptides normally produced by other cells. Second, ectopic hormones may be produced by neoplastic cells embryologically related to precursors of normal endocrine cells. Most of the ectopic hormones are secreted by oat cell carcinoma with one exception; squamous cell carcinoma causes most cases of ectopic parathyroid hormone oversecretion.

ACTH and precursors of ACTH are produced by some malignant lung tumors. When biologically active ACTH is synthesized, an acute Cushing's syndrome is present; the patient usually dies before the classical manifestations of Cushing's syndrome, "moon face," "buffalo hump," are present. The major abnormalities are due to excessive corticosteroid and mineralocorticoid secretion stimulation by the ACTH: hyperglycemia, hypokalemia, and metabolic alkalosis.

Parathyroid hormone (*PTH*) causes release of calcium from bone, which elevates calcium concentration of the blood. Antidiuretic hormone (*ADH*) secretion causes resorption of water from the distal convoluted tubules and the collecting ducts. The excessive water resorption dilutes serum sodium. Because of the reduced serum osmotic pressure, water will go into cells. When cerebral cells become overhydrated, seizures and coma may occur. *Gonadotropin* secretion may cause gynecomastia. *5-Hydroxytryptamine* and other vasoactive compounds may be secreted by lung malignancies, as well as by bronchial adenomas (carcinoid tumor), and cause the *carcinoid syndrome* characterized by diarrhea, flushing, and sometimes bronchoconstriction.

Abnormal Function Due to Unknown Effects of Lung Cancer

In people with cancer, some of the major symptoms such as tiredness, loss of appetite, and weight loss cannot be easily explained. These symptoms are common in most malignancies. In lung cancer, there may develop abnormality of neuromuscular function or abnormal growth of bone and connective tissue in the absence of metastatic disease. Removal of the tumor may reverse the problems.

Neuromuscular Abnormalities

The peripheral nerves (motor and sensory), the cerebellum, and the spinal cord may be affected. In one syndrome, progressive multifocal leukoencephalopathy, in which there is widespread loss of neural function, a slow virus has been implicated.

Muscle may be involved in two ways. With one type, the Eaton-Lambert syndrome, rested muscle is weak and it strengthens with repeated stimulation (the *"myasthenic" syndrome*). In contrast, in true myasthenia gravis (which is not caused by lung cancer), the rested muscle is strong and it weakens with use. The second muscle abnormality seen with lung cancer is diffuse muscle inflammation, polymyositis.

Bone and Connective Tissue

Subperiosteal new bone formation in the long bones produces severe pain, the syndrome of *hypertrophic pulmonary osteoarthropathy.* Some patients with this syndrome also have clubbing of the fingers; this latter finding may be present without osteoarthropathy. These findings may be caused by elevated levels of growth hormone produced by the tumor. It is of interest that removal of the cancer or cutting the vagus nerve may reverse these findings.

Is the Patient Operable?

The results from surgical resection for lung cancer are not encouraging but offer the patient the only chance of cure. At present, chemotherapy cannot be considered curative. There are two separate considerations when deciding treatment.

Is the Surgical Treatment Going to Cure the Disease?

In general, when the malignancy has metastasized (to bone marrow, liver, brain, pleura, or lymph nodes), it is incurable by surgery. Even spread into the lymph nodes of the mediastinum makes the patient surgically incurable.

Will the Patient Survive Surgical Treatment?

Many patients with lung cancer also have chronic airflow obstruction, since both diseases share a common etiology, cigarette smoking. With surgical therapy, there is removal of functioning lung tissue as well as the tumor. It is important that the patient be left with sufficient lung function, so that he or she will not be disabled. In general, if the patient is hypoventilating or has pulmonary hypertension, he will not be able to survive a major procedure. If the FEV_1 anticipated postoperatively is less than .5 liters, the patient may be anticipated to develop severe hypoventilation and to be incapacitated.

METASTATIC DISEASE IN THE THORAX

The thorax is a common location of metastatic disease for neoplasms arising from other organs. Most metastatic lesions in the lung are blood borne and do not disturb lung function. Slowly growing (e.g. renal) metastatic nodules may be removed as part of the treatment of the primary malignancy. Metastatic lesions in the pleural space cause a protein-rich exudative effusion.

BIBLIOGRAPHY

Blackman MC, Rosen SW, Weintraub BD: Ectopic hormones. *Adv Intern Med* 23:85, 1978.

Chovil AC: Occupational lung cancer and smoking: A review in the light of current theories of carcinogenesis. *Can Med Assoc J* 121:548, 1979.

Fraser RG, Paré JAP: *Diagnosis of Diseases of the Chest.* Philadelphia, WB Saunders, 1978, p 1102.

Odell WD, Wolfsen AR: Humoral syndromes associated with cancer. *Annu Rev Med* 29:379, 1978.

Fishman AP (ed): Tumors of the lung and pleura: in *Pulmonary Diseases and Disorders.* New York, McGraw-Hill, 1980, p 1383.

15

Respiratory Infections

Bruce Light

Infections of the lung and airways are among the commonest causes of abnormal ventilation and gas exchange. An infectious process of the upper airways or bronchi can cause airway obstruction; an infection of the lung itself causes acutely disturbed gas exchange and severe illness (pneumonia). In this chapter, we will consider the ways in which the normal lung protects itself from infection and how these protective mechanisms may fail.

LUNG DEFENSE MECHANISMS

The lung and airways are exposed in a particularly vulnerable way to our microbiological environment. Several thousand liters of air are inhaled and exhaled each day, and every breath contains suspended particles, which are contaminated with microorganisms. Before reaching the lungs, inspired gas passes through the nose and pharynx. This region, which is heavily colonized with a complex menagerie of microorganisms, is directly continuous with the lower respiratory tract along a pathway that is usually widely open. Because part of the upper respiratory tract is also the upper gastrointestinal tract, everything put in the mouth, all contaminated with microorganisms, is directly exposed to the mucosa of the upper airway and, when swallowed, passes within millimeters of the entrance to the lower respiratory tract.

The lung, unlike the skin, does not have a thick horny covering and layers of subcutaneous tissue to defend itself from microbial invasion. The alveoli, unlike the mucous membranes, do not have mucous layers, multiple columnar cell layers, and a lamina propria filled with phagocytic cells and lymphocytes. The function of the lung is to place large volumes of air in intimate contact with blood, a function that would be difficult if these kinds of defenses were relied on. Instead, there is a complex series of mechanisms that serve first to minimize contamination of the lower respiratory tract from above, second to clear the lung of any materials that do penetrate the airways, and finally, to kill or otherwise neutralize any contaminants that remain.

Upper Airway Mechanisms that Prevent Contamination of the Lung

Leaving aside for the present the possibility of organisms entering the lung via the blood stream, microbes can reach the lower respiratory tract by being carried on particles in the inspired air or by aspiration of fluid or solid material from the upper airway. The upper airway defenses against pulmonary infection include removing particulate matter from the inspired air, minimizing the microbial population on the mucous membranes of the upper airway, and finally, minimizing the possibility of aspiration.

Conditioning of Air

Particles that become suspended in air tend to settle back onto surfaces, if larger than about 20 μm in diameter; smaller particles from .1 to 10 μm can remain suspended for prolonged periods and account for most of the material inhaled with air. Nearly all inhaled particles larger than 10 μm and most of those between 5 and 10 μm are deposited in the nose by *inertial impaction.* This occurs because the air flowing through the narrow, sharply turning nasal passages has a high velocity of flow and is extremely turbulent. The larger particles have inertia proportional to their mass, and since they cannot change direction as easily as the air stream, they impact on the mucous membranes. Most particles between 1 and 5 μm escape removal in the nose and are deposited in the tracheobronchial tree and alveoli by *sedimentation* (Figure 15.1). They simply settle on the membrane surfaces as the velocity of the gas decreases in the small airways. Still smaller particles are deposited by Brownian motion and diffusion, though many of this size will not deposit in the lung but pass out again with exhalation.

Although the upper airway is extremely efficient in protecting the lung from larger particles, a substantial proportion of particles between 1 and 5 μm in diameter are deposited in the lung. *Droplet nuclei* are particles of about 2 to 4 μm in diameter and consist of the dried remnants of moist particles produced during sneezing, coughing, or talking. They may contain viruses or bacteria and are important in their spread from person-to-person. Microbe-containing particles of less than 10 μm diameter may also be produced by a variety of other activities that produce dusts from clothing, skin, and from surfaces in the environment.

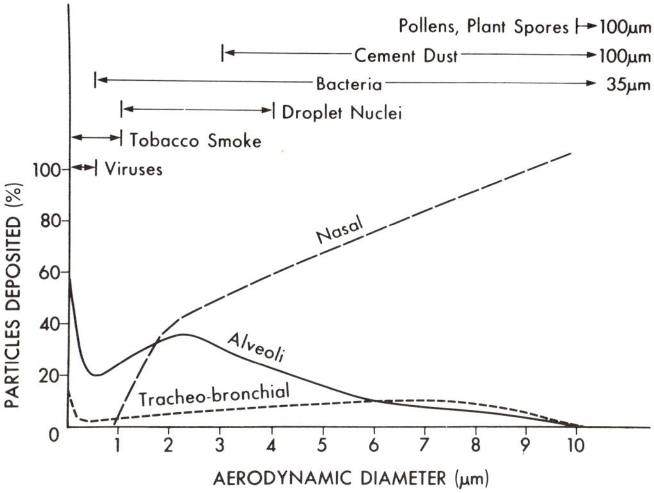

Figure 15.1. Particle deposition in the respiratory tract. The percentage of inhaled particles deposited in the nose, bronchial tree, and alveoli plotted against the aerodynamic diameter of the particles. Note that nearly 100% of particles 10 μm or larger are deposited in the nose, and almost none reach the lung. On the other hand, only half of the particles 3 μm in diameter are deposited in the nose, and a substantial percentage do reach the lung.

Upper Airway Mucociliary Clearance

The particulate matter that is continually deposited on the mucous membranes must be removed to avoid local tissue damage and prevent build-up of the microbe population. The major mechanism performing this function is *mucociliary transport.* The posterior two-thirds of the nasal cavity, the sinuses, and the nasopharynx are lined by ciliated epithelium covered with a thin layer of mucus. Beneath these layers there is a dense concentration of small blood vessels that, by changes in vasomotor tone and blood flow, can alter the size of the airway, surface temperature, and the amount of surface fluid. Mucus and fluid are produced by this membrane (about 1000 cc/24 hours in normal people) and carried at a rate of 5 to 10 mm/minute back into the hypopharynx on the tips of the beating cilia. The accumulations of mucus, fluid, and inhaled debris are then swallowed. This continuous flow minimizes the opportunity for build-up of large populations of pathogenic microbes or for their penetration into tissues. A similar process occurs in the mouth where saliva is continuously produced and swallowed.

Clearance is aided by substances in the local secretions that inhibit microbial growth and prevent organisms from sticking to the mucous membrane. Among these are *immunoglobulins* (especially secretory IgA), *lysozyme* (an antibacterial enzyme derived from leucocytes), and *complement.*

Motor Function of the Upper Airway

Despite the clearance mechanisms described above, the microflora of the nose, mouth, and pharynx is both varied and numerous. But the lung and airways below the larynx are virtually sterile in normal people. This fact is itself remarkable, considering the proximity of the heavily contaminated mucous membranes to the larynx, the high pressures developed in the pharynx during swallowing, and the direction of flow of material (downward from the mouth toward the larynx).

The key to this efficiency is the *laryngeal mechanism.* When the pharynx is empty of fluids, as during normal respiration, the relaxed larynx is widely open allowing free entry and exit of air. During swallowing, there is first a coordinated contraction of the muscles of the larynx that bring together the structures forming the walls of the larynx. This firmly closes off the airway by obliterating the laryngeal cavity (also called the *glottis*). The pharyngeal muscles can then force the swallowed bolus into the esophagus without danger of aspiration.

Another important reflex, the *gag,* also results in closure of the laryngeal mechanism, but it is coupled with contraction of many other muscles of the pharynx and so closes off the entire upper airway and pharynx, a defensive reflex to exclude material from the upper airway and prevent choking.

There are many other motor mechanisms useful for clearing specific parts of the upper airway. Some of these are throat-clearing, hawking, spitting, nose-blowing, and sneezing. The sneeze, like the cough or gag, is almost purely reflex; but the rest are done voluntarily and so depend both on sensation and on an alert level of consciousness to be functional as clearance mechanisms.

Contamination of the Lower Respiratory Tract

Disorders that disrupt any of the upper airway defenses we have discussed can result in an increased potential for contamination of the lower respiratory tract and increase the risk of lower respiratory tract infection. We have already seen that the ability of the upper airway to remove particles from inhaled air is not perfect and that many potentially infective particles do penetrate to the lung. This is important in such diseases as tuberculosis and viral pneumonia, which require only a small number of microbes to enter the lung to cause disease. Deposition of particles in the upper airway is also a major route for spread of upper respiratory infection (e.g., colds, streptococcal sore throat). This is probably important in the spread of bacteria that may colonize the upper airway and cause disease at a later time, either in the respiratory tract (e.g., *Streptococcus pneumoniae* pneumonia) or elsewhere in the body (e.g., *Staphylococcus aureus* skin infections, *Neisseria meningititis* meningitis).

Impaired clearance of the upper respiratory tract also predisposes to both upper and lower respiratory tract infection by allowing accumulation of debris and microbes, which may then penetrate tissues or be aspirated into the trachea. Examples of the first include sinusitis and otitis media; both of which occur when drainage of the area is partially or completely blocked. Lung abscess due to anaerobic bacteria found in the mouth is often associated with severe gingival disease and is an example of a build-up of infected material in the upper airway leading to a lower respiratory infection.

Finally, the most important upper airway defense, the larynx, is also the most frequently disturbed. To function properly, the larynx requires accurate sensation of materials within the pharynx and adequate motor control to perform both voluntary clearing maneuvers and maneuvers that are largely involuntary, such as swallowing. Even minor disruptions, such as being distracted or intoxicated while swallowing, can lead to material "going down the wrong way." Normal sleep is known to result in minor aspiration, and any abnormal disturbance of consciousness further increases the risk. Other, more specific neurological lesions involving any of the sensory or motor pathways subserving the swallowing or gag reflexes may also do this, as may anatomic abnormalities that impair these functions. Although it is usually not the only factor involved in pathogenesis, aspiration of pharyngeal contents is the route of entry to the lung for organisms causing most cases of bacterial pneumonia.

Lower Respiratory Tract Clearance Mechanisms

The next lines of defense are the mechanisms that remove contaminants that have managed to elude the defenses of the upper airway. These are of two general kinds: those that physically clear contaminant material and those that primarily kill microbes in situ.

Pulmonary Reflexes

It is common experience that when a faulty swallow has resulted in aspiration, the immediate response is a violent cough. Cough is an involuntary reflex elicited by stimulation of irritant receptors located in the subepithelium of the hypopharynx, larynx, and tracheobronchial tree. It is mediated by the vagus nerve. A typical cough sequence, following stimulation of the irritant receptors is as follows. A sharp inspiration is followed by closure of the glottis. The glottis remains closed for a brief period (about .2 sec), while muscles of the chest wall and abdomen contract, generating very high pressures in the thorax and still greater pressure in the abdomen. The glottis then opens abruptly, allowing a rapid flow of air out of the thorax. Coinciding with this rush of air out of the lungs, there is collapse of airways in the lung causing still higher gas velocities within airways and propelling mouthward any material in the tracheobronchial tree or larynx. Under ordinary circumstances, the larynx allows very little to pass into the trachea and the mucociliary clearance mechanism (below) is highly efficient. Cough, therefore, is generally believed to be of importance mainly as a facilitator of mucociliary clearance and as an aid in dealing with gross contamination from above the larynx. However, in circumstances that combine impaired upper airway defenses with an absent or decreased cough mechanism, as in patients with stupor or coma, the risk of pneumonia is greatly increased.

Bronchoconstriction is another reflex response to airway irritants, which normally aids clearance. By reducing the cross-sectional area of the bronchus, forced expiration and cough become more effective in pushing mouthward any debris in the bronchial lumen, an effect that has been compared to a peashooter. On the other hand, excessive bronchoconstriction, as in asthma, decreases expiratory airflows, causes air trapping in the lungs, and can make an effective cough difficult.

Mucociliary Clearance

In normal man, each day between 10 and 100 ml of mucus passes up the trachea into the hypopharynx and is swallowed. This material will contain most of the particulate matter deposited in the lung during the day and any pharyngeal material that may have slipped by the larynx.

Mucus. Mucus is secreted by epithelial goblet cells and from submucosal glands. It covers the tracheobronchial ciliated epithelium as a thin, discontinuous blanket. The blanket consists of at least two layers. The uppermost layer is composed of fluid and high molecular weight viscous mucopolysaccharides forming a "gel." Beneath this, surrounding the beating epithelial cilia, is the periciliary fluid layer (Figure 15.2).

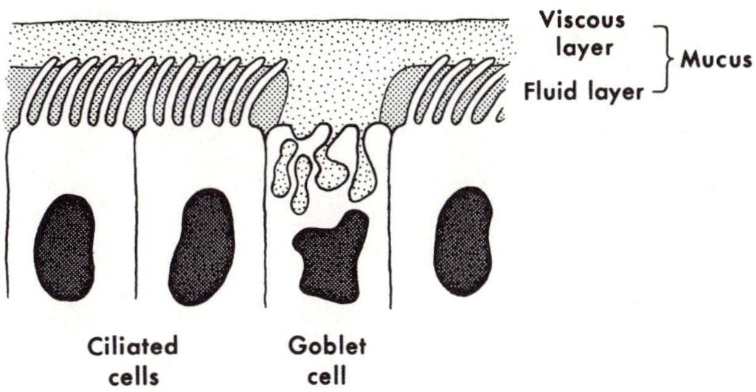

Figure 15.2. The tips of the beating cilia propel the high-viscosity upper mucus layer up the airways. In addition to the goblet cells, mucus is also secreted by submucosal glands just beneath the epithelium.

Cilia. The lower respiratory tract epithelium is ciliated from the larynx to the terminal bronchioles (Figure 15.3). The surface of each cell has about 200 cilia all beating rhythmically at a rate of about 1200 beats/min, with each ciliary beat occurring as part of a wave of mouthward beats, which begins at the terminal bronchioles and ends at the larynx. The beating tips of the cilia come into contact with the gel portion of the overlying mucus layer and propel it mouthward at a rate of .5 mm/min in small airways, increasing to about 10 mm/min in major bronchi.

The normal mucociliary mechanism can clear particles deposited in the tracheobronchial tree extremely rapidly, removing half of a given number of particles within minutes. Further out in the alveoli where there are no cilia, clearance is much slower (half-time of about 20 hours). Overall efficiency of mucociliary clearance depends on the complex interaction between ciliary motion and the amount and nature of secreted mucus. The physiological mechanisms that control cilia remain largely unknown, but there are a variety of pharmacological and environmental agents that can modify mucociliary clearance rates by affecting ciliary activity. The amount and nature of mucus secreted is, in part, controlled by the parasympathetic nervous system and can also be affected by neurohumoral stimulation (adrenergic or cholinergic) and by direct mucosal irritation. In general, mucociliary clearance rates vary inversely with the mucus viscosity and directly with the amount of ciliary activity.

Clearance is increased by bronchodilator drugs such as β-adrenergic agents and the methylxanthines. Adrenergic drugs do this primarily by stimulating transport of water and salt into mucus, so decreasing viscosity, while the methylxanthines increase both mucus production and ciliary activity. Cholinergic drugs directly stimulate both ciliary activity and mucus production and so increase clearance rates, though the applicability of this in patients

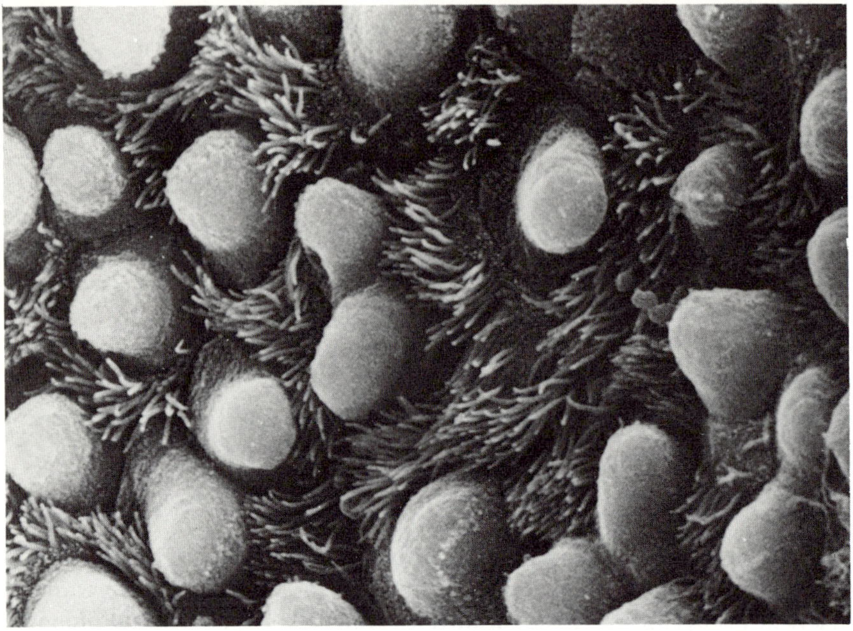

Figure 15.3. Scanning electronmicroscopic view of the surface of ciliated bronchial epithelium. Interspersed among the ciliated epithelial cells are the tops of secretory goblet cells, which cover the cilia with a thin layer of mucus (magnification ×4250). (The author acknowledges the work of Dr. J.M. Papadimitriou, Pathologist, Sir Charles Gairdner Hospital, The Queen Elizabeth II Medical Centre, Nedlands, Western Australia, 6009.)

is limited, since they also stimulate bronchoconstriction. Irritation of mucous membranes by inhaled pollutants has variable effects on transport since, though they may acutely increase mucus secretion and decrease mucus viscosity, they may also have toxic effects on cilia.

Among the factors that can depress ciliary function are chronic exposure to airway irritants (e.g., cigarette smoke and other pollutants), pharmacological agents (e.g., 100% oxygen, anticholinergic agents, alcohol), and infection (e.g., viral bronchitis). Some of these factors may also depress mucociliary function by affecting the characteristics of mucus. With chronic irritation of the respiratory tract, there is an increase in the number of mucus-secreting goblet cells in the epithelium, thus increasing amounts of mucus. Along with this, there is an inflammatory response to irritation, which increases the numbers of phagocytic cells and amount of cellular debris in the mucus. The increased amount of material in the mucus, especially cellular DNA, causes the mucus to be more viscous and less readily moved along by ciliary motion.

Immotile Cilia. Rarely, cilia function can be impaired on a congenital basis as occurs in the *Kartagener syndrome.* Patients with this syndrome have deficient

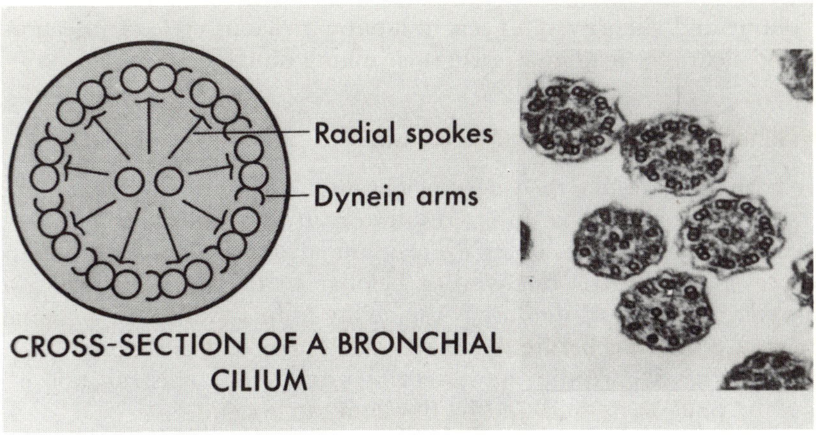

Figure 15.4. This electronmicrograph and schematic diagram of bronchial cilia in cross section show the 9 pairs of outer microtubules and 2 central microtubules that run the length of the cilium. Bending of cilia is due to sliding between the outer microtubules, an active process mediated by the dynein "arms" projecting from the outer microtubules. The sliding motion is translated into bending of the cilium by the radial spokes connecting the outer to the central microtubules. (The author acknowledges the work of Dr. David Ostrow, Department of Respiratory Medicine, Vancouver General Hospital, Vancouver, B.C. V52 1M9.)

dynein arms (see Figure 15.4) in cilia throughout their body, rendering the cilia immotile. The resulting ineffective mucociliary transport leads to sinusitis, recurrent lung infection, and bronchiectasis. The syndrome also includes infertility in males (due to immotile sperm) and situs inversus (right to left transposition of abdominal viscera, probably due to failure of embryonic cilia responsible for rotation of the midgut). Some patients with deficient dynein arms do not have situs inversus but show the rest of the syndrome, and a further group of patients have a similar "immotile cilia syndrome" caused by a different congenital abnormality, defective radial spokes in cilia. Some of the cilia in these disorders are not actually immotile; however, the beats may be vastly abnormal. Instead of the coordinated whiplike action, only part of the cilia may move, or the middle of the cilia may twirl around in an eggbeaterlike motion.

Cystic fibrosis is another congenital disorder causing impaired mucociliary transport. The nature of the primary defect is not known. Although at one time it was thought that production of abnormally viscid mucus was the cause, it now seems likely that this is not the whole story. Other, more subtle defects have been suggested (e.g., production of factors that inhibit ciliary motion) but have not yet been proven. Whatever the cause, consequent to the impaired ability to clear foreign material, infection is more likely to occur, which in turn causes chronic inflammatory increases in the respiratory mucus volume and viscosity. This sets in motion a vicious cycle of infection and impaired clearance leading to progressive lung damage.

Intrapulmonary Detoxification Mechanisms

As we have seen, despite the very efficient mechanisms that prevent materials from the environment or upper respiratory tract from entering the lung, some contamination does occur even under ideal conditions. Although the major responsibility for removing it belongs to the mucociliary clearance system, the final line of defense is the ability to inactivate toxic materials or pathogenic organisms before damage to the lung occurs and to combat pathological processes once they have become established. This function is performed by phagocytic cells and by the immune system.

Phagocytes

The predominant phagocytic cell in the lung is the *alveolar macrophage.* This cell originates in the bone marrow and is transported to the lung as a blood monocyte. Once in the lung, it remains in the interstitium or within alveoli until it is needed. Its major function is phagocytosis of particles, which may be inhaled particulate debris, bacteria, or cell constituents. It is capable of killing most kinds of microbes that it may ingest and performs this more efficiently if its lysosomal enzymes and other intracellular bacteriocidal mechanisms have been activated by interaction with sensitized lymphocytes (see below).

The other important phagocyte is the blood *polymorphonuclear neutrophil,* which is normally present in the lung only in small numbers. Even more than the macrophage, it is an avid phagocytic cell and is capable of killing microbes. Neutrophils are of most importance in the lung in defending against infectious processes that have become established. Once an infection has begun in tissue, some of the products of inflammation originating from lymphocytes, macrophages, and activation of the complement system have the ability to attract neutrophils to the site of the infection (chemotaxis). Thus, any beginning inflammatory process immediately results in an influx of large numbers of these cells, which then aid the macrophages already present in phagocytosing and destroying the offending agents. This is of particular importance, because phagocytes are the major defense against the more pathogenic invasive bacteria. If even small numbers of organisms such as *Streptococcus pneumonia, Staphylococcus aureus*, or aerobic gram-negative rods penetrate into the lung, they are capable of rapid multiplication and invasion of tissues unless immediately neutralized by phagocytic cells. Therefore, even moderate impairment or deficiency of these cells is an important risk factor.

In order to perform their function, phagocytic cells must be capable of movement using amoebalike pseudopods (diapedesis), phagocytosis, and finally of producing the lysosomal enzymes and other materials used to digest particles that they have phagocytosed. There are a number of factors that can interfere with some or all of these functions. Cigarette smoke is known to inhibit alveolar macrophage function, as are other inhaled pollutants (ozone, nitrogen dioxide, oxygen) and drugs such as corticosteroids, anticancer and anti-inflammatory cytotoxic agents, and ethanol. Several metabolic derangements are also known to impair phagocyte function, the most common being uremia (renal failure) and the hyperglycemia of diabetes mellitus.

In addition, there are rare congenital disorders that limit the ability of neutrophils to kill bacteria (e.g., chronic granulomatous disease) as well as congenitally low numbers of blood neutrophils (granulocytopenia).

Finally, of major and increasing importance in recent years is acquired granulocytopenia. This may occur because of rare, unexpected bone marrow toxicity associated with any one of a large number of drugs, but is more commonly due to dose-related bone marrow toxicity complicating treatment of cancer with cytotoxic drugs.

Immunoglobulins (see p. 136)

Immunoglobulins are proteins produced by bone-marrow derived lymphocytes (B-lymphocytes) after the lymphocyte has been sensitized by antigen. Only one kind of immunoglobulin is produced by each lymphocyte, and that one is structured in a way that enables it to bind only to foreign antigens identical or very similar to the original sensitizing antigen. Immunoglobulins function in host defense in several ways. First, many immunoglobulins serve as opsonins. That is, they have the ability, once bound to the surface of foreign material, to stimulate phagocytic cells to engulf the antigen more avidly. Some immunoglobulins also have the ability to fix (or bind to) complement and so initiate the complement cascade, a complex series of enzymatic reactions leading to the release of compounds that can attract more phagocytes and lymphocytes, increase blood flow to the area, and even attack directly the cell surfaces to which the immunoglobulins are bound.

Of the five classes of immunoglobulins, the most important for lung defense are IgG and IgA, since they are present not only in the blood but also in the secretions of the respiratory tract. Secretory IgA is the predominant immunoglobulin secreted by the B-lymphocytes and plasma cells in the mucosal lamina propria of the upper respiratory tract and from the tonsils, adenoids, and aggregates of lymphoid tissue around major bronchi.

IgA antibodies specific for viral antigens are able to neutralize viruses and prevent infection. This local immunity is probably more important for host defense against respiratory viruses than are serum antibodies. But unlike IgG and IgM, IgA is not a very active opsonin and does not fix complement. Killing invading bacteria is, therefore, not a major IgA function. Its main contribution to defense against bacteria is due to its ability to inhibit multiplication and mucosal adherence by bacteria, so aiding mucociliary clearance.

In the terminal lung units, IgA concentrations are much lower and IgG predominates. Antigen specific IgG is a good opsonin and usually fixes complement; therefore, it can contribute directly to local defense against bacterial infection as well as neutralizing viruses. In addition to locally produced antibody, serum immunoglobulins also contribute to respiratory defense, in part because some are present in respiratory secretions due to transudation and in part because they, along with other blood components, are released and participate in the inflammatory response to tissue invasion.

IgG antibody (and to some extent IgM), like phagocytes, is most important in defense against invasive pathogenic bacteria. These proteins do not penetrate into host cells; therefore, they are less valuable in dealing with acute infection due to microbes that multiply inside cells (e.g., viruses, *Mycobacterium tuberculosis*). But along with IgA, they do contribute to immunity against reinfection with viruses, since the preformed antibody is then able to bind to the virus before it can penetrate cells. This is the reason for the effectiveness of immunizations.

IgA Deficiency. Although some people with congenital absence of mucosal secretory IgA appear to have an increased frequency of respiratory infections and allergic disorders, the majority have no such problem suggesting that, by itself, it is not crucial to the defense of the respiratory tract. In many such patients, IgM appears to replace IgA on the respiratory mucosa and perform its function in host defense.

Other Immunoglobulin deficiencies. As we have noted, IgG is the major immunoglobulin in the lung that can act as an opsonin and complement fixer. This makes it especially important in neutralizing the few highly pathogenic encapsulated bacteria (especially *Streptococcus pneumoniae* and *Hemophilus influenza*), which may penetrate the lung, since these types of bacteria are especially resistant to phagocytosis. Deficiency of this important immunoglobulin can occur congenitally or associated with a variety of acquired systemic diseases affecting the reticuloendothelial system. More commonly, most or all of the immunoglobulins are decreased together, and there is an overall increased susceptibility to infection attributable largely to decreased IgG and IgM.

Cell-Mediated Immunity (CMI)

About half the lymphocytes in and around airways are thymus-derived lymphocytes or *T-cells*. They are found in the lymphoid aggregates adjacent to bronchi (bronchus-associated lymphoid tissue or BALT) and are also present in the mucosal lamina propria. Their function depends on the local tissue macrophages, which ingest and process foreign antigens and pass them along to uncommitted T-cells in the local lymphoid tissue. This sensitizes lymphocytes to that antigen. Thereafter, they can respond to that antigen by producing a variety of proteins (*lymphokines*) that inhibit macrophages from leaving the area, attract phagocytes, increase macrophage phagocytic and bactericidal activity, and stimulate the sensitization of still more T-cells. They are also able to attack directly and lyse both foreign cells and host cells that have foreign antigen on their surface. It is this ability to increase the host response to foreign antigen, particularly those located within cells, that makes

T-cells especially important in resistance to some viral infections, most fungal infections, and infections caused by organisms that can survive and multiply inside host cells, as occurs in infections due to *Mycobacterium tuberculosis, Brucella* species, *Listeria monocytogenes,* and *Pneumocystis carinii.*

There are congenital forms of CMI deficiency that may occur alone or in association with deficient humoral immunity. Both result in marked increases in the susceptibility to infection. More common is deficient T-cell function (called *anergy*) associated with neoplasms such as lymphoma, with cytotoxic or corticosteroid therapy, or related to various systemic diseases such as sarcoidosis and malnutrition. All of these can render the host much more susceptible to the kinds of infection mentioned above. Indeed, there are many lung infections (e.g., pneumonia due to *Cytomegalovirus, Herpes zoster, Aspergillus* species or *Pneumocystis carinii*) that occur almost exclusively in the setting of severely impaired CMI, though in most such patients all components of the immune system are abnormal.

PATHOGENESIS OF LOWER RESPIRATORY TRACT INFECTIONS

In order for an infection of the lung to occur, pathogenic microbes must gain access to the lower respiratory tract, escape the clearance mechanisms of the lung, survive the immunological and phagocytic cell defenses, and multiply within the tissues and air spaces. Thus, the likelihood of an infection occurring at any time depends on an interaction among many factors, which include the number and virulence of the microbes, the nature of the inoculum reaching the lower respiratory tract (aerosol, aspiration of oral contents, etc.), the efficiency of the clearance mechanisms, and the state of the phagocytic cell system and immune defenses. The ways in which these factors interact can be related to some of the common patterns of respiratory tract infection (Figure 15.5).

Viral Respiratory Tract Infections

Most of the viruses commonly affecting the respiratory tract are highly infectious. That is, only a few virus particles are required to produce infection in the absence of specific preformed antibody against them. Once the virus has entered host cells and has begun to multiply, it spreads from cell to cell via intercellular connections or in respiratory secretions. Thus, nearly everyone gets viral respiratory infections and host defenses other than antibody-mediated immunity are of much less importance in determining incidence. The severity and extent of disease produced depend on the virulence characteristics of the virus and on the efficiency of the host factors responsible for limiting the acute infection. We have already discussed the importance of the cell-mediated immune system in this regard, and patients with a deficient CMI response will often have a more severe or protracted infection. *Interferon* is

	HOST FACTORS		MICROBIAL FACTORS	
Likelihood of Infection	Mucociliary Clearance	Intrapulmonary Defenses (phagocytes, antibody)	Inoculum Size	Organism Invasiveness
HIGH	IMPAIRED	DEFICIENT	LARGE	HIGH
↑	Cystic Fibrosis Immotile Cilia Syndrome Chronic Bronchitis Acute viral respiratory infection Atmospheric pollutants Ethanol	Granulocytopenia Hypogammaglobulinemia Uremia Diabetes Mellitus Ethanol	Major aspiration Endotracheal tube with microbial colonization Minor aspiration Inhaled aerosols Droplet nuclei	Influenza viruses Mycobacterium Tuberculosis Streptococcus Pneumoniae Enteric gram-negative aerobic bacteria Oral anaerobic bacteria
LOW	NORMAL	NORMAL	SMALL	LOW

Figure 15.5. A simplified chart of some of the host and microbial factors involved in the pathogenesis of pulmonary infection. Among the host factors are mucociliary clearance, immunoglobulins, and phagocytes. Note that inoculum size (the number of microbes reaching the lung) is itself the result of an interaction of many factors, including the type of inhaled or colonizing upper airway microflora, the upper airway clearance mechanisms, and the efficiency of the larynx. Organism "invasiveness" includes characteristics such as microbial multiplication time, enzymes that promote invasion or protect the organism from host defenses, extracellular capsules, and the ability to penetrate and survive within cells.

another host factor helping to limit disease. This substance is a small protein produced and released by all host cells infected with virus. It has the property of rendering other host cells relatively resistant to penetration by virus, serving to limit and delay spread of the infection. Antibody in amounts that are not completely protective, formed during past exposure to the virus or an antigenically similar one, also serves to limit disease.

The "cold" (upper respiratory infection or URI) is the most common manifestation of viral respiratory infections and frequently precedes or goes along with infection involving other levels of the respiratory tract. This is because virus usually first contacts the upper respiratory mucus membrane in the nose via droplet nuclei carried in the air or by direct contact (hand-to-hand-to-eye or nose, etc.). The symptoms are mainly those of irritation and inflammation of the mucus membrane, increased fluid secretion and mucus membrane swelling producing the characteristic runny nose and plugged nasal and sinus passages. If the infection involves the pharynx, a sore, red throat results. This complex of symptoms is characteristic of virus infection, occurs in all age groups, and is produced by a wide range of viruses.

Viral spread into the larynx, trachea, and major bronchi produce different syndromes depending mainly on age. In adults, the symptoms are mainly hoarse voice (due to inflammatory mucosal thickening in the larynx), cough with increased lower respiratory tract secretions, and sometimes burning retrosternal chest pain due to tracheitis. In adults, the *acute bronchitis* syndrome is often caused by influenza viruses, coronaviruses, and rhinoviruses but may also be due to adenovirus or *Mycoplasma pneumoniae.*

Young children (ages about 3 to 36 months) may have acute bronchitis symptoms but frequently develop the *croup* syndrome. The syndrome is due to inflammation of the larynx, trachea, and bronchi producing significant obstruction to air flow. There is usually cough, dyspnea, and stridor often combined with URI symptoms. It is characteristically caused by parainfluenza virus (types 1 and 3) but can be caused by many other viruses and *Mycoplasma pneumoniae.*

Spread of infection to the small airways and airspaces produces viral pneumonia in adults. The symptoms are similar to acute bronchitis, but dyspnea and systemic symptoms (fever, prostration) may be more prominent, and significant gas-exchange abnormalities can result due to impaired ventilation of alveoli. Although many nonbacterial pathogens may produce pneumonia, the most characteristic ones are influenza A viruses, adenoviruses, and *Mycoplasma pneumoniae.*

Infection and inflammation to the level of the small bronchi do not produce a characteristic syndrome distinguishable from bronchitis and pneumonia in adults and older children, but in infants (up to 24 months of age) *bronchiolitis* may occur. As with the other respiratory infection syndromes, the symptoms begin with a URI and then progress to include cough and severe dyspnea. The usual cause here is *respiratory syncytial virus,* but again nearly any of the respiratory viral pathogens or *Mycoplasma pneumoniae* can be responsible. One of the reasons for the characteristic syndrome in this age group is the very small size of the terminal bronchioles. The reaction to infection might thus more easily produce significant obstruction to gas flow and ventilation-perfusion inequality. In many such cases, pneumonia is also present.

Most viral infections do involve the entire respiratory epithelium to varying degrees and some, especially influenza viruses, are really systemic infections producing a wide range of systemic symptoms (e.g., fever, headache, myalgia, and gastrointestinal symptoms). Any of the disease syndromes mentioned can occur in people with unimpaired defense mechanisms. The acute infection is controlled by the CMI and macrophage systems, and as might be expected, patients with deficient CMI are at increased risk for protracted and severe viral infection. Immunity to reinfection depends largely on development of specific antibody, which gives varying degrees of protection for varying periods of time. In some cases (e.g., a particular strain of influenza A), immunity may be complete and lifelong. In many others, reinfection may not be prevented but only reduced in severity.

Chronic Bronchitis

Chronic bronchial irritation, usually by cigarette smoke, is a cause of persistent cough, sputum production, and dyspnea. The symptoms are due to thickening of bronchial mucosa and increases in the number of mucus-secreting goblet cells, bronchoconstriction, and in some cases, destruction of lung tissue. Episodes of increased symptoms may be brought on by environmental irritants, but many are due to infection. The usual infectious agents are the common viral pathogens, which cause colds and acute bronchitis in normal people. In chronic bronchitis, the symptoms produced are more severe because the inflammation of mucosal surfaces produced increases airway obstruction that was already significant. In patients who have severe chronic airway obstruction, any additional obstruction can be critical and can even precipitate acute respiratory failure.

The chronic bronchial irritation also causes impaired mucociliary clearance and leads to an increase in the bacterial microflora of the lower respiratory tract, often including potential pathogens such as *Streptococcus pneumoniae* and less pathogenic unencapsulated strains of *Hemophilus influenza.* As might be expected, this leads to an increased risk of pneumococcal pneumonia. These bacteria may also have a role in increasing the duration and severity of bronchitis symptoms from viral infection or perhaps be responsible for exacerbations in their own right, but this remains largely speculative.

Classic Bacterial Pneumonia

The most common cause of acute bacterial pneumonia in nonhospitalized patients is *Streptococcus pneumoniae. Klebsiella pneumoniae, Staphylococcus aureus,* and *Hemophilus influenza,* among others, are also occasional causes. These organisms occasionally colonize the upper respiratory tract of even normal people, though colonization is certainly more frequent with an upper respiratory tract abnormality. Further, they can gain access to the lower respiratory tract by aspiration, an event that also occurs to some degree even in normal people. Since all of these species are highly invasive in man and are relatively resistant to phagocytosis, it is perhaps surprising that acute pneumonia is not more common than it is. Nevertheless, acute bacterial pneumonia almost never occurs in people with fully intact defenses, demonstrating the ability of the normal clearance mechanisms to deal with small numbers of even quite virulent bacteria.

Pneumococcal pneumonia is typically a secondary pneumonia. That is, it occurs when there is a dysfunction of the mucociliary clearance system or of phagocyte cells. An acute viral respiratory infection can cause both of these, and accordingly, a viral infection frequently precedes cases of pneumococcal pneumonia. Ethanol is also known to impair mucociliary clearance and phagocytosis and may depress consciousness, making larger scale aspiration more likely. These factors account for the many cases of bacterial pneumonia in alcoholics. Impaired opsonization and killing of bacteria of the disorders discussed in the previous section, among them metabolic disorders and immunoglobulin deficiency, also predispose patients to pneumonia. The general principle is that any significant impairment of the clearance or bactericidal mechanisms of the lung may be sufficient to allow highly pathogenic organisms to invade, once they have reached the lower respiratory tract.

Streptococcus pneumoniae, once it has begun to multiply within the lung interstitium and air spaces, produces an exudation of edema fluid, which fills alveoli and carries the multiplying pneumococci into adjacent lung units. This pattern of contiguous spread is the reason that pneumococcal pneumonia classically produces the dense localized infiltrate called *lobar pneumonia*, though the infected exudate may also spread along bronchi yielding a bronchopneumonic infiltrate. Dilatation of blood vessels and damage to them due to the infection leads to local hemorrhage, and the inflammatory response brings polymorphonuclear leukocytes in large numbers and hence the purulent "rusty" sputum. The developing lesion consists of the older central area where the air space is filled with erythrocytes and neutrophils and very few remaining pneumococci, an area bordering this where hyperemia and hemorrhage predominate and pneumococci present are still viable, and an outer border of edema filled with large numbers of rapidly multiplying organisms.

The inflammatory exudate fills alveoli and impairs ventilation by reducing compliance (making the lung "stiff") and by partially obstructing air flow. In addition, if the inflammation extends to the pleural surface, there may be pain caused by respiratory movements and ventilation reduced on that basis. This reduced local ventilation causes ventilation-perfusion inequality and hypoxemia. Further, many of the exudate-filled units receive no ventilation at all or are collapsed. Blood perfusing these areas represents intrapulmonary shunt and also contributes to hypoxemia.

Nosocomial Bacterial Pneumonia

In general, the pathogenesis of nosocomial (hospital-acquired) bacterial pneumonia is similar to acute pneumonia acquired outside of the hospital. It is usually due to relatively small numbers of highly pathogenic organisms reaching the lower respiratory tract at a time when clearance and bactericidal mechanisms are impaired.

About one-half of cases of in-hospital pneumonia are due to *Streptococcus pneumoniae*. Other common causes are *Klebsiella* species, *Pseudomonas* species, and *Staphylococcus aureus*. The increased frequency of disease due to enteric Gram-negative organisms is due to changes in the upper respiratory tract flora. Hospitalized patients often have metabolic disorders or a depressed level of consciousness, which impair the nasopharyngeal clearance mechanism permitting the mucous membranes to become colonized with organisms that usually originate from the patients' own gut microflora. Colonizing organisms can also be acquired from the hospital environment. *Pseudomonas* colonization of respiratory treatment equipment is one common example of this. Antimicrobial therapy for existing infections also contributes to the problem, since the antimicrobial may reduce the normal nonpathogenic flora of mucosal surfaces and allow overgrowth of antibiotic resistant microorganisms.

The ability of the larynx to prevent contamination of the lung is often impaired in sick patients (e.g., decreased level of consciousness from disease, sedation, anaesthesia), and many have deficient lung clearance and bactericidal defenses. The pneumonia that results can be catastrophic. The mortality rate of Gram-negative pneumonia occurring in the hospital is about 50%, partly because of the debilitated state of many of the patients and partly because of the nature of the pathogens, which are often more resistant to antimicrobials and typically produce a pneumonia that is more destructive than pneumococcal pneumonia.

Anaerobic Pneumonia and Lung Abscess

In contrast to the usual bacterial pneumonias, most lung abscesses are caused by anaerobic organisms that are noninvasive normal inhabitants of the mouth and pharynx. A moderate impairment of clearance or bactericidal mechanisms alone seldom results in this kind of disease. Rather, the defenses are overwhelmed by a large inoculum and fail to clear the contamination even though the organisms are relatively nonpathogenic. For example, many cases of lung abscess or anaerobic pneumonia occur in people who have severe periodontal or gingival disease. Anaerobic pneumonia can then occur if the increased amount of infected debris in the mouth is aspirated during sleep. Another group of patients at risk are those who have had a decreased level of consciousness due to alcohol or other drug overdosage, epileptic seizures, or intracranial disease. These interfere with the laryngeal mechanism allowing frank aspiration of oral contents.

Bronchial obstruction, as in bronchogenic carcinoma, occasionally causes anaerobic pneumonia without preceding abnormal aspiration. In this situation, the severe local impairment of clearance allows a build-up of mouth organisms originating from normal amounts of aspiration. Without mucociliary clearance, the local cellular defenses are overwhelmed and pneumonia occurs.

These relatively noninvasive organisms typically produce an indolent, localized anaerobic pneumonia, which may last days to weeks before coming to medical attention. Usually the patient is only moderately ill, has a low-grade fever, and often is coughing up large amounts of foul smelling sputum. The pneumonia does destroy lung tissue and often, at the time of presentation, an abscess cavity has already formed. A few patients, often those with severely deficient bactericidal defenses, depart from this typical pattern and develop a rapidly progressive necrotizing pneumonia and severe systemic toxicity.

Tuberculosis

M. tuberculosis is an example of an organism with a special virulence characteristic, which causes it to interact with the host defenses in special ways. The bacillus usually gains access to the lower respiratory tract in relatively small numbers as inhaled droplet nuclei from other infected subjects. These nuclei are deposited in the bronchi and air spaces. The organisms are then subject to clearance and phagocytosis in the usual manner, but they have the special characteristics of being able not only to survive but also to multiply within macrophages. Therefore, a very small number of organisms may cause a primary infection even in a host with normal defenses. The bacilli multiply locally, are carried in the lymphatics to the regional lymph nodes, and often are disseminated throughout the body by the circulation. The primary infection is usually halted before significant disease occurs as the macrophage-processed antigen sensitizes T-lymphocytes and the full cell-mediated immune response is activated. If the response is for any reason not adequate, there may be locally invasive disease (pneumonia or pleuritis), systemic disease due to dissemination of organisms throughout the body (miliary tuberculosis), or tuberculous meningitis.

Even in that majority who respond adequately and control the primary infection, *Mycobacterium tuberculosis* organisms survive in a quiescent state within some cells. At a later time, especially if cell-mediated immunological defenses become deficient, these organisms can again cause invasive disease. This is called *reactivation,* and it can occur from months to years to decades after the primary infection. Reactivation in the lung often occurs in the upper lobes, probably because the bacilli are strictly aerobic organisms and so have a better growth environment in these hyperventilated areas. Disease occasionally reactivates at an extrapulmonary site to which the organisms were carried during the primary infection. The more common sites include bone (often the spine), meninges, peritoneum, or the urogenital tract, though no organ is exempt.

Pulmonary Infections in the Compromised Host

In recent years there have been increasing numbers of patients who, because of neoplastic disease, multisystem disease, multiple trauma, organ transplantation, or the medical treatments for these problems, have substantially deficient defenses against infection. The respiratory system is prominently exposed to the microbial environment and so is by far the most commonly involved organ when defenses against infection fail. In patients treated with antineoplastic drugs, there may be damage to the mucus membranes of the upper airway leading to decreased clearance, decreased antimicrobial defenses, and colonization with pathogenic organisms, frequently aerobic Gram-negative bacilli. A depressed level of consciousness may impair the ability of the larynx to prevent aspiration and suppress the cough reflex. Mucociliary clearance may be decreased by metabolic abnormalities, cytotoxic drugs and other drugs, or by the presence of an endotracheal tube used for mechanical ventilation. Macrophage function may be impaired by similar problems, and there may be concurrent abnormally low numbers of leucocytes. Finally, there may be deficient cell-mediated or humoral immunity in such patients. Since some or all of the major pulmonary defenses may be deficient, there is both an increased risk of severe disease from highly pathogenic microbes and an increased risk of disease from organisms not ordinarily considered pathogenic. In order to determine the relative likelihood of any particular type of infection, it is therefore necessary to decide which mechanisms are significantly deficient and to have some knowledge about which kinds of organisms are most likely to gain an opportunistic advantage from the deficiency.

BIBLIOGRAPHY

Brain JD, Proctor DF, Reid LM, (eds): *Respiratory Defense Mechanisms*, Vol 5 (Parts 1 and 2). Lung Biology in Health and Disease. New York, Marcel Dekker Inc, 1977.

Green GM, Jakab GJ, Low RB, et al: Defense mechanisms of the respiratory membrane. *Am Rev Resp Dis* 115:479, 1977.

Kaltreider HB: Expression of immune mechanisms in the lung. *Am Rev Resp Dis* 113:347, 1976.

Newhouse M, Sanchis J, Bienenstock J: Lung defense mechanisms. *N Eng J Med* 295:990 and 1045, 1976.

Proctor DF: The upper airways. I Nasal physiology and defense of the lungs. *Am Rev Resp Dis* 115:97, 1977.

Proctor DF: The upper airways. II The larynx and trachea. *Am Rev Resp Dis* 115:315, 1977.

Rossman CM, Forrest JB, Lee, RMKW, Newhouse, MT: The dyskinetic cilia syndrome. *Chest* 78:580, 1980.

Wanner A: Clinical aspects of mucociliary transport. *Am Rev Resp Dis* 116:73, 1977.

16

High Altitude

Meir H. Kryger

The vast majority of humans live at the top of an ocean of water and at the bottom of an ocean of air. The higher one ascends in this ocean of air, the more rarified the air and the lower the oxygen pressure.

The atmosphere extends about 2000 kilometers (1200 miles) above the surface of the earth. Up to about 120 km there is a mixture consisting of mainly oxygen (20.93%), nitrogen (78.09%), and trace quantities of argon, carbon dioxide, neon, and other gases. This height and beyond is indeed inhospitable; the air is so rarified, it neither scatters light nor propagates sound; it is dark and silent. Beyond are layers of atomic oxygen, helium, and then hydrogen before reaching "empty" interplanetary space.

Because humans require oxygen, they are limited by the reduced oxygen pressure of altitude and can only function normally in the lowest kilometers of the atmosphere. In spite of these limitations, or perhaps because of them, humans climb mountains, fly airplanes, and explore interplanetary space. These activities are possible only because we can modify the oxygen pressure in our environment and, if necessary, put ourselves in a sealed hospitable environment that travels with us.

People are exposed to the hypoxia of high altitude on aircraft and on mountains (Figure 16.1). On aircraft the hypoxic exposure is usually short. On mountains, problems occur in persons who have recently ascended to high altitude (acute mountain sickness) or in persons resident at high altitude in whom the physiological responses to hypoxia have failed (chronic mountain sickness).

ALTITUDE AND INSPIRED OXYGEN PRESSURE

Since air is basically 21% O_2 and 79% N_2, it is easy to calculate the pressure of oxygen in air entering the trachea. We must remember that air is humidified before reaching the trachea. The total pressure for O_2 and N_2 is, therefore, the barometric pressure minus the water vapor pressure, which is 47 mmHg. Thus, inspired oxygen pressure is $.21 \times (Pb - 47)$. The relationship between altitude and inspired Po_2 is shown in Figure 16.1. Alveolar Po_2 is calculated from inspired Po_2, alveolar Pco_2, and the respiratory exchange ratio (R) by the alveolar gas equation:

$$P_{A_{O_2}} = P_{I_{O_2}} - \frac{P_{ACO_2}}{R}$$

Although modern commercial aircraft cruise at altitudes well in excess of 6.2 km (about 20,000 feet), the pressure inside the cabin is maintained at pressure equivalent to that found at 1.5 to 2.5 km (5000 to 8000 ft) altitude. Thus in aircraft there is present a reduction in inspired oxygen pressure. This reduction is not physiologically important, since the resultant drop in Po_2 is associated with only a small drop in Sa_{O_2}, being on the flat portion of the oxyhemoglobin dissociation curve. However, in a patient with pre-existing

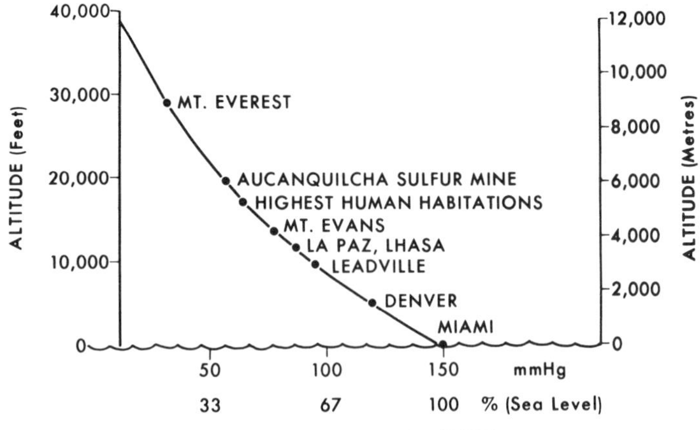

Figure 16.1. Relationship between altitude and inspired oxygen pressure.

hypoxemia from lung disease, the reduction in inspired Po_2 can cause serious hypoxemia.

The major manifestations of acute hypoxemia are due to its effect on the system most sensitive to oxygen lack, the central nervous system. As was mentioned on page 201, cerebral blood flow increases with hypoxemia, which tends to maintain O_2 delilvery to the brain. Several mechanisms can interfere with this compensatory response. Hyperventilation, a normal response to hypoxemia lowers Pco_2, which can then lead to reduced cerebral blood flow and also induces alkalemia, which left shifts the oxyhemoglobin dissociation curves and thus interferes with oxygen unloading. With very severe hypoxemia the cardiovascular system may fail causing a marked reduction in cerebral blood flow. These effects can all interfere with oxygen unloading.

Impairment can be detected with fairly mild hypoxemia, at levels of Po_2 that are not likely to interfere with aerobic metabolism (Figure 16.2). It is likely that with mild hypoxemia, disturbed neural function is in fact due to interference in neurotransmitter synthesis, a failure in communication between neurons, rather than failure of energy generation of neurons.

Acclimatization and Adaptation to High Altitude

Because humans evolved at low altitude, the "machinery" for gas exchange and oxygen delivery functions best at high inspired Po_2. When people ascend to high altitudes, a series of physiological adjustments occur to compensate for

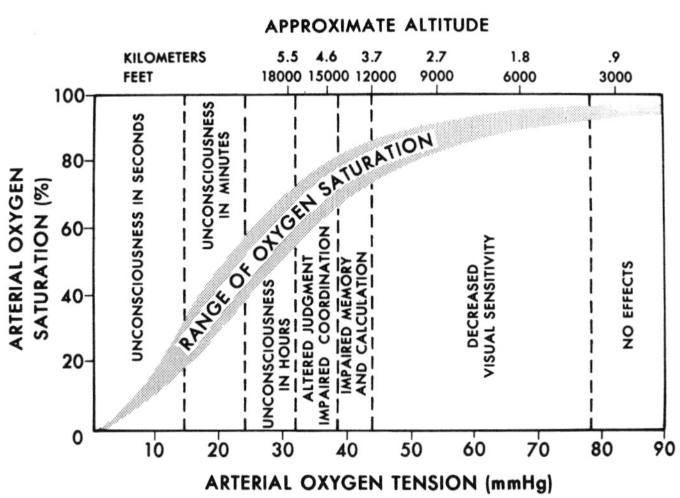

Figure 16.2. Cerebral cortical function, altitude, and oxygenation. Impairment may be detected with acute exposure to even mild hypoxemia. $Po_2 < 30$ mmHg severely impairs cerebral function. (Modified with permission, *Bioastronautics Data Book*, Figure 2-3. National Aeronautics and Space Administration, Washington, 1973.)

the low inspired P_{O_2}. This reversible series of physiological changes is called *acclimatization.*

The major changes occurring with acclimatization involve the organs taking part in oxygen delivery, the respiratory system, the cardiovascular system, and the hematopoietic system.

Ventilation

With acute exposure to high altitude, ventilation abruptly increases but increases further over the ensuing 7 to 14 days. When a person has acclimatized, hyperventilation persists, even when P_{O_2} is acutely increased to normal levels. Deacclimatization, the return of ventilation to sea level values on return to sea level, is actually a slow process.

In spite of intensive study over 3 decades, the process of acclimatization of ventilation is not well understood. The initial hyperventilation is probably mediated by hypoxemia stimulating the carotid bodies. Indeed, the carotid bodies enlarge with hypoxemia and regress when hypoxemia is reversed in acclimatizing animals. The cause of the persistent hyperventilation is not clear. It was once believed that the stimulus was $[H^+]$ in the cerebrospinal fluid. It is now clear the changes in cerebrospinal fluid $[H^+]$ follow, rather than cause, the change in ventilation. Perhaps an increase in intraneural $[H^+]$ or brain interstitial space $[H^+]$ caused by changes in neuronal metabolism induced by hypoxemia is responsible.

The increase in ventilation after acute ascent is primarily due to an increase in tidal volume, not breathing frequency. During sleep, however, a Cheyne-Stokes breathing pattern commonly develops, which may cause severe hypoxemia.

After many years at high altitude, ventilatory response to hypoxia becomes blunted. In spite of this, hyperventilation persists. Thus, paradoxically, although they hyperventilate, natives of high altitude have blunted hypoxic drive to breathe.

Increased ventilation cannot, of course, return Pa_{O_2} to normal at altitude. What is gas exchange like on Mt. Everest (8848 m altitude)? Barometric pressure on top of the mountain is about 250 mmHg, and so inspired P_{O_2} is about $.2093 \times (250 - 47) = 42.5$ mmHg. Alveolar P_{CO_2} and alveolar P_{O_2} have been predicted to be about 10 mmHg and 31 mmHg respectively. As was discussed previously (Chapter 9), diffusion limitation occurs when $P_{A_{O_2}}$ is low, and thus hemoglobin does not fully equilibrate with alveolar P_{O_2}. Thus at rest, Pa_{O_2} will only be about 25 mmHg. The least exercise will increase red blood cell velocity, worsen diffusion, and lower Pa_{O_2} below 25 mmHg. Oxygen is thus commonly used by climbers at high altitude.

Hematopoietic System

Within 2 hours of high altitude exposure, there occurs an increase in erythropoietin-mediated red blood cell production. Within weeks there has occurred an increase in red blood cell mass, hemoglobin, and hematocrit. The values obtained after chronic exposure are shown in Figure 9.25.

With acute altitude exposure there occurs an acute increase in 2,3 diphosphoglycerate concentration in cells. This reduces hemoglobin-oxygen affinity and thus facilitates O_2 unloading in the tissues. This response may be inappropriate at great altitudes where the problem is loading oxygen in the lung, not unloading it in the tissues.

Cardiovascular System

Initially on ascent to high altitude, there occurs an increase in cardiac output, which returns to normal within a few days. However, blood flow is redistributed to maintain oxygen delivery to vital tissues. In longtime residents at high altitude, an increased number of capillaries is also present in tissues, facilitating gas transfer. Pulmonary arterioles constrict with airway hypoxia; thus, mild pulmonary hypertension is common at high altitude. It is unclear whether pulmonary vasoconstriction offers any advantage and certainly may cause problems. The terminal pulmonary arterioles may become muscularized. The pulmonary arterial pressure usually decreases when airway Po_2 is increased.

Adaptation vs Acclimatization

Humans must acclimatize to survive at high altitude; a series of physiological changes occur with the hypoxic exposure. Races that have resided at high altitude for thousands of years have acclimatized very effectively and appear to have changed by natural selection. For example, the lungs of Indians in the Andes are larger than those of sea level residents, a mechanism which increases the gas-exchanging surface. In addition, the work capacity of high altitude natives is much higher than that of people who visit or have moved to high altitude. The physiological responses to hypoxia may not always be advantageous. Natives of high altitude and newcomers to altitude, regardless of how well they were acclimatized, may develop a disease caused by loss of acclimatization, mountain sickness.

Some animals who have evolved at high altitude were "designed" to live in a hypoxic environment, their normal environment. These animals are born with inherited biochemical, physiological, and anatomic machinery to thrive at high altitude. They require no physiological adjustments to cope with hypoxia, since that is their normal habitat. This is *adaptation* to high altitude. These animals are markedly different from acclimatized high altitude human natives.

A comparison of acclimatization in humans and adaptation of animals indigenous to altitude is useful. The llama is the high altitude animal which has been studied in the most detail.

Respiratory System. Acclimatized individuals hyperventilate and have enlarged carotid bodies. Llamas do not.

Cardiovascular System. Acclimatized individuals have pulmonary hypertension. Llamas do not.

Hematopoietic System. Acclimatized individuals have an increased red cell mass (polycythemia), an increased 2,3 DPG concentration in red cells that reduces hemoglobin-oxygen affinity. Llamas have a low hematocrit, the red cells being small and ellipsoid. Their blood contains no 2,3 DPG. Hemoglobin-oxygen affinity is increased, which helps O_2 uptake in the lungs.

The major problem at altitude is not to unload O_2 to the tissues but is to trap O_2 from the air. The best way to solve this problem is to *increase* hemoglobin-oxygen affinity. The llama with its left-shifted oxyhemoglobin dissociation curve can saturate its hemoglobin with oxygen at a low Po_2 and can unload it in the tissues at a very low Po_2. It can thus thrive without hyperventilation or polycythemia at extreme altitude.

DISORDERS OCCURRING AFTER ACUTE ASCENT TO HIGH ALTITUDE

Problems after acute ascent to altitude were once most often associated with military operations. Today with armies of tourists trekking in the Himalayas, skiing at extreme altitudes, and attempting to climb mountains with and without oxygen, most of the cases occur in civilians.

Acute Hypoxia of Altitude

Immediately on acute exposure to hypoxia, many people notice breathlessness, dizziness, and palpitations, particularly during exercise. These symptoms, which may occur at altitudes as low as 1500 m (about 5000 ft), represent physiological adjustments and are not to be considered a disease.

Acute Mountain Sickness

The features of acute mountain sickness do not occur immediately after acute exposure; instead, they usually become evident 6 or more hours later and may begin days later. The main manifestations are due to edema in the skin, lungs, and brain, and patients have symptoms of edema in one or more of these organs. Acute mountain sickness is more common in younger people and in those who ascend to altitude rapidly rather than slowly.

Edema around the eyes, in the hands, and in the feet is often associated with pulmonary edema and cerebral edema. The cause is not clear but may be related to right ventricular failure.

The pathogenesis of *high altitude pulmonary edema* (HAPE) is not well understood. Pulmonary edema can be caused by increased pressure in the pulmonary circulation and/or increased permeability. One possible explanation is that in the presence of hypoxia, there occurs uneven pulmonary arterial vasoconstriction. This may cause the less constricted vessels to be overdistended and overperfused. The high velocity of blood in these vessels may cause endothelial injury. Thus, the edema may be caused by injured vessels "seeing" high pressures. It has been shown that left heart failure does not contribute significantly. HAPE may occur at altitudes as low as 2300 m (7500 ft). Patients may have findings ranging from just fine crackles in the bases without symptoms, to fulminant fatal edema with frothy edema fluid emanating from the respiratory tract.

Cerebral edema causes severe symptoms and may cause death. Headaches, nausea and vomiting, ataxia, irrational behavior, and coma are all manifestations of increased intracranial pressure. Retinal hemorrhages are also commonly found. Hypoxemia causes the problem. In spite of low P_{CO_2} caused by hyperventilation, there is probably an increase in cerebral blood flow (caused by hypoxemia) together with a flux of water into neurons. The latter event may be due to abnormality in the way neurons maintain intracellular Na^+ and K^+ concentrations when hypoxemia is present. Severe cerebral edema rarely occurs at altitudes below 3,700 m (12,000 ft).

The only definitive treatment of acute mountain sickness is for the patient to descend to lower altitude. Oxygen breathing, of course, should be done until this is possible. Acetazolamide, a carbonic anhydrase inhibitor that induces loss of HCO_3^- in the urine and thus may speed up acclimatization, may prevent some cases of acute mountain sickness.

DISORDERS OCCURRING IN RESIDENTS OF HIGH ALTITUDE

The vast majority of people living at high altitude have no medical problems. The process of acclimatization allows them to function in a hypoxic environment. Humans can live up to an altitude of about 5300 m (about 17,500 ft) and can work at slightly higher altitudes. A small number of people, mostly men, appear to lose acclimatization and develop *chronic mountain sickness,* which has also been called Monge's disease and chronic mountain polycythemia. The disease is common in the Andes and in Leadville, Colorado, but does not occur in the Himalayas. This may be due to the fact that people in the Himalayas have been living at altitude for thousands of years longer than those in the Andes and may be more suited by natural selection to life in a hypoxic environment.

The major difference between patients with chronic mountain polycythemia and normals residing at altitude is that the patients are much more hypoxemic. Excessive hypoxemia at altitude is usually caused by hypoventilation, mismatching of ventilation, diffusion defect, or a combination of these.

Hypoventilation. As mentioned on p. 302, normals at high altitude hyperventilate. Yet when ventilatory response to hypoxia is measured, it is found to be blunted! It is not clear what "drives" breathing in high altitude residents. In any case, hypoventilation occurs in patients with chronic mountain sickness. Patients have a shallow breathing pattern that increases ventilation of dead space, which results in alveolar hypoventilation.

$\dot{V}/\dot{Q}$ Mismatching. In some instances, the excessive hypoxemia can be adequately explained by the ventilation-perfusion mismatching of lung disease. Chronic airflow obstruction due to cigarette smoking or interstitial disease due to dust inhalation (from mining) are common in some high altitude communities. In other words, the combination of lung disease and high altitude causes the severe hypoxemia.

Because these patients have blunted hypoxic drive to breathe, they do not respond to the hypoxemia, which is thus allowed to persist.

The hypoxemia leads to increased red blood cell production, which causes marked polycythemia, and hypoxic pulmonary vasoconstriction, which causes pulmonary hypertension.

The major symptoms are caused by the effect of polycythemia on cerebral function. The patients complain of headaches, inability to think clearly, and sleepiness. The quality of these patients' blood is molasseslike and one can visualize how thick blood flowing through the cerebral circulation could cause problems.

Reducing blood volume by phlebotomy (withdrawing blood) usually results in prompt but temporary relief of symptoms. Moving to low altitude cures the disease with regression of the polycythemia and the pulmonary hypertension. Respiratory stimulation with a progestational agent has been used with positive results: increase of ventilation, improvement in arterial Po_2, and reduction in red blood cell production.

The mechanism of chronic mountain sickness in humans can be distinguished from that of *brisket disease*, a disorder of cattle at high altitude. The major problem in these cattle, usually European breeds evolved at low altitude, is that their pulmonary circulation is hyperactive to hypoxia. The intense pulmonary vasoconstriction causes pulmonary hypertension, which leads to right ventricular failure and venous hypertension. Edema in cattle often collects in the area between the front legs and neck, the brisket, hence the name brisket disease. Thus, whereas the main defect in human mountain sickness is in the respiratory system, in cattle it is in the cardiovascular system.

BIBLIOGRAPHY

Hackett PH: Acute mountain sickness—the clinical approach. *Adv Cardiol* 27:6, 1980.

Hackett PH, Rennie D, Levine HD: The incidence, importance, and prophylaxis of Acute Mountain Sickness. *Lancet* 2:1149, 1976.

Heath D, Williams DR: *Man at High Altitude.* London, Churchill Livingstone, 1977.

Houston CS: High Altitude Illness. *JAMA* 236:2193, 1976.

Kryger M, McCullough R, Doekel R, et al: Excessive polycythemia of high altitude. *Am Rev Resp Dis* 118:659, 1978.

Lenfant C, Sullivan K: Adaptation to High Altitude. *New Engl J Med* 284:1298, 1971.

Sutton JR, Gray GW, Houston CS, et al: Effects of duration at altitude and acetazolamide on ventilation and oxygenation during sleep. *Sleep* 3:455, 1980.

Ward M: *Mountain Medicine.* London, Crosby Lockwood Staples, 1975.

17

Symptoms and Signs

David Ostrow

Patients seek medical help because of symptoms. In order to best treat patients, we must first diagnose their illness using information gathered from the history and physical examination. Laboratory tests are then done to confirm the diagnosis and to document the degree of physiological impairment. The first and most crucial step remains the unravelling of the cause of the patients' symptoms and physical findings. In this chapter, we will review the physiological mechanisms that produce the cardinal symptoms and signs of respiratory disease.

Cough and Expectoration

The production of mucus in the bronchial tree and the act of coughing with the subsequent expectoration of that mucus and any trapped foreign material constitute the first line in the lung's defenses to potential toxic inhaled agents. The pathophysiological conditions that lead to increased coughing and excessive sputum production involve a number of complex neurological and chemical mechanisms.

Cough

The lungs are innervated by the vagus nerves and by fibers from the upper thoracic sympathetic ganglia. The receptors for the cough reflex are located in the tracheal and bronchial mucosa. The receptors are rapidly adapting end organs that are inhibited by local anesthesia. The impulses from these receptors travel to the respiratory center, which integrates the information and then sends back impulses via the vagus nerves, the efferent part of the reflex arc, to the glottis, bronchial smooth muscles, and the expiratory muscles.

The act of coughing consists first of a deep inspiration followed by a maximum expiratory effort against the closed glottis. This produces a tremendous increase in intrathoracic pressure. As the glottis opens, air is forced out of the airways at very high velocity, carrying with it mucus and inhaled particles. Associated with this increase in intrathoracic pressure is reflex bronchoconstriction. The narrowed airway, acting like a peashooter, helps to increase the velocity of the expelled air, so that it is nearly at the speed of sound.

Coughing can be initiated by a number of factors, including mechanical contact of the nose and upper airways, inert dusts, or irritant gases. Inhalation of certain chemicals such as histamine or methacholine can initiate both coughing and bronchoconstriction.

Sputum

Sputum is material coughed up or expectorated from the bronchial tree. It originates as secretions from the mucus glands and goblet cells present in the airways. The mucus coats the normal respiratory epithelium in a uniform fashion. Mucus is an extremely complex substance being a polymer of mucopolysaccharide. Its production is increased with cholinergic stimulation.

There are two layers to the mucus blanket. One, the outside layer in contact with the lumen of the airways, has the property of a gel. The inside layer is less viscid and surrounds the cilia of the epithelial cells. This thin layer allows the cilia to beat. The cilia reach into the thick mucous gel only at the very apex of their beat (see Figures 15.2, 15.3).

When seen in cross section, these cilia are a series of nine vertical pairs of filaments located circumferentially around a pair of central filaments. It is presumed that these filaments slide over each other to give rise to the ciliary motion. There is a familial condition of bronchiectasis and infertility in which the ciliary filaments lack their radial spokes. Another syndrome of sinusitis, bronchiectasis, and situs inversus (*Kartagener's*) is associated with loss of the dynein side arms of the cilia. It is clear then that structural abnormalities of cilia can be associated with a predisposition to suppurative lung disease.

Contained in the mucus are a number of bacteriostatic substances such as lysozyme, complement, secretory IgA, and lactoferrin. Cells that originate as pulmonary alveolar macrophages and migrate up the bronchial tree are also present. Eosinophils or neutrophils are not normally present in large amounts.

Clinical Factors

Coughing may or may not be associated with sputum production (Table 17.1). Cough unassociated with sputum is most commonly seen in upper respiratory infections or in cigarette smokers. It may also be associated with irritation of the upper airways from *tumor, goiter*, or vascular abnormality such as an *aortic aneurysm.* Lower respiratory tree factors are also important, though the pathophysiological mechanism is not clear. *Pulmonary fibrosis*, for example, may be associated with a nonproductive cough.

Table 17.1. An Approach to Cough

- **Nonproductive**
  - Acute
    - Infection (viral laryngitis, tracheitis, bronchitis)
    - Inhalation of irritants
    - Pleural irritation
      - pneumothorax
  - Chronic
    - Extrinsic irritation (goiter, aortic aneurysm, mediastinal nodes)
    - Inhalation of irritants (smoking)
    - Bronchial tumors
    - Interstitial lung disease
    - Asthma
- **Productive**
  - Acute
    - Infections
      - pneumonia
      - bronchitis
    - Inhalation of irritants
  - Chronic
    - Chronic bronchitis
    - Bronchiectasis
    - Abscess
    - Asthma
    - Tumor
      - bronchogenic carcinoma
      - alveolar cell carcinoma

Persons presenting with cough and sputum production are a more common problem for the physician. Infections of the bronchi (*bronchitis*) or lung (*pneumonia*) are considered an acute event. The sputum is usually purulent and contains an increased number of polymorphonuclear leukocytes. Bacteria may be found in the sputum and, if present in large amounts, may have etiological significance. Sputum is not always a good specimen for bacteriological study, because it is contaminated by the bacterial content of the mouth and pharynx.

The color and consistency of sputum may give helpful information. In chronic bronchitis, sputum usually has the consistency of the mucus secreted by the respiratory secretory cells; the sputum is clear and of low viscosity. In the presence of infection, a change in both the color and the viscosity of the sputum occurs. The large quantity of DNA from neutrophils results in an increase in the viscosity of the sputum; it becomes sticky or tenacious and more difficult to cough up. Purulent sputum may be rusty or yellow. When sputum has been in the airways for a while, it turns green or grey because of the action of an enzyme liberated from neutrophils, verdoperoxidase. Frothy pink sputum is found in pulmonary edema. The bubbles in the froth are stable because of surfactant. The pink color is due to the presence of red blood cells.

Inhalation of irritant gases such as phosgene, NO_2, or SO_2 may give rise to acute inflammation of the tracheobronchial tree with production of sputum.

Chronic cough and sputum production is the sine qua non of *chronic bronchitis.* The sputum in such patients varies from mucoid, containing few, to purulent, containing many, polymorphonuclear leukocytes. Persons with *bronchiectasis* also may produce large quantities of sputum, up to 200 cc per day. It also may vary in constitution from mucoid to purulent. The amount of sputum production in such persons is sometimes related to positioning, since gravitational factors are important for mucus drainage when the normal bronchial tree anatomy is modified. *Lung abscess* is associated with purulent sputum production, and because there is often a large growth of anaerobic organisms, the sputum may have a putrid odor to it.

Bronchogenic carcinoma, because it so often occurs in smokers, is associated with cough and sputum, though most tumors do not actually produce an increase in sputum unless there is bronchial obstruction and infection. In one particular type of carcinoma, namely alveolar cell carcinoma, there may be a copious amount of watery sputum arising from the tumor.

Asthma is commonly associated with wheezing, but cough and sputum production may be important symptoms. Recent studies have shown that cough may be the only presenting symptom of persons with asthma. The sputum of persons with asthma may look purulent to the naked eye, but simple microscopic studies will reveal that the predominant cell type present is the eosinophil. In addition, the mucus may contain Curshman's spirals, which are fibrils of elastic fiber, fibrin, mucopolysaccharide, and cellular debris or Charcot-Leyden crystals, which appear to derive from the degenerated granules of the eosinophils.

Hemoptysis

The lungs and bronchial tree have two separate vascular supplies, the high pressure bronchial system and the low pressure pulmonary system. The bronchial system supplies the airways to the level of the terminal respiratory bronchiole. There are a complex series of arterial and venous plexes on either side of the bronchial smooth muscle layer leading to the bronchial mucosa. The blood supply to the bronchial mucosa can thus be modified by bronchial smooth muscle contraction.

The pulmonary arteries are elastic vessels but contain much less elastic tissue, in adults, than the aorta. They branch into muscular arteries, and then these lead to the pulmonary alveolar-capillary bed. There are anastomoses between pulmonary arteries and veins, which bypass the capillaries. There are also anastomoses between the bronchial veins and pulmonary veins.

When patients complain of coughing up blood, the nose and upper respiratory tree must be searched carefully to be certain that the bleeding is not coming from that region, a much less serious problem.

Generally, we think of the location first, when approaching the problem of hemoptysis and then a pathological process (Table 17.2). In the bronchial tree, inflammatory processes are by far the most common causes. Of these, the most common cause is chronic bronchitis. The bleeding in *bronchitis* is due to rupture of vessels in the bronchial mucosa often associated with the increased cough seen with a respiratory infection. The sputum in such bronchitic patients often appears purulent with bright red streaks in it. *Bronchiectasis* is a

Table 17.2. An Approach to Hemoptysis

Bronchial tree
- Inflammation
  - Bronchitis, bronchiectasis, tuberculosis
- Tumors
  - Benign, (Adenoma)
  - Malignant, (Carcinoma)
- Congenital
  - Sequestrations

Lung
- Inflammatory diseases
  - Pneumonia, abscess, tuberculosis
- Vascular abnormalities
  - Pulmonary embolism (with infarction)
  - Vasculitis, Goodpasture's syndrome
  - A-V anastomosis
  - Mitral stenosis
- Congenital factors
  - Cysts
  - A-V malformation

chronic severe inflammatory process of the bronchial tree, leading to distorted anatomy of the tree. Episodes of hemoptysis associated with bronchiectasis are also often associated with an increased growth of bacteria, which are ever-present in the distorted bronchi. The sputum here may be very purulent, perhaps foul smelling. The bleeding in bronchiectasis originates in dilated vessels in the bronchial mucosa and may be much more severe than in bronchitis.

Cancer is now the disease that patients think of when they expectorate blood, just as it was tuberculosis 50 years ago. Both benign *bronchial adenomas* and malignant *carcinomas* may be associated with hemoptysis. Recurrent bleeding is often the only symptom of the slow growing bronchial adenoma.

Congenital pulmonary sequestrations may be entirely asymptomatic before they bleed or they may be associated with a history of chronic infections similar to bronchiectasis.

Blood emanating from the lungs may also be associated with inflammatory diseases. The sputum of *pneumococcal pneumonia* is classically described as "rusty" in appearance. *Tuberculosis* may cause hemoptysis by both endobronchial disease or from pulmonary cavities whose centers are full of caseous necrosis. Old healed tuberculous cavities may be infected with the fungus *Aspergillus,* and this organism can locally invade tissues leading to massive hemoptysis. Hemoptysis from a *lung abscess* may be associated with putrid smelling sputum, since many of these are associated with anaerobic bacterias.

Conditions affecting the blood vessels of the lung are also associated with hemoptysis. A *pulmonary embolism* often begins as a clot in the veins of the legs or pelvis. It arises in the setting of bedridden and debilitated patients, perhaps in congestive heart failure or perhaps in the setting of a woman on birth control pills. Inflammation of the pulmonary vessels related to such diseases as *polyarteritis nodosa* or *Wegener's granulomatosis* are less common causes of bleeding as is *Goodpasture's disease,* in which antibasement membrane antibodies are found to both kidney glomeruli and to the alveolar endothelium. The pink frothy sputum associated with pulmonary venous hypertension (mitral stenosis, left ventricular failure, etc.) is made up of plasma and erythrocytes that have leaked out of the pulmonary capillaries and that have mixed with surfactant. *Arteriovenous malformations* in the lung may be either congenital or acquired. The latter, which are associated with cirrhosis, are not often associated with hemoptysis.

Dyspnea and Lack of Dyspnea

Dyspnea or breathlessness is the uncomfortable awareness of difficulty in breathing. It is a sensation and, therefore, a subjective phenomenon. While there are no models that explain all aspects of dyspnea, a useful one is that of E.J.M. Campbell and J. Howell. According to their model, the brain is continuously assessing both the body's metabolic demand for ventilatory activity and the actual ventilation performed. These are monitored by impulses from the respiratory muscles, which respond to changes in their length and tension. This process of assessment normally is carried out on an unconscious level. Inappropriateness in these relationships ("length-tension inappropriateness") raise the sensation into the level of a conscious perception. In other words, dyspnea is sensed when a discrepancy exists between the *drive to breathe* and *ventilation actually attained* (Table 17.3).

The afferent receptors for these sensations are thought to be located in the muscle spindle or the Golgi tendon organs of the intercostal muscles. An increased load will cause a misalignment of the intrafusal and extrafusal muscle fibers. This will cause stimulation of the muscle spindles, which will be relayed to the brain via intercostal nerves and the spinal cord.

It is also possible that the J-receptors that are believed to be in the interstitial space play a role in sensing inappropriate work, in particular in some of the interstitial lung diseases.

The time course of the onset of this inappropriateness cannot be too heavily emphasized. Patients with a gradually progressive disease, such as chronic

Table 17.3. An Approach to Dyspnea

Increased drive to breathe
- Chemical
  - Hypoxia
  - Hypercapnia, acidemia
  - Increased metabolic rate
    - fever
    - hyperthyroidism
- Lung Reflexes
  - Interstitial diseases
  - Pulmonary edema
  - Pneumothorax
  - Pneumonia
  - Pulmonary vascular disease
- Cerebral cortex
  - "Neurogenic" hyperventilation

Hindrance to ventilation
- Increased airway resistance
  - Asthma
  - Chronic airflow obstruction
- Intrapulmonary restriction
  - Interstitial lung disorders
- Extrapulmonary restriction
  - Obesity
  - Kyphoscoliosis
  - Pleural effusion
  - Respiratory muscle paralysis

bronchitis, may perform much greater work breathing than a mild asthmatic, whose airway obstruction develops over a few minutes. Yet the asthmatic will be found to have a much stronger perception of breathlessness than the bronchitic.

Since dyspnea appears to be related to the discrepancy between drive to breathe and the ventilation achieved, dyspnea may be due to increased neural drive to breathe with or without an impediment in the breathing apparatus.

Increased drive may thus be present when the respiratory center is bombarded with impulses from the chemoreceptors, from reflexes arising in the lungs, and from the cerebral cortex.

An *impediment to breathe* may arise where there occurs airflow obstruction or lung restriction. Restriction of lung movement may be due to disease of structures surrounding the lung or disease of the lung itself. Causes of extrapulmonary restriction include kyphoscoliosis, obesity, and ankylosing spondylitis. Intrapulmonary restriction is caused by many disorders, which are reviewed in Chapter 3.

When both increased drive and impediment to breathe are present, the dyspnea can be intense. Perhaps the most severe unrelenting dyspnea in medicine occurs in patients with severe interstitial lung disease in whom breathing is driven by the lung reflexes described in Chapter 6.

Another complication in our understanding of dyspnea is that in some conditions of increased hindrance to breathing, there may occur a reduction in drive to breathe. This occurs in some patients with airflow obstruction, obesity, and kyphoscoliosis. In these patients dyspnea is not prominent. Thus, the absence of dyspnea in patients in whom there should be dyspnea suggests that drive to breathe is reduced. For example, when a patient has severe hypoxemia and hypercapnia but is not short of breath, reduced drive to breathe is likely. The causes of reduced drives to breathe are reviewed in Chapter 6 and include abnormalities in the various components of the respiratory control system, especially central nervous system disorders.

Chest Pain

As with pain in most regions of the body, the problem of chest pain is best approached along anatomical lines. While pain from organs outside the chest can cause the sensation of chest pain, this discussion will be confined to conditions in the chest (Table 17.4).

Pain may originate in the chest wall, the pleura, the structures in the mediastinum, and the heart, in particular the pericardium and presumably myocardium. The lung itself and the visceral pleura are relatively free of pain fibers. Lung disease causing the sensation of pain does so by irritating the pleura, for example, pneumonia and pulmonary embolism. Sometimes pulmonary hypertension is associated with a peculiar type of chest pain.

Pain in the chest wall often originates in the *intercostal muscle fibers* and may be associated with episodes of severe coughing. Unlike pleuritic pain, it is present during breath-holding. Pain from the ribs may be due to fractures or

Table 17.4. An Approach to Chest Pain

Chest wall
Muscles (trauma, stretching)
Ribs (tumor, fracture)
Costochondral junction (inflammation)
Pleura
Inflammation (infection, tumor)
Trauma
Mediastinum
Esophagus
Heart (ischemic, pericardial)
Pulmonary vessels

invasion by malignant tissue. *Costochondritis* is an inflammation of the costochondral junctions of the ribs and is associated with a persistent anterior ache. Chest wall pain from all sources is made worse by palpation of the area involved.

Pain from the pleura arises from afferents in the parietal pleura. These join to branches of the intercostal nerves and are stimulated by inflammation, tumors, and stretching. Since the intercostals feed the pleura located directly beneath them, pleural pain in this region accurately reflects the site of irritation. Pain over the diaphragmatic pleura is, however, mediated via the phrenic nerve (C3, 4, 5), and so pleural irritation in this region is perceived as pain in the neck or upper shoulders. The pain of pleural origin is characteristically worse on inspiration and often occurs at a consistent lung volume, preventing further inspiration.

It is not difficult to imagine that infections or malignant infiltrations of the pleura might cause chest pain. It is, however, difficult to explain the pain associated with a simple *pneumothorax,* although pain with this condition is not uncommon.

The most important organ in the mediastinum that is associated with chest pain is the heart. *Ischemic cardiac* pain is "squeezing" and not pleuritic and is brought on by exercise or emotion and relieved by nitroglycerine. *Pericardial* pain may be similar, but this pain is often modified by position, especially decreased by leaning forward. *Esophagitis* may simulate cardiac pain but is relieved by antacids and is typically related to food intake.

Both the acute pulmonary hypertension of *pulmonary embolism* and the chronic hypertension in *cor pulmonale* may be associated with a dull retrosternal pain. The mechanism for this pain is yet unclear.

Somnolence and Sleep Apnea

Until recently somnolence was not considered a symptom of respiratory disease. In literature, there is the reference to the very obese Joe, the fat boy, in Charles Dickens' *Pickwick Papers.* Joe is described as a "young opium eater" in reference to his pathological sleepiness, and Dickens implied a relationship between the obesity and somnolence.

We now know that *Pickwickian* (obesity-hypoventilation) patients have a depression in their control of ventilation and have a depressed response to hypoxia and hypercapnia. Study of Pickwickian and other somnolent patients has provided us with some dramatic new manifestations of respiratory disease, the sleep apnea syndrome (see p. 118).

Normal adults have periods of cessation of airflow at the mouth and nose (apnea) lasting as long as 15 seconds during sleep. Some somnolent patients, however, have hundreds of longer apneic periods during sleep. These may be associated with dramatic hypercapnia and hypoxemia. Each of these episodes is terminated by a short awakening, hence the daytime sleepiness.

Central apnea is characterized by an abnormality in the central nervous system such as a *brainstem infarction* or *bulbar polio*. *Ondine's curse* (idiopathic hypoventilation) is a syndrome of obscure etiology in which primary alveolar hypoventilation is exacerbated by sleeping. The patients are like the mythical Paracelsus who had to remain awake in order to breathe.

Obstructive sleep apnea is associated with upper airway obstruction. An electromyogram attached to the jaw often shows relaxation of the musculature of the tongue and pharynx just before a period of apnea. There appears to be upper airway obstruction that may be partial and associated with snoring or grunting or that may be complete leading to apnea. Conditions associated with this form of apnea include *obesity, hypertrophy of the adenoids and tonsils, acromegaly* (enlarged tongue), and *myxedema*. Sometimes there is no obvious reason found for the apnea. Sometimes patients demonstrate evidence of both forms of sleep apnea.

Sleepiness then is an important clue to respiratory disease and requires close investigation. This is especially so if a family member can provide a history of snoring or unusual breathing pattern or if the patient has evidence of prolonged hypoxia, such as pulmonary hypertension or erythrocytosis.

Other Neurological Symptoms

We must remember that the brain is very sensitive to hypoxemia and hypercapnia. Hypercapnia causes cerebral acidosis and increases cerebral blood flow, which may increase intracerebral pressure. Thus severe headache, which often awakens the patient during sleep, is a common symptom.

Neural tissue is exquisitely sensitive to oxygen lack. Thus, hypoxemia can cause a variety of symptoms ranging from mild confusion to stupor to coma.

Cor Pulmonale

The excessive afterload faced by the right ventricle due to the pulmonary vasoconstriction of lung disease can cause it to fail. This causes increased right ventricular end diastolic pressure, increased atrial pressure, and then increased venous pressure. The latter may lead to a *tender liver*, the patient complaining of vague upper abdominal pains, and the development of *peripheral edema*, the patient complaining of swollen feet. The increased venous pressure can be detected by the presence of jugular venous distension. Such patients often develop excessive red blood cell production, *erythrocytosis* (also often called polycythemia).

Sounds from the Chest

The nomenclature used for sounds generated by the airways is subject to great debate and sometimes confusion. Much of the problem arises from a poor English translation of the original papers of Laennec. He used the word *râle* to describe any abnormal or new sound in the chest and translated the word from French to Latin where it became rhonchus. We commonly use *rale* and *rhonchus* to mean two sounds quite different from each other. Table 17.5 contains the terms commonly used to describe breath sounds.

Wheezes

The two most important and commonly heard sounds are best thought of as either continuous or discontinuous. The continuous sounds go by the name of *wheeze* in the British and *rhonchus* in the American literature. This continuous sound is associated with increased airway resistance. It was once thought that the particular pitch of a wheeze was determined by the position in the bronchial tree where the obstruction occurred, hence from which the sound was generated. However, recent cogent arguments point out that the pitch of a wheeze is independent of gas density and, therefore, is independent of the length of the tube and more dependent on the actual physical properties of the bronchus itself. It appears to be due to the air moving at high velocity as it flows through a nearly closed bronchus. This gives rise to the continuous sound, which we recognize as the wheeze.

The adage, "All that wheezes is not asthma," is of practical importance. Causes for increased airway resistance and wheezing include endobronchial factors such as *tumors* or *foreign bodies,* bronchial wall factors such as *asthma,* and extrabronchial compression as by enlarged *tuberculous lymph nodes* (Table 17.6).

Crackles

With the development of sophisticated recorders and audio filters, more accurate studies have been made of discontinuous breath sounds. These sounds have been variously called rales, crepitations, and crackles. The latter seems the most acceptable. These sounds are heard most often during the inspiratory cycle, and their place in that cycle is of importance. Patients with early inspiratory crackles have been found to have evidence of airways obstruction secondary to *chronic bronchitis* or *asthma* or *emphysema.* Persons with late inspiratory or paninspiratory crackles have evidence of interstitial lung

Table 17.5. Terms Commonly Used to Describe Breath Sounds

Acoustic Characteristics	*British Usage*	*Terms in Some Textbooks*	*Recommended ATS[a] Nomenclature*	*Laennec's Original Term*
Discontinuous, interrupted explosive sounds Loud, low in pitch.	Crackle	Coarse rale	Coarse crackle	Râle muquex ou gargouillement
Discontinuous, interrupted explosive sounds Less loud than above and of shorter duration; higher in pitch than coarse rales or crackles.	Crackle	Fine rale	Fine crackle	Râle humide ou crepitation
Continuous sounds Longer than 250 msec, high pitched; dominant frequency of 400 Hz or more, a hissing or whistling sound.	High-pitched wheeze	Sibilant rhonchus	Wheeze	Râle sibilant sec ou sifflement
Continuous sounds Longer than 250 msec, low pitched; dominant frequency about 200 Hz or less; a snoring sound.	Low-pitched wheeze	Sonorous rhonchus	Rhonchus	Râle sec sonore ou ronflement

[a] American Thoracic Society

Table adapted, with permission, from "A Simplified Introduction to Lung Sounds" by R.L.H. Murphy, published by Stethophonics, P.O. Box 122, Wellesley Hills, MA 02181.

Table 17.6. An Approach to Factors Causing Wheezing

Endobronchial
Tumors
Foreign bodies
Mucus (bronchitis)
Bronchial wall
Increased mucosal thickness (chronic bronchitis)
Increased bronchial muscle tone (asthma)
Extrabronchial
Compression (tumors, lymph nodes)
Loss of elastic recoil of surrounding lung (emphysema)

disease or of diseases of the terminal airway unit. These may include *idiopathic pulmonary fibrosis, pneumonia, congestive heart failure* or *sarcoidosis.* The etiology of the late crackles is probably due to the opening of closed peripheral airways and deflated lung units. This may be gravity dependent; thus late inspiratory crackles are related to patient position in some conditions (e.g., congestive heart failure).

Stridor

Stridor is a high pitched, continuous crowing sound that is maximal on inspiration and flow dependent. It is characteristic of an extrathoracic obstruction in the trachea or above.

Causes of stridor include *tumors* of the tracheal mucosa, compression of the trachea (from lymph nodes or thyroid), postinflammatory *stricture* of the trachea, and acute inflammations such as *acute epiglottitis.*

Physiologically, upper airway obstruction can be differentiated from lower airway obstruction by tests described on page 40.

Pleural Rub

The pleural rub or pleural crackle is due to friction between the visceral and parietal pleura. This is usually a discontinuous sound heard in both inspiration and expiration. It can be simulated by rubbing the thumb very firmly against the distal portion of the first finger. It is characteristic of an inflammatory process of the pleura and may be brought on by many conditions ranging from *parapneumonic* inflammation to *pulmonary embolism* with infarction of the underlying lung.

Clubbing and Hypertrophic Pulmonary Osteoarthropathy

While both clubbing and hypertrophic pulmonary osteoarthropathy (HPOA) may occur in the absence of the other, it is common to group these two

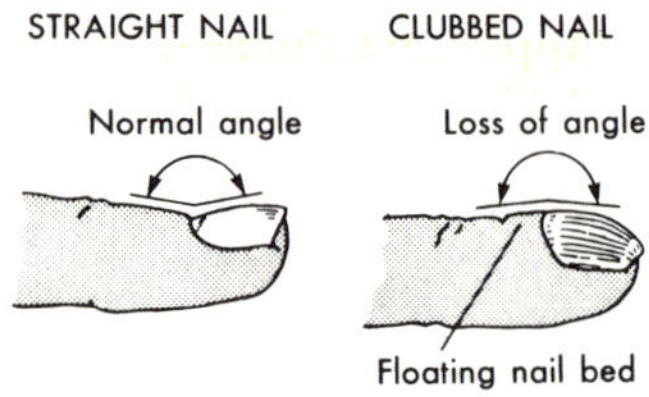

Figure 17.1. Nail bed angle.

peripheral manifestations of cardiopulmonary disease together, because they are believed to have a similar pathogenic mechanism.

Considerable controversy exists about the means to detect clubbing, especially during its early stages (Figure 17.1). There are two important criteria. A change in the nail bed angle is the earliest visual sign. This angle is normally 180° or less. A more accurate way of defining clubbing appears to be by assessment of the bulk and sponginess or floating of the nail bed. It is important to note that many people have "beaked" nails, and this phenomenon does not have the same pathophysiological significance as clubbing.

Hypertrophic pulmonary osteoarthropathy is characterized by either joint symptoms (stiffness, pain, swelling) and/or pain in the distal portion of the long bones. An x-ray film of these bones will usually show evidence of subperiosteal new bone formation.

The pathophysiological basis of both clubbing and HPOA are not clear. In both instances, it appears that there is increased blood flow to the digits. No single hypothesis has been put forward to explain all instances of the phenomena.

In some instances neurogenic factors are important. For example, surgeons, by performing a vagotomy in association with surgery for bronchogenic carcinoma, have at times been able to promptly relieve the clubbing and HPOA. Sometimes the HPOA can be seen to regress completely after such procedures.

Hypoxia has also been postulated as an etiological factor. However, while it is true that cyanotic lung and heart disease have been associated with clubbing, the phenomenon can also be seen in noncyanotic lung disease, and there is no good correlation between degree of oxygen desaturation and degree of clubbing. In fact, clubbing is unusual in hypoxemic patients with chronic airflow obstruction.

Neither neurogenic nor hypoxic hypotheses will explain the clubbing found in some patients with cirrhosis, or those with inflammatory bowel disease such as *ulcerative colitis,* or in suppurative pulmonary diseases such as *bronchiectasis* (Table 17.7). Increased levels of growth hormone, estrogens, and gonadotrophic hormones have been postulated despite the fact that cross circulation experiments using dogs have failed to confirm this hypothesis. It may turn out that no single hypothesis can be used and that different conditions produce clubbing through different mechanisms.

Table 17.7. An Approach to Some Conditions Associated with Clubbing and HPOA

Pulmonary
Carcinoma
Idiopathic pulmonary fibrosis
Suppurative lung disease (bronchiectasis, abscess)
Cardiac
Cyanotic heart disease
Bacterial endocarditis
Gastrointestinal
Carcinoma (stomach, esophagus)
Inflammatory bowel (regional enteritis, ulcerative colitis)
Cirrhosis
Familial clubbing (benign)
Idiopathic clubbing and HPOA

Cyanosis

Cyanosis is a bluish discoloration of the skin, nail beds, and mucous membranes. Clinically, it is commonly looked for in the nail beds, conjunctivae, or tongue and buccal mucosa. It is assessed better under daylight conditions than where fluorescent or tungsten lighting are used.

Cyanosis is due to the amount of unoxygenated or reduced hemoglobin visible in the tissues. Generally, approximately 5 gm of reduced hemoglobin per 100 cc blood must be present before cyanosis is detectable. Since cyanosis depends on the concentration of reduced hemoglobin, it is apparent that it is not a terribly accurate reflection of the oxygen tension of the blood. For example, if an oxygen saturation of about 80% produces cyanosis in a normal person, a much lower saturation will be needed to produce the same amount of reduced hemoglobin in a person with anemia. Conversely, persons with increased numbers of red blood cells, erythrocytosis, may have amounts of reduced hemoglobin in the 5 gm/100 cc range at oxygen saturations considerably above 80%. This is of some importance, since erythrocytosis is a response to chronic hypoxia. Thus some patients with lung disease and longstanding hypoxia will appear very cyanotic, out of proportion to their actual oxygen saturation.

Central Versus Peripheral Cyanosis

A useful approach to the pathophysiological basis for cyanosis in a particular patient is the concept of central versus peripheral cyanosis. Central cyanosis is due usually to pulmonary or cardiac diseases that cause arterial hypoxemia or may be associated with abnormalities of hemoglobin (see Table 17.8). The pulmonary causes of cyanosis will operate through the mechanisms of defects of diffusion, alveolar hypoventilation, right to left shunts, or ventilation-perfusion mismatching, or a combination of these. Acute cyanosis may occur

Table 17.8. An Approach to Central Versus Peripheral Cyanosis

Central
Cardiac factors
Right to left shunts
Pulmonary factors
Alveolar hypoventilation
Low $\dot{V}/\dot{Q}$ areas
Right to left shunts
Diffusion defects
Abnormal hemoglobin
Methemaglobin
Sulfhemoglobin
Peripheral
Peripheral vasoconstriction
Venous obstruction
Arterial obstruction

in *pneumothorax, pulmonary embolism, pulmonary edema* or *pneumonia.* Causes of chronic forms of cyanosis include *chronic bronchitis* and *emphysema, idiopathic pulmonary fibrosis,* and *obesity-hypoventilation.*

Peripheral cyanosis is distinguished by bluish skin over the extremities and nail beds but relatively good color in the conjunctiva and buccal mucous membranes. The extremities are often cold and clammy. Peripheral cyanosis is seen in states of vasoconstriction such as *shock, Raynaud's phenomenon,* or exposure to cold. Localized arterial disease (embolism) or venous obstruction also may cause cyanosis.

BIBLIOGRAPHY

Campbell EJM: *The Relationship of the Sensation of Breathlessness to the Act of Breathing.* Oxford, Blackwell, 1966.

Cherniack NS, Fishman AP: Abnormal breathing patterns. *Dis Month,* July 1975, p 3.

Comroe JH Jr: Some theories of the mechanism of dyspnea, in Howell JBL, Campbell EJM (eds): *Breathlessness.* Oxford, Blackwell, 1966.

Crocco JA, Rooney JJ, Fankushen DS, et al: Massive Hemoptysis. *Arch Intern Med* 121:495, 1968.

DeGowin EL, DeGowin RL: *Bedside diagnostic examination.* London, Macmillan, 1969.

Fishman AP: Manifestations of Pulmonary Disorders in Fishman AP (ed): *Pulmonary Diseases and Disorders.* New York, McGraw-Hill, 1980, pp 44–83.

Forgacs P: *Lung Sounds.* London, Tindall, 1978.

Fraser RG, Paré JAP: Methods in clinical, laboratory, and functional investigations, in Fraser RG, Pare JAP: *Diagnosis of Diseases of the Chest,* ed 2. Philadelphia, Saunders, 1977.

Murphy RLH Jr, Holford SK: Lung Sounds. *Basics of RD* 8(4):1–6, 1980.

APPENDIX 1

A Note on Système International (SI) Units

Many nations have adopted Système International (SI) units as the only legally accepted system of measurement. Some have not. At present there is general agreement on the use of most SI units including meter (m) for length, kilogram (kg) for mass, second (s) for time. Volume in SI units should be expressed as cubic meters (m^3); however liters (l), and milliliters (ml) are still widely used.

Pressure (force per unit area) in SI units is newtons (the force unit) per square meter. This pressure unit is called the pascal (Pa): 1 kPa = 7.5 mmHg. Conversion between the older pressure units (mmHg and cmH_2O) and the SI units is given in Tables I and II.

Volume of gas in SI units is expressed in mmol instead of ml (STPD). Conversion Table III is used to convert ml to mmol. The conversion between the two units is:

for oxygen 1 mmol = 22.39 ml (STPD)
for carbon dioxide 1 mmol = 22.26 ml (STPD)

For a further discussion of the SI system see Rose JC: Pressures on the millimeter of mercury. *N Engl J Med* 298:1361, 1978.

Table I. Conversion of mmHg to kPa[a]

mmHg	*kPa*	*mmHg*	*kPa*	*mmHg*	*kPa*	*mmHg*	*kPa*	*mmHg*	*kPa*
1	0.133	25	3.333	49	6.533	73	9.733	97	12.933
2	0.267	26	3.467	50	6.667	74	9.867	98	13.067
3	0.400	27	3.600	51	6.800	75	10.000	99	13.200
4	0.533	28	3.733	52	6.933	76	10.133	100	13.333
5	0.667	29	3.867	53	7.067	77	10.267	110	14.667
6	0.800	30	4.000	54	7.200	78	10.400	120	16.000
7	0.933	31	4.133	55	7.333	79	10.533	130	17.333
8	1.067	32	4.267	56	7.467	80	10.667	140	18.667
9	1.200	33	4.400	57	7.600	81	10.800	150	20.000
10	1.333	34	4.533	58	7.733	82	10.933	160	21.333
11	1.467	35	4.667	59	7.867	83	11.067	170	22.666
12	1.600	36	4.800	60	8.000	84	11.200	180	24.000
13	1.733	37	4.933	61	8.133	85	11.333	190	25.333
14	1.867	38	5.067	62	8.267	86	11.467	200	26.666
15	2.000	39	5.200	63	8.400	87	11.600	250	33.333
16	2.133	40	5.333	64	8.533	88	11.733	300	40.000
17	2.267	41	5.467	65	8.667	89	11.867	350	46.666
18	2.400	42	5.600	66	8.800	90	12.000	400	53.333
19	2.533	43	5.733	67	8.933	91	12.133	450	59.999
20	2.667	44	5.867	68	9.067	92	12.267	500	66.666
21	2.800	45	6.000	69	9.200	93	12.400	550	73.333
22	2.933	46	6.133	70	9.333	94	12.533	600	79.999
23	3.067	47	6.267	71	9.467	95	12.667	650	86.666
24	3.200	48	6.400	72	9.600	96	12.800	700	93.332
								760	101.332

[a] 1 mmHg = 0.133332 kPa
1 kPa = 7.5006 mmHg

Table II. Conversion of cmH_2O to kPa[a]

cmH_2O	kPa
1	.098
2	.196
3	.294
4	.392
5	.490
6	.588
7	.686
8	.784
9	.882
10	.980
15	1.471
20	1.961
25	2.451
30	2.941
35	3.431
40	3.922
45	4.412
50	4.902

[a] 10.2 cmH_2O = 1 kPa

Table III. Conversion of ml of a Dry Gas to mmol[a]

ml	*mmol* O_2	*mmol* CO_2	*ml*	*mmol* O_2	*mmol* CO_2
1	.045	.045	150	6.699	6.739
2	.089	.090	160	7.146	7.188
3	.134	.135	170	7.593	7.637
4	.179	.180	180	8.039	8.086
5	.223	.225	190	8.486	8.535
6	.268	.270	200	8.933	8.985
7	.313	.314	210	9.379	9.434
8	.357	.359	220	9.826	9.883
9	.402	.404	230	10.272	10.332
10	.447	.449	240	10.719	10.782
20	.893	.898	250	11.166	11.231
30	1.340	1.347	260	11.612	11.680
40	1.787	1.797	270	12.059	12.129
50	2.233	2.246	280	12.506	12.579
60	2.680	2.695	290	12.952	13.028
70	3.126	3.145	300	13.399	13.477
80	3.573	3.594	400	17.865	17.969
90	4.020	4.043	500	22.331	22.462
100	4.466	4.492	1000	44.66	44.9
110	4.913	4.942	2000	89.3	89.8
120	5.360	5.391	3000	134.0	134.8
130	5.806	5.840	4000	178.7	179.7
140	6.253	6.289	5000	223.3	224.6

[a] For O_2 1 mmol = 22.39 ml (STPD)
For CO_2 1 mmol = 22.26 ml (STPD)

APPENDIX 2

Abbreviations Used in This Volume

The abbreviations used in this volume are based on those recommended in Pappenheimer JR, Comroe JH, Cournand A, Ferguson JKW, Filley GF, Fowler WS, Gray JS, Helmholtz HF, Otis AB, Rahn H, and Riley RL: Standardization of definitions and symbols in respiratory physiology. *Fed Proc* 9:602, 1950. A few of the abbreviations used in this volume differ in minor ways from those recommended.

The abbreviations involve the linkage of a letter that indicates a type of measurement (large capital letters) and a letter that represents an adjective term referring to gases (small capital letters) or blood (small letters). A dot over a letter symbolizes "per unit time." A bar over a letter indicates "mean." An apostrophe following a letter symbolizes "end."

For Gases

Type of Measurement (large capitals)	*Adjective Term* (small capitals)
V = gas volume	A = alveolar gas
P = gas pressure	E = expired gas
D = diffusing capacity	I = inspired gas
F = fractional concentration	T = tidal gas
	D = dead space gas
	B = barometric

Examples

$\dot{V}$	= gas volume per minute
V_D	= dead space volume
V_D/V_T	= dead space tidal volume ratio
$\dot{V}_A$	= alveolar ventilation per minute
P_B	= barometric pressure
$P_{A_{O_2}}$	= alveolar oxygen pressure
$P_{\bar{E}_{CO_2}}$	= mean or mixed expired carbon dioxide pressure
P_{O_2}	= oxygen pressure
D_{CO}	= diffusing capacity for carbon monoxide
$F_{I_{O_2}}$	= fractional oxygen concentration in inspired gas

For Blood

Type of Measurement (large capitals)	*Adjective Term* (small letters)
Q = volume of blood	a = arterial blood
P = pressure	v = venous blood
C = concentration or content	c = capillary blood
S = saturation	s = shunted blood
	t = total blood

Examples

$\dot{Q}$ = blood flow per minute
$\dot{Q}s/\dot{Q}t$ = ratio of shunt blood flow to total blood flow
Ca_{O_2} = arterial oxygen content
$C\bar{v}_{O_2}$ = mean venous oxygen content
$C\acute{c}_{O_2}$ = oxygen content of end capillary blood
Sa_{O_2} = saturation of hemoglobin with oxygen in arterial blood
Pa_{CO_2} = partial pressure of carbon dioxide in arterial blood
$\dot{V}/\dot{Q}$ = ventilation-perfusion ratio; also written $\dot{V}_A/\dot{Q}$

Abbreviations Commonly Used in the Pulmonary Function Laboratory

VC = vital capacity
FRC = functional residual capacity
TLC = total lung capacity
RV = residual volume
ERV = expiratory reserve volume
FVC = forced vital capacity; obtained during forced expiratory maneuver
FEV_1 = volume expired in first second of forced expiration
MMEF or MMEFR = maximum midexpiratory flow rate; also called $FEF_{25-75\%}$, forced expiratory flow between 25% and 75% of the vital capacity
CV = closing volume; volume at which airway closure begins to occur

APPENDIX 3

Normal Values for Blood Gases

Sa_{O_2}	>95%
Pa_{O_2}	80 to 100 mmHg (10.7 to 13.3 kPa) subtract about 1 to 1.5 mmHg (.1 to .2 kPa) for every decade of age. subtract about 3 to 4 mmHg (.4 to .5 kPa) for every 1000 feet (.3 km) altitude. >600 mmHg (80 kPa) breathing O_2
Pa_{CO_2}	35 to 45 mmHg (4.7 to 6.0 kPa) subtract about .5 to 1 mmHg (.07 to .13 kPa) for every 1000 feet altitude. subtract 5 to 10 mmHg (.7 to 1.33 kPa) in pregnancy.
$(A - a)\ Po_2$ difference	<20 mmHg (2.67 kPa)
pH	7.39 to 7.42

APPENDIX 4

Commonly Used Equations

To Calculate Shunt

$$\frac{\dot{Q}s}{\dot{Q}t} = \frac{C\acute{c}_{O_2} - Ca_{O_2}}{C\acute{c}_{O_2} - C\bar{v}_{O_2}}$$

$\dot{Q}s$ = shunt flow
$\dot{Q}t$ = total flow
Ca_{O_2} = oxygen content of arterial blood
$C\acute{c}_{O_2}$ = oxygen content of end capillary blood; i.e., blood fully equilibrated with alveolar O_2. This content is calculated from ideal $P_{A_{O_2}}$.
$C\bar{v}_{O_2}$ = oxygen content of mixed venous blood
O_2 content = (hemaglobin concentration $\times$ Sa_{O_2} $\times$ 1.34) + (Po_2 $\times$ .003)

To Calculate Dead Space Tidal Volume Ratio (V_D/V_T)

$$V_D/V_T = \frac{Pa_{CO_2} - P_{E_{CO_2}}}{Pa_{CO_2}}$$

$P_{E_{CO_2}}$ = mixed expired Pco_2
V_D/V_T is normally less than .3.

To Calculate Ideal Alveolar Po_2 ($P_{A_{O_2}}$)

$$P_{A_{O_2}} = P_{I_{O_2}} - P_{A_{CO_2}}\left[F_{I_{O_2}} + \frac{1 - F_{I_{O_2}}}{R}\right]$$

when $F_{I_{O_2}}$ = 1 (100% O_2) the equation simplifies to

$$P_{A_{O_2}} = P_{I_{O_2}} - P_{A_{CO_2}}$$

when $F_{I_{O_2}} < 1$ the equation simplifies to

$$P_{A_{O_2}} = P_{I_{O_2}} - \frac{P_{A_{CO_2}}}{R} + \left[\frac{F_{I_{O_2}}(1 - R)}{R} \times P_{A_{CO_2}}\right]$$

The portion of the above equation in the square brackets is small and the $P_{A_{O_2}}$ is closely approximated by

$$P_{A_{O_2}} = P_{I_{O_2}} - \frac{P_{A_{CO_2}}}{R}$$

R = respiratory exchange ratio
$P_{I_{O_2}}$ = inspired P_{O_2}

To Calculate Alveolar Ventilation

$$\dot{V}_A = \frac{\dot{V}_{CO_2}}{P_{A_{CO_2}}} \times .863$$

$\dot{V}_A$ = alveolar ventilation, liters/min, the volume at body temperature saturated with water vapor.
$\dot{V}_{CO_2}$ = CO_2 production, ml/min, the volume measure as a dry gas at standard temperature and pressure.
.863 = a correcting factor to compensate for the different units used.

APPENDIX 5

Normal Values for Commonly Used Pulmonary Function Tests

The following nomograms are widely used and are those of Morris (adapted from Morris JF: Spirometry in the evaluation of pulmonary function. *West J Med* 125:110–118, Aug 1976, with permission). To obtain the predicted values for an individual, use a ruler to join height and age. The point that this line intersects the other lines indicates normal values for the tests.

MALES

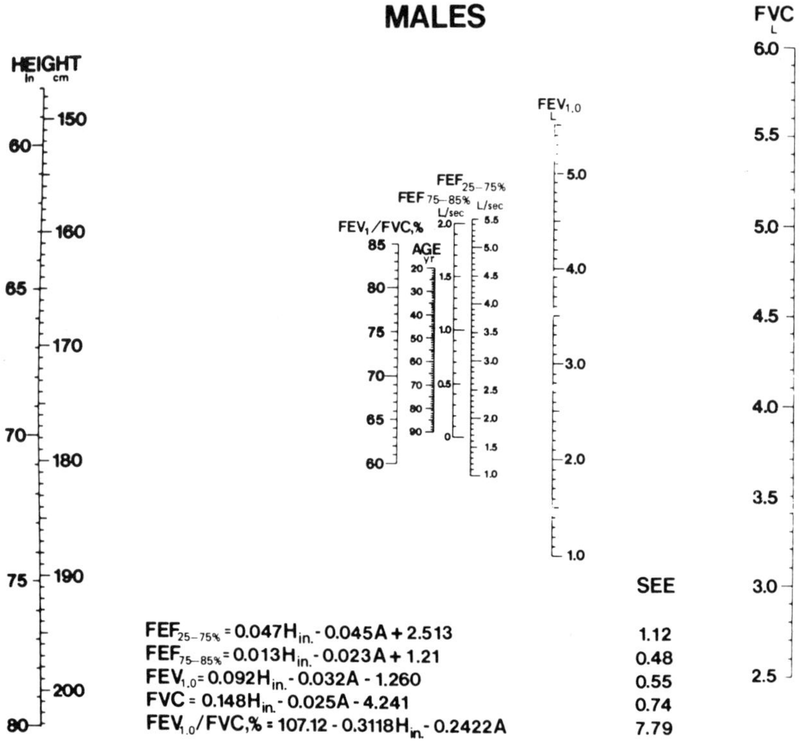

	SEE
$FEF_{25-75\%} = 0.047H_{in.} - 0.045A + 2.513$	1.12
$FEF_{75-85\%} = 0.013H_{in.} - 0.023A + 1.21$	0.48
$FEV_{1.0} = 0.092H_{in.} - 0.032A - 1.260$	0.55
$FVC = 0.148H_{in.} - 0.025A - 4.241$	0.74
$FEV_{1.0}/FVC,\% = 107.12 - 0.3118H_{in.} - 0.2422A$	7.79

FEMALES

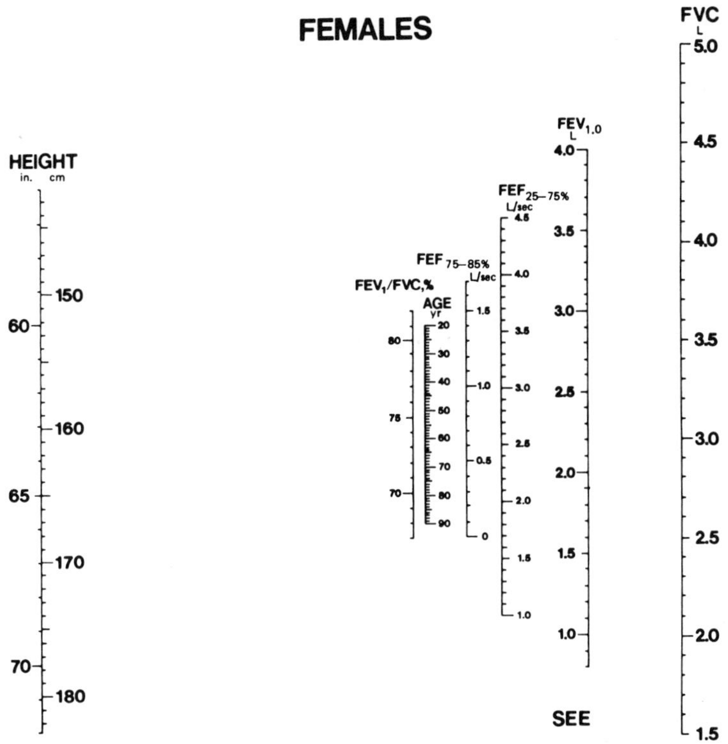

	SEE
$FEF_{25-75\%} = 0.060H_{in.} - 0.030A + 0.551$	0.89
$FEF_{75-85\%} = 0.025H_{in.} - 0.021A + 0.321$	0.45
$FEV_{1.0} = 0.089H_{in.} - 0.025A - 1.932$	0.47
$FVC = 0.115H_{in.} - 0.024A - 2.852$	0.52
$FEV_{1.0}/FVC,\% = 88.70 - 0.0679H_{in.} - 0.1815A$	6.84

Index